Medical Nutrition Therapy in Critically Ill and COVID-19 Patients

Medical Nutrition Therapy in Critically Ill and COVID-19 Patients

Editors

Dimitrios T. Karayiannis
Zafeiria Mastora

MDPI • Basel • Beijing • Wuhan • Barcelona • Belgrade • Manchester • Tokyo • Cluj • Tianjin

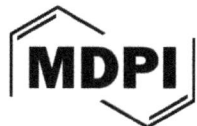

Editors
Dimitrios T. Karayiannis
Evangelismos General Hospital of Athens
Greece

Zafeiria Mastora
National and Kapodistrian University of Athens
Greece

Editorial Office
MDPI
St. Alban-Anlage 66
4052 Basel, Switzerland

This is a reprint of articles from the Special Issue published online in the open access journal *Nutrients* (ISSN 2072-6643) (available at: https://www.mdpi.com/journal/nutrients/special_issues/critical_care_nutrition).

For citation purposes, cite each article independently as indicated on the article page online and as indicated below:

LastName, A.A.; LastName, B.B.; LastName, C.C. Article Title. *Journal Name* **Year**, *Volume Number*, Page Range.

ISBN 978-3-0365-4803-6 (Hbk)
ISBN 978-3-0365-4804-3 (PDF)

© 2022 by the authors. Articles in this book are Open Access and distributed under the Creative Commons Attribution (CC BY) license, which allows users to download, copy and build upon published articles, as long as the author and publisher are properly credited, which ensures maximum dissemination and a wider impact of our publications.

The book as a whole is distributed by MDPI under the terms and conditions of the Creative Commons license CC BY-NC-ND.

Contents

About the Editors vii

Preface to "Medical Nutrition Therapy in Critically Ill and COVID-19 Patients" ix

Dimitrios Karayiannis, Sotirios Kakavas, Zoi Bouloubasi and Zafeiria Mastora
COVID-19 Disease and Outcomes among Critically Ill Patients: The Case of Medical Nutritional Therapy
Reprinted from: *Nutrients* **2022**, *14*, 1416, doi:10.3390/nu14071416 1

Michał Czapla, Raúl Juárez-Vela, Vicente Gea-Caballero, Stanisław Zieliński and Marzena Zielińska
The Association between Nutritional Status and In-Hospital Mortality of COVID-19 in Critically-Ill Patients in the ICU
Reprinted from: *Nutrients* **2021**, *13*, 3302, doi:10.3390/nu13103302 5

Pin-Kuei Fu, Chen-Yu Wang, Wei-Ning Wang, Chiann-Yi Hsu, Shih-Pin Lin and Chen-Tsung Kuo
Energy Achievement Rate Is an Independent Factor Associated with Intensive Care Unit Mortality in High-Nutritional-Risk Patients with Acute Respiratory Distress Syndrome Requiring Prolonged Prone Positioning Therapy
Reprinted from: *Nutrients* **2021**, *13*, 3176, doi:10.3390/nu13093176 21

Dimitrios Karayiannis, Sotirios Kakavas, Aikaterini Sarri, Vassiliki Giannopoulou, Christina Liakopoulou, Edison Jahaj, Aggeliki Kanavou, Thodoris Pitsolis, Sotirios Malachias, George Adamos, Athina Mantelou, Avra Almperti, Konstantina Morogianni, Olga Kampouropoulou, Anastasia Kotanidou and Zafeiria Mastora
Does Route of Full Feeding Affect Outcome among Ventilated Critically Ill COVID-19 Patients: A Prospective Observational Study
Reprinted from: *Nutrients* **2022**, *14*, 153, doi:10.3390/nu14010153 35

Francisco Arrieta, Victoria Martinez-Vaello, Nuria Bengoa, Marta Rosillo, Angélica de Pablo, Cristina Voguel, Rosario Pintor, Amaya Belanger-Quintana, Raquel Mateo-Lobo, Angel Candela and José I. Botella-Carretero
Stress Hyperglycemia and Osteocalcin in COVID-19 Critically Ill Patients on Artificial Nutrition
Reprinted from: *Nutrients* **2021**, *13*, 3010, doi:10.3390/nu13093010 45

Lourdes Herrera-Quintana, Yenifer Gamarra-Morales, Héctor Vázquez-Lorente, Jorge Molina-López, José Castaño-Pérez, Juan Francisco Machado-Casas, Ramón Coca-Zúñiga, José Miguel Pérez-Villares and Elena Planells
Bad Prognosis in Critical Ill Patients with COVID-19 during Short-Term ICU Stay regarding Vitamin D Levels
Reprinted from: *Nutrients* **2021**, *13*, 1988, doi:10.3390/nu13061988 57

Marine Gérard, Meliha Mahmutovic, Aurélie Malgras, Niasha Michot, Nicolas Scheyer, Roland Jaussaud, Phi-Linh Nguyen-Thi and Didier Quilliot
Long-Term Evolution of Malnutrition and Loss of Muscle Strength after COVID-19: A Major and Neglected Component of Long COVID-19
Reprinted from: *Nutrients* **2021**, *13*, 3964, doi:10.3390/nu13113964 71

Paul Muhle, Karen Konert, Sonja Suntrup-Krueger, Inga Claus, Bendix Labeit, Mao Ogawa, Tobias Warnecke, Rainer Wirth and Rainer Dziewas
Oropharyngeal Dysphagia and Impaired Motility of the Upper Gastrointestinal Tract—Is There a Clinical Link in Neurocritical Care?
Reprinted from: *Nutrients* **2021**, *13*, 3879, doi:10.3390/nu13113879 83

José Ignacio Ramírez Manent, Bárbara Altisench Jané, Pilar Sanchís Cortés, Carla Busquets-Cortés, Sebastiana Arroyo Bote, Luis Masmiquel Comas and Ángel Arturo López González
Impact of COVID-19 Lockdown on Anthropometric Variables, Blood Pressure, and Glucose and Lipid Profile in Healthy Adults: A before and after Pandemic Lockdown Longitudinal Study
Reprinted from: *Nutrients* **2022**, *14*, 1237, doi:10.3390/nu14061237 95

Phil-Robin Tepasse, Richard Vollenberg, Manfred Fobker, Iyad Kabar, Hartmut Schmidt, Jörn Arne Meier, Tobias Nowacki and Anna Hüsing-Kabar
Vitamin A Plasma Levels in COVID-19 Patients: A Prospective Multicenter Study and Hypothesis
Reprinted from: *Nutrients* **2021**, *13*, 2173, doi:10.3390/nu13072173 113

Amelia Faradina, Sung-Hui Tseng, Dang Khanh Ngan Ho, Esti Nurwanti, Hamam Hadi, Sintha Dewi Purnamasari, Imaning Yulia Rochmah and Jung-Su Chang
Adherence to COVID-19 Nutrition Guidelines Is Associated with Better Nutritional Management Behaviors of Hospitalized COVID-19 Patients
Reprinted from: *Nutrients* **2021**, *13*, 1918, doi:10.3390/nu13061918 125

Sotirios Kakavas, Dimitrios Karayiannis and Zafeiria Mastora
The Complex Interplay between Immunonutrition, Mast Cells, and Histamine Signaling in COVID-19
Reprinted from: *Nutrients* **2021**, *13*, 3458, doi:10.3390/nu13103458 137

Elena Gangitano, Rossella Tozzi, Orietta Gandini, Mikiko Watanabe, Sabrina Basciani, Stefania Mariani, Andrea Lenzi, Lucio Gnessi and Carla Lubrano
Ketogenic Diet as a Preventive and Supportive Care for COVID-19 Patients
Reprinted from: *Nutrients* **2021**, *13*, 1004, doi:10.3390/nu13031004 151

About the Editors

Dimitrios T. Karayiannis

Dimitrios T. Karayiannis earned his Bachelor's, Master's and Doctoral degrees in Clinical Nutrition from the Department of Nutrition and Dietetic at Harokopio University of Athens. He also received the European Society for Clinical Nutrition and Metabolism Diploma in Clinical Nutrition and Metabolism. Currently, he serves in the largest hospital in Greece (Evangelismos General Hospital, Athens) and has been there for the last 10 years as a Clinical Dietitian; he is also a member of the ICU, Internal Medicine, and Neurosurgery Nutrition Support Team. Having 16 years of experience in the field of Nutrition and Clinical Dietetics, Dimitrios has been involved in numerous trials and projects related to the effects of diet and malnutrition on parameters influencing survival, length of hospital stay and human fertility. He has experience in the field of Dietetics and Metabolism, and has worked in five different hospitals and community settings. Currently, he also serves as a Research Associate of the Department of Nutrition and Dietetic at Harokopio University. He worked closely with students from local internship programs and was responsible for graduate students' practice placements for almost 10 years. He participated for almost 12 years in the activities of the Hellenic Dietetic Association, as a member of the organizing committee of conferences, seminars and practice working groups. In 2012, he became a Member and Life Long Learning Teacher of the Hellenic Society of Medical Nutrition, a certified instructor of the European Society of Clinical Nutrition and Metabolism and a board Member of the Hellenic Society of Hospital Dietitians (2010-2014). He is a reviewer in the *Nutrients, Nutrition, Human Reproduction, Clinical Nutrition, Clinical Nutrition ESPEN, British Journal of Nutrition* among other nutrition and cancer journals, coeditor of 2 Nutrition text books, co-author of 11 text-book chapters and contributed to 17 peer-reviewed publications in international scientific journals.

Zafeiria Mastora

Zafeiria Mastora is a Physician specialized in Intensive Care Medicine at the University of Athens Medical School and served as Pulmonologist - Intensivist in the First Department of Critical Care Medicine and Pulmonary Services, Evangelismos General Hospital under the auspices of the National and Kapodistrian University of Athens. She has published more than 35 original scientific manuscripts and editorials, she has edited 12 books in the area of Critical Care Medicine and Nutrition.

Preface to "Medical Nutrition Therapy in Critically Ill and COVID-19 Patients"

The COVID-19 pandemic, in addition to the enormous challenges that were placed on the scientific community when responding to the situation, was accompanied by many questions regarding the nutritional management of these cases. In particular, the increase in the number of patients admitted to Intensive Care Units gave rise to a number of questions. The nutritional support of the critically ill patient who is hospitalized in the Intensive Care Unit is one of the most important factors for planning treatment and the rehabilitation of dysfunctions.

The present summary attempted to present the basic principles of nutritional support of patients admitted to the ICU with COVID-19. The purpose of this Special Issue is to provide a comprehensive approach regarding the factors of a proper and effective nutrition support plan among patients treated in the ICU, but also to provide scientific studies that provide updates on the importance of nutritional evaluation and nutritional support in patients with serious cardiorespiratory diseases. The importance of malnutrition and the complications of artificial nutrition in the clinical picture of the patient and in the course of his disease, demonstrate the severity of the effects of diet in critically ill patients in the ICU.

Dimitrios T. Karayiannis and Zafeiria Mastora
Editors

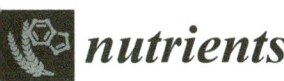

Editorial

COVID-19 Disease and Outcomes among Critically Ill Patients: The Case of Medical Nutritional Therapy

Dimitrios Karayiannis [1,*], Sotirios Kakavas [2], Zoi Bouloubasi [1] and Zafeiria Mastora [3]

1. Department of Clinical Nutrition, "Evangelismos" General Hospital of Athens, Ypsilantou 45-47, 10676 Athens, Greece; zoippp@yahoo.com
2. Intensive Care Unit, Center for Respiratory Failure, "Sotiria" General Hospital of Chest Diseases, 152 Mesogeion Avenue, 11527 Athens, Greece; sotikaka@yahoo.com
3. First Department of Critical Care Medicine and Pulmonary Services, Evangelismos General Hospital, National and Kapodistrian University of Athens, 11527 Athens, Greece; zafimast@yahoo.gr
* Correspondence: jimkar_d@yahoo.com

The recent COVID-19 pandemic, which resulted from SARS CoV-2 coronavirus infection, contributed to a rapid increase in hospital and intensive care unit (ICU) admissions [1]. Although during the last 3 years there have been numerous research publications on patient care, data concerning the role of the dietary approach in the overall treatment of the disease are minimal. Moreover, with regard to the dietary approach during COVID-19 critical illness, practice guidelines are based on data which were developed too quickly and were based on targeted recommendations on feeding the critically ill [2]. Since then, new sources of data have emerged, which clearly display significant nutritional challenges.

In relation to the organization of the provision of nutritional care, data from the USA proclaim that only about 1 in 5 centers (21%) have developed a specialized protocol for the provision of nutritional treatment [3]. Among these centers, some of the key issues raised by feeding staff included the difficulty of feeding awake patients and the reluctance to add additional PN in cases of inadequate EN administration. The results of this study reported that the emphasis given to the exclusive administration of food through the gastric tract was rarely effective in this group of patients.

Why are we so interested in providing individualized nutritional therapy to critically ill patients with COVID-19? Firstly, these patients tend to exhibit a significantly higher length of hospital stay compared to other subcategories of critically ill patients, while simultaneously they will need nutritional support for longer periods, according to the data of Arrieta et al., as presented in the current Special Issue (SI) [4]. In addition, according to recent findings, about 8 in 10 patients will leave the ICU at high nutritional and sarcopenia risk [5]. This finding supports the hypothesis that these patients obviously do not receive optimal nutritional care. Additionally, disease symptoms and de-arrangement of the nutritional status persists until 6 months after hospital discharge, as an interesting French study published in this SI informed us [6]. The authors supported the hypothesis that COVID-19 patients had a much higher risk of developing muscle weakness, malnutrition and functional loss. On the other hand, the presence of obesity or overweight seems to be positively related to the likelihood of death during hospitalization among COVID-19 patients [7].

In relation to the energy requirements of the critically ill COVID-19 patients, studies report that there are substantial differences compared to other groups of critically ill patients, characterized by a prolonged hypermetabolic state [8]. The hyperinflammatory response during COVID-19 disease is a systemic phenomenon leading to a cytokine storm with an increase in systemic markers such as C-reactive protein (CRP) and erythrocyte sedimentation rate (ESR) [9]. This prolonged period of hyperinflammation causes several metabolic disorders and extremely high levels of energy expenditure, and secondarily other changes, such as severe insulin resistance, tumor overload and hypernatremia secondary to

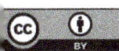

Citation: Karayiannis, D.; Kakavas, S.; Bouloubasi, Z.; Mastora, Z. COVID-19 Disease and Outcomes among Critically Ill Patients: The Case of Medical Nutritional Therapy. *Nutrients* **2022**, *14*, 1416. https://doi.org/10.3390/nu14071416

Received: 7 March 2022
Accepted: 8 March 2022
Published: 29 March 2022

Publisher's Note: MDPI stays neutral with regard to jurisdictional claims in published maps and institutional affiliations.

Copyright: © 2022 by the authors. Licensee MDPI, Basel, Switzerland. This article is an open access article distributed under the terms and conditions of the Creative Commons Attribution (CC BY) license (https://creativecommons.org/licenses/by/4.0/).

imperceptible loss and osmotic diuresis [10]. Patients usually present with hypocalcaemia, hyperkalaemia or hypokalaemia, hyperphosphataemia (secondary to muscle breakdown and mitochondrial insufficiency), and hypertriglyceridaemia.

Are there any data on best nutrition support practices? Unfortunately, there are no data from randomized clinical trials, with the exception of some micronutrient supplementation studies with immunomodulating actions [11]. Although reduced levels of vitamin C, D, Zinc and selenium may be considered as a risk factor for patients with COVID-19, data from published studies so far highlight the lack of well-designed clinical intervention, evaluating the effect of the administration of either individual nutrients or their combination [11]. Kakavas et al., in the present SI hypothesized that immunonutrient administration could be associated with a reduction in the de novo synthesis and/or release of histamine and other mast cell mediators that could mediate, at least in part, the immune and microvascular alterations present in COVID-19 [12].

When it comes to the feeding route, retrospective data from 176 patients suggest that the majority of patients tend to reach protein and caloric requirements through the use of Parenteral Nutrition during the first week of hospitalization [13]. One recent prospective monocentric study conducted in a large Greek ICU and published in this SI evaluated the influence of feeding practices on patient outcomes. In this study, the route for delivery of full nutritional support (enteral vs. parenteral nutrition) during the second week of hospitalization was not associated with mortality risk [14]. However, there was a significant difference in length of hospital stay and duration of mechanical ventilation support, both being lower in the enteral feeding group.In relation to the macronutrient composition of the diet, fragmentary reports show a tendency for lower mortality in those who receive adequate amounts of protein, but these data do not come from high-quality studies [15]. Regarding more critical questions, such as the optimal macronutrient ratio, when to use parenteral nutrition, when to start enteral nutrition in patients with vasopressors, how tofeed prone ventilated patients, how to consider extubation phase and whether there is utility tousing special feeds (fish oil, immunonutrition), there are choices, but no answersyet.

In conclusion, the key concept identified in this SI was that optimizing dietary practices for patients both during their ICU stay and beyond is crucial. Clinicians should be capable of managing their patients both during their hospitalization and rehabilitation phase, in order to confirm the continuous care and to minimize the susceptibility of adverse events due to malnutrition.

Author Contributions: Writing—original draft preparation, D.K.; writing—review and editing, D.K., S.K., Z.B. and Z.M. All authors have read and agreed to the published version of the manuscript.

Conflicts of Interest: The authors declare no conflict of interest.

References

1. Zhou, F.; Yu, T.; Du, R.; Fan, G.; Liu, Y.; Liu, Z.; Xiang, J.; Wang, Y.; Song, B.; Gu, X.; et al. Clinical course and risk factors for mortality of adult inpatients with COVID-19 in Wuhan, China: A retrospective cohort study. *Lancet* **2020**, *395*, 1054–1062. [CrossRef]
2. Barazzoni, R.; Bischoff, S.C.; Breda, J.; Wickramasinghe, K.; Krznaric, Z.; Nitzan, D.; Pirlich, M.; Singer, P. ESPEN expert statements and practical guidance for nutritional management of individuals with SARS-CoV-2 infection. *Clin. Nutr.* **2020**, *39*, 1631–1638. [CrossRef] [PubMed]
3. Suliman, S.; McClave, S.A.; Taylor, B.E.; Patel, J.; Omer, E.; Martindale, R.G. Barriers to nutrition therapy in the critically ill patient with COVID-19. *JPEN J. Parenter. Enteral Nutr.* **2021**. [CrossRef] [PubMed]
4. Arrieta, F.; Martinez-Vaello, V.; Bengoa, N.; Rosillo, M.; de Pablo, A.; Voguel, C.; Pintor, R.; Belanger-Quintana, A.; Mateo-Lobo, R.; Candela, A.; et al. Stress Hyperglycemia and Osteocalcin in COVID-19 Critically Ill Patients on Artificial Nutrition. *Nutrients* **2021**, *13*, 3010. [CrossRef] [PubMed]
5. Cuerda, C.; Sánchez López, I.; Gil Martínez, C.; Merino Viveros, M.; Velasco, C.; Cevallos Peñafiel, V.; Maíz Jiménez, M.; Gonzalo, I.; González-Sánchez, V.; Ramos Carrasco, A.; et al. Impact of COVID-19 in nutritional and functional status of survivors admitted in intensive care units during the first outbreak. Preliminary results of the NUTRICOVID study. *Clin. Nutr.* **2021**. [CrossRef] [PubMed]

6. Gérard, M.; Mahmutovic, M.; Malgras, A.; Michot, N.; Scheyer, N.; Jaussaud, R.; Nguyen-Thi, P.L.; Quilliot, D. Long-Term Evolution of Malnutrition and Loss of Muscle Strength after COVID-19: A Major and Neglected Component of Long COVID-19. *Nutrients* **2021**, *13*, 3964. [CrossRef] [PubMed]
7. Czapla, M.; Juárez-Vela, R.; Gea-Caballero, V.; Zieliński, S.; Zielińska, M. The Association between Nutritional Status and In-Hospital Mortality of COVID-19 in Critically-Ill Patients in the ICU. *Nutrients* **2021**, *13*, 3302. [CrossRef] [PubMed]
8. Karayiannis, D.; Maragkouti, A.; Mikropoulos, T.; Sarri, A.; Kanavou, A.; Katsagoni, C.; Jahaj, E.; Kotanidou, A.; Mastora, Z. Neuromuscular blockade administration is associated with altered energy expenditure in critically ill intubated patients with COVID-19. *Clin. Nutr.* **2021**. [CrossRef] [PubMed]
9. Whittle, J.; Molinger, J.; MacLeod, D.; Haines, K.; Wischmeyer, P.E. Persistent hypermetabolism and longitudinal energy expenditure in critically ill patients with COVID-19. *Crit. Care* **2020**, *24*, 581. [CrossRef]
10. Kovacevic, M.P.; Dube, K.M.; Lupi, K.E.; Szumita, P.M.; DeGrado, J.R. Evaluation of Hypertriglyceridemia in Critically Ill Patients With Coronavirus Disease 2019 Receiving Propofol. *Crit. Care Explor.* **2021**, *3*, e0330. [CrossRef] [PubMed]
11. Pedrosa, L.F.C.; Barros, A.; Leite-Lais, L. Nutritional risk of vitamin D, vitamin C, zinc, and selenium deficiency on risk and clinical outcomes of COVID-19: A narrative review. *Clin. Nutr. ESPEN* **2022**, *47*, 9–27. [CrossRef] [PubMed]
12. Kakavas, S.; Karayiannis, D.; Mastora, Z. The Complex Interplay between Immunonutrition, Mast Cells, and Histamine Signaling in COVID-19. *Nutrients* **2021**, *13*, 3458. [CrossRef]
13. Miguélez, M.; Velasco, C.; Camblor, M.; Cedeño, J.; Serrano, C.; Bretón, I.; Arhip, L.; Motilla, M.; Carrascal, M.L.; Morales, A.; et al. Nutritional management and clinical outcome of critically ill patients with COVID-19: A retrospective study in a tertiary hospital. *Clin. Nutr.* **2021**. [CrossRef]
14. Karayiannis, D.; Kakavas, S.; Sarri, A.; Giannopoulou, V.; Liakopoulou, C.; Jahaj, E.; Kanavou, A.; Pitsolis, T.; Malachias, S.; Adamos, G.; et al. Does Route of Full Feeding Affect Outcome among Ventilated Critically Ill COVID-19 Patients: A Prospective Observational Study. *Nutrients* **2021**, *14*, 153. [CrossRef]
15. Silvah, J.H.; de Lima, C.M.M.; Nicoletti, C.F.; Barbosa, A.C.; Junqueira, G.P.; da Cunha, S.F.C.; Marchini, J.S. Protein provision and lower mortality in critically ill patients with COVID-19. *Clin. Nutr. ESPEN* **2021**, *45*, 507–510. [CrossRef] [PubMed]

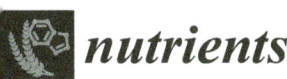

Article

The Association between Nutritional Status and In-Hospital Mortality of COVID-19 in Critically-Ill Patients in the ICU

Michał Czapla [1,2], Raúl Juárez-Vela [3,*], Vicente Gea-Caballero [4], Stanisław Zieliński [5,6] and Marzena Zielińska [5,7]

1. Department of Public Health, Faculty of Health Sciences, Wroclaw Medical University, 51-618 Wroclaw, Poland; michal.czapla@umed.wroc.pl
2. Institute of Heart Diseases, University Hospital, 50-566 Wroclaw, Poland
3. Biomedical Research Centre of La Rioja (CIBIR), Research Group GRUPAC, Research Unit on Health System Sustainability (GISSOS), University of La Rioja, 26004 Logroño, Spain
4. Faculty of Health Sciences, International University of Valencia, 46002 Valencia, Spain; vicenteantonio.gea@campusviu.es
5. Department and Clinic of Anaesthesiology and Intensive Therapy, Faculty of Medicine, Wroclaw Medical University, 50-556 Wroclaw, Poland; stanislaw.zielinski@umed.wroc.pl (S.Z.); marzena.zielinska@umed.wroc.pl (M.Z.)
6. Department of Anaesthesiology and Intensive Care, University Hospital, 50-556 Wrocław, Poland
7. Department of Paediatric Anaesthesiology and Intensive Care, University Hospital, 50-556 Wrocław, Poland
* Correspondence: raul.juarez@unirioja.es

Abstract: Background: Coronavirus disease 2019 (COVID-19) has become one of the leading causes of death worldwide. The impact of poor nutritional status on increased mortality and prolonged ICU (intensive care unit) stay in critically ill patients is well-documented. This study aims to assess how nutritional status and BMI (body mass index) affected in-hospital mortality in critically ill COVID-19 patients Methods: We conducted a retrospective study and analysed medical records of 286 COVID-19 patients admitted to the intensive care unit of the University Clinical Hospital in Wroclaw (Poland). Results: A total of 286 patients were analysed. In the sample group, 8% of patients who died had a BMI within the normal range, 46% were overweight, and 46% were obese. There was a statistically significantly higher death rate in men (73%) and those with BMIs between 25.0–29.9 ($p = 0.011$). Nonsurvivors had a statistically significantly higher HF (Heart Failure) rate ($p = 0.037$) and HT (hypertension) rate ($p < 0.001$). Furthermore, nonsurvivors were statistically significantly older ($p < 0.001$). The risk of death was higher in overweight patients (HR = 2.13; $p = 0.038$). Mortality was influenced by higher scores in parameters such as age (HR = 1.03; $p = 0.001$), NRS2002 (nutritional risk score, HR = 1.18; $p = 0.019$), PCT (procalcitonin, HR = 1.10; $p < 0.001$) and potassium level (HR = 1.40; $p = 0.023$). Conclusions: Being overweight in critically ill COVID-19 patients requiring invasive mechanical ventilation increases their risk of death significantly. Additional factors indicating a higher risk of death include the patient's age, high PCT, potassium levels, and NRS $\geq$ 3 measured at the time of admission to the ICU.

Keywords: COVID-19; malnutrition; SARS-CoV-2; nutritional status; intensive care unit

1. Introduction

On 30 August 2021, 216 million people were infected, and 4.5 million had died of severe coronavirus disease 2019 (COVID-19) [1]. The impact of poor nutritional status on increased mortality and prolonged ICU (intensive care unit) stays in critically ill patients is well known and well-documented [2]. Old age, male sex, comorbidities, being overweight, obesity and malnutrition are some of the known risk factors for severe COVID-19 cases [3]. Moreover, COVID-19 infection lasting several days or even weeks prior to ICU admission enhances patient malnutrition, which in turn leads to increased pathogenicity of the infecting agent and disease progression [4,5]. Furthermore, published studies show a risk of malnutrition in COVID-19 patients. The incidence of malnutrition in patients hospitalised for COVID-19 is 50% [6,7]. Due to malnutrition observed in mechanically ventilated patients even months after discharge from the ICU, both the examination of the nutritional status of critically ill patients at the beginning of hospitalisation and early initiation of nutritional treatment are of great importance [8]. Being overweight and obesity are also factors that worsen prognosis. Individuals coping with these conditions have a higher risk of CVD (cardiovascular disease) and DM (diabetes mellitus). In addition, overweight and obese individuals may experience respiratory complications due to increased ventilatory demand, increased work during breathing, respiratory muscle insufficiency and decreased respiratory compliance [9].

Patients who require treatment in the ICU should be assessed for nutritional status [10]. According to the criteria for diagnosing malnutrition set out by the Global Leadership Initiative on Malnutrition (GLIM), every patient at increased risk for malnutrition should be screened. GLIM indicates that tools such as NRS 2002 (Nutritional Risk Score), SGA (Subjective Global Assessment), MUST (Malnutrition Universal Screening Tool), or MNA (Mini Nutritional Assessment) can be used for screening. In Poland, every person admitted to a hospital ward should undergo a screening test performed using NRS 2002 or SGA (the test does not apply to patients in a hospital Emergency Department; ED) [11,12]. According to ESPEN (European Society for Clinical Nutrition and Metabolism) experts, at-risk patients with more severe COVID-19 should be screened with NRS 2002 if hospitalised [13].

This study aims to assess how nutritional status and BMI (body mass index) affected in-hospital mortality in critically ill COVID-19 patients.

2. Materials and Methods

2.1. Study Design and Setting

A retrospective study was performed based on an analysis of medical records of active COVID-19 patients (ICD10: U07) admitted to the ICU of the University Clinical Hospital in Wroclaw (Poland) between September 2020 and June 2021. The study followed the STROBE (Strengthening the Reporting of Observational Studies in Epidemiology) guidelines.

2.2. Study Population

All the patients who met the following inclusion criteria were analysed: primary diagnosis of COVID-19 (confirmed by RT-PCR), age $\geq$ 18 years, mechanical ventilation (invasive ventilation), hospitalisation in the ICU.

A final group of 286 patients' medical records was analysed. The analysis included data (collected at the time admission) concerning patients' age, sex and BMI; test results such as total cholesterol (TC), triglycerides (TGs), albumins, lymphocytes, potassium, sodium, C-reactive protein (CRP), procalcitonin (PCT); data concerning medical history and comorbidities, as well as assessment of the patients' nutritional status using NRS 2002.

2.3. Nutritional Screening

The NRS 2002 is one of the screening tools recommended by GLIM for risk assessment of nutritional status. The scale consists of two parts.

1. Impaired nutritional status, in which weight loss and BMI are assessed. The same applies to the percentage of food intake compared to its requirements within the last week. The rating scale is 0–3 points, where 0 is lack of deterioration of health status, and 3 is severe deterioration of health status.
2. Severity of disease (an increase in requirements), in which, depending on the disease, patients may receive 0–3 points, where 0 is normal nutritional requirements and 3 is high disease severity (e.g., head injury, bone marrow transplant). Moreover, if patients are over 70, they get an additional point. Thus, patients can score 0–7 points. Nutritional therapy is indicated in patients with NRS $\geq$ 3 [14]. The WHO criteria were used for classifying patients as underweight (BMI < 18.5 kg/m^2), with normal weight (BMI: 18.5–24.9 kg/m^2), pre-obese (BMI: 25–29.9 kg/m^2) and obese (BMI $\geq$ 30 kg/m^2).

A physician measured the NRS 2002 and BMI at the time of admission to the ICU.

2.4. Statistical Analysis

Statistical analysis was performed using Statistica 13.1 software (TIBCO, Inc., Palo Alto, CA, USA). First, arithmetic means and standard deviations were calculated for measurable variables. Next, quantitative variables were examined using the Shapiro-Wilk test to determine the distribution type. Then, intergroup comparisons were made using the t-test or the Mann-Whitney U test (if assumptions were met). Finally, the comparison of results of more than two groups was performed using one-way analysis of variance (ANOVA) or the Kruskal-Wallis test (if assumptions were met).

Survival analysis was carried out using the Kaplan-Meier method and refers to ICU mortality. The log-rank test was used for comparing patient survival against selected clinical variables. The Cox proportional hazards model was used for assessing the influence of qualitative or quantitative variables on patient survival. The analysis included both categorical variables and continuous variables. The categorical variables included sex, BMI (18.5–24.9, <18.5, 25.0–29.9, ≥30), NRS (<3 vs. ≥3), HF (heart failure, yes/no), HT (hypertension, yes/no), DM (diabetes mellitus, yes/no), CVD (cardiovascular disease, yes/no), CKD (chronic kidney disease, yes/no), CRD (chronic respiratory disease, yes/no), TGs (triglycerides, <135, 135–200, >200), TC (total cholesterol, <40, >40). The continuous variables included age, BMI [kg/m^2], height [m], body weight [kg], TGs [mg/dL], TC [mg/dL], CRP [mg/L], albumins [g/dL], lymphocytes [%], PCT [ng/mL], potassium [mmol/l], sodium [mmol/L].

Variables such as BMI, TC, or NRS were analysed as continuous and categorical variables in the univariate model. Variables were included in the multivariate model in accordance with the adopted criteria. Those criteria included the outcome of $p < 0.30$ in a univariate model, a lack of correlation of variables, and clinical recommendations. Multivariate analysis was performed using backwards elimination to stay in the model. For the final multivariate model, the variables were selected according to the better fit of the model based on the assessment of the goodness of fit (AIC). The results were considered statistically significant at $p < 0.05$.

3. Results

3.1. Characteristics of the Group

The profile of the whole group with a comparison of the analysed characteristics of the survivors and nonsurvivors is shown in Table 1. A total of 286 patients were analysed. Due to a lack of data for some parameters, those numbers are smaller and are provided for each variable. There was a statistically significantly higher death rate in men (73%, $n = 142$) and those with BMI between 25.0–29.9 (46% vs. 26%; $p = 0.011$). Nonsurvivors had a statistically significantly higher HF rate (9% vs. 2%; $p = 0.037$) and HT rate (55% vs. 24%; $p < 0.001$). Furthermore, nonsurvivors were statistically significantly older ($\bar{x} = 63.6$ vs. $\bar{x} = 53.8$ years; $p < 0,001$), taller ($\bar{x} = 175.9$ vs. $\bar{x} = 172.1$ cm; $p = 0.008$). Considering laboratory test parameters, PCT levels were statistically significantly higher in nonsurvivors. TC levels were statistically significantly lower in nonsurvivors (Table 1).

Table 1. Characteristics of the group with a comparison of survivors and nonsurvivors.

Variables		Total (n = 286)		Death				p-Value *
				No (n = 92)		Yes (n = 194)		
		n	%	n	%	N	%	
Sex (n = 286)	M	194	67.8	52	56.5	142	73.2	0.005
BMI (n = 194)	<18.5	-	-	-	-	-	-	0.011
	18.5–24.9	22	11.3	11	19.3	11	8.03	
	25.0–29.9	78	40.2	15	26.3	63	45.9	
	≥30	94	48.5	31	54.4	63	45.9	
NRS (n = 286)	<3	28	9.8	9	9.8	19	9.8	0.991
	≥3	258	90.2	83	90.2	175	90.2	
HF (n = 286)	Yes	19	6.64	2	2.2	17	8.8	0.037
HT (n = 286)	Yes	145	50.7	38	41.3	107	55.2	0.029
DM (n = 286)	Yes	92	32.2	25	27.2	67	34.5	0.214
CVD (n = 286)	Yes	99	34.6	30	32.6	69	35.6	0.622
CRD (n = 286)	Yes	24	9.4	6	6.52	18	9.3	0.433
CKD (n = 286)	Yes	8	2.8	1	1.1	7	3.6	0.232
TC (n = 232)	>190	49	21.1	20	24.4	29	19.3	0.900
TGs (n = 251)	>150	183	72.9	58	73.4	125	72.7	0.372
Variables		$\bar{x}$	SD	$\bar{x}$	SD	$\bar{x}$	SD	p-value **
Age (n = 286)		60.5	13.2	53.8	13.5	63.6	11.8	<0.001
ICU length stay (n = 286)		14.2	14.4	20.2	16.0	11.0	12.6	<0.001
NRS (n = 286)		3.3	1.1	3.1	1.1	3.4	1.1	0.061
BMI (n = 194)		31.0	5.7	31.6	6.4	30.7	5.4	0.291
TGs [mg/dL] (n = 251)		250.3	148.3	236.7	160.5	256.5	142.5	0.333
TC [mg/dL] (n = 232)		144.2	50.7	155.8	47.9	137.9	51.2	0.010
Albumins [g/dL] (n = 276)		2.9	0.4	2.9	0.4	2.9	0.4	0.652
Lymphocytes [%] (n = 271)		9.3	10.4	9.4	7.7	9.3	11.5	0.981
Potassium [mmol/L] (n = 280)		4.4	0.8	4.3	0.7	4.5	0.9	0.092
Sodium [mmol/L] (n = 280)		139.6	5.4	140.2	4.2	139.2	5.8	0.141
CRP [mg/L] (n = 281)		140.1	100.2	132.7	87.1	143.5	105.7	0.400
PCT [ng/mL] (n = 280)		2.1	8.7	0.5	0.8	2.9	10.4	0.030

Abbreviations: n, number of participants; x̄ mean; SD, standard deviation; M, males; p, level of significance; BMI, body mass index; NRS, nutritional risk screening; HF, heart failure; HT, arterial hypertension; DM, diabetes mellitus; CVD, cardiovascular disease; CRD, chronic respiratory disease; CKD, chronic kidney disease; TGs, triglycerides; TC, total cholesterol; CRP, C-reactive protein; PCT, procalcitonin; * χ^2 test; ** t-test.

3.2. Subgroup Analysis According to BMI

A comparison of the assessed variables between groups according to BMI is shown in Tables 2 and 3. Men showed a statistically significantly higher percentage in the BMI ranges of 18.5–24.9 kg/m², 25.0–29.9 and above 30 kg/m², compared to women. The highest percentage of deaths was observed in patients with BMI between 25.0 and 29.9 kg/m² (Table 2). The highest (statistically significant) CRP levels were observed in the group of patients with BMI between 18.5 and 24.9 kg/m².

Table 2. Comparison of assessed parameters (qualitative variables) and BMI range (WHO criteria) values.

Variables		\multicolumn{6}{c}{BMI}	p-Value *
		18.5–24.9 n = 22		25.0–29.9 n = 78		≥30 n = 94		
		n	%	n	%	n	%	
Sex	M	21	95.5	65	83.3	53	56.4	<0.001
NRS	<3	2	9.09	8	10.26	4	4.26	0.300
	≥3	20	90.91	70	89.74	90	95.74	
Death	Yes	11	50.00	63	80.77	63	67.02	0.011
HF	Yes	1	4.55	6	7.69	6	6.38	0.861
HT	Yes	9	40.91	41	52.56	55	58.51	0.311
DM	Yes	5	22.73	28	35.90	35	37.23	0.433
CVD	Yes	6	27.27	27	34.62	28	29.79	0.722
CRD	Yes	0	0.00	9	11.54	10	10.64	0.261
CKD	Yes	1	4.55	2	2.56	2	2.13	0.811
TC	>190	4	21.05	10	16.13	16	20.25	0.792
TGs	>150	11	57.89	53	74.65	67	81.71	0.081

Abbreviations: n, number of participants; M, males; p, level of significance; BMI, body mass index; NRS, nutritional risk screening; HF, heart failure; HT, arterial hypertension; DM, diabetes mellitus; CVD, cardiovascular disease; CRD, chronic respiratory disease; CKD, chronic kidney disease; TGs, triglycerides; TC, total cholesterol; CRP, C-reactive protein; PCT, procalcitonin; * χ^2 test.

Table 3. Comparison of assessed parameters (quantitative variables) and BMI range (WHO criteria) values.

Variables	\multicolumn{9}{c}{BMI}	p-Value **
	18.5–24.9 n = 22			25.0–29.9 n = 78			≥30 n = 94			
	n	$\bar{x}$	SD	n	$\bar{x}$	SD	n	$\bar{x}$	SD	
Age	22	56.6	17.2	78	62.8	10.0	94	60.2	12.2	0.081
NRS	22	3.4	1.4	78	3.4	1.2	94	3.4	1.0	1.001
TGs [mg/dL]	19	215.8	160.8	71	242.9	123.7	82	259.4	128.7	0.392
TC [mg/dL]	19	143.1	46.1	62	131.2	50.7	79	149.7	48.8	0.091
Albumins [g/dL]	21	3.0	0.4	76	2.9	0.5	91	3.0	0.4	0.202
Lymphocytes [%]	18	6.0	3.7	76	10.2	14.3	90	9.3	6.7	0.322
Potassium [mmol/L]	21	4.4	0.9	77	4.5	0.9	92	4.3	0.6	0.281
Sodium [mmol/L]	21	138.8	4.0	77	140.6	5.4	92	139.4	5.8	0.242
CRP [mg/L]	21	183.5	115.9	77	122.3	100.8	92	133.8	89.5	0.040
PCT [ng/mL]	21	2.5	8.6	76	1.7	4.7	92	1.9	9.3	0.913

Abbreviations: n, number of participants; $\bar{x}$, mean; SD, standard deviation; p, level of significance; BMI, body mass index; TGs, triglycerides; TC, total cholesterol; CRP, C-reactive protein; PCT, procalcitonin; ** t-test.

3.3. Subgroup Analysis According to NRS

Comparisons of the assessed parameters between groups according to NRS scores are shown in Tables 4 and 5. Based on the NRS score, two groups were distinguished: NRS <3 and ≥3. There were no statistically significant differences between the groups.

Table 4. Comparison of assessed parameters (qualitative variables) and NRS scores.

Variables		NRS <3 n = 28		NRS ≥3 n = 258		p-Value *
		n	%	n	%	
Sex	M	18	64.39	176	68.22	0.671
BMI	<18.5	2	14.29	20	11.11	0.301
	18.5–24.9	8	57.14	70	38.89	
	25.0–29.9	4	28.57	90	50.00	
Death	Yes	19	67.86	175	67.83	0.994
HF	Yes	1	3.57	18	6.98	0.493
HT	Yes	11	39.29	134	51.94	0.202
DM	Yes	9	32.14	83	32.17	0.992
CVD	Yes	13	46.43	86	33.33	0.171
CRD	Yes	4	14.29	20	7.75	0.244
CKD	Yes	0	0.00	8	3.10	0.343
TC	>190	7	30.43	42	20.10	0.253
TGs	>150	17	68.00	166	73.45	0.561

Abbreviations: n, number of participants; M, males; p, level of significance; BMI, body mass index; NRS, nutritional risk screening; HF, heart failure; HT, arterial hypertension; DM, diabetes mellitus; CVD, cardiovascular disease; CRD, chronic respiratory disease; CKD, chronic kidney disease; TGs, triglycerides; TC, total cholesterol; CRP, C-reactive protein; PCT, procalcitonin; * χ^2 test.

Table 5. Comparison of assessed parameters (quantitative variables) and NRS scores.

Variables	NRS <3 n = 28			NRS ≥3 n = 258			p-Value **
	n	$\bar{x}$	SD	n	$\bar{x}$	SD	
Age	28	57.3	13.2	258	60.8	13.2	0.181
BMI	14	29.6	6.7	180	31.1	5.7	0.362
Height [cm]	13	174.5	8.2	180	174.8	9.1	0.901
Body Mass [kg]	13	85.6	13.1	181	94.8	17.7	0.071
TGs [mg/dL]	25	240.1	150.0	226	251.4	148.5	0.722
TC [mg/dL]	23	148.9	61.1	209	143.7	49.6	0.644
Albumins [g/dL]	27	2.8	0.5	249	2.9	0.4	0.071
Lymphocytes [%]	26	8.2	3.9	245	9.5	10.9	0.551
Potassium [mmol/L]	27	4.6	1.1	253	4.4	0.8	0.242
Sodium [mmol/L]	27	141.1	5.4	253	139.4	5.4	0.121
CRP [mg/L]	28	123.5	93.7	253	141.9	100.9	0.364
PCT [ng/mL]	28	3.6	16.0	252	2.0	7.5	0.351

Abbreviations: n, number of participants; $\bar{x}$, mean; SD, standard deviation; p, level of significance; BMI, body mass index; TGs, triglycerides; TC, total cholesterol; CRP, C-reactive protein; PCT, procalcitonin; ** t-test.

3.4. Survival Analysis

Survival analysis is shown in Kaplan-Meier survival curves (Figure 1). The median survival was 14 days (Table 6). Total survival was 32.2% (n = 92).

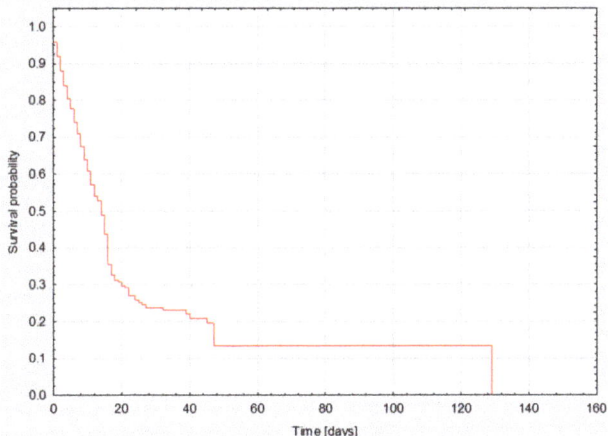

Figure 1. Analysis of survival of the whole group.

Table 6. Survival time.

		Survival Time [Days]
	25 percentiles (lower quartile)	6.0
Percentiles	50 percentiles (median)	14.3
	75 percentiles (upper quartile)	25.3

3.5. Survival Analysis—Group Comparisons

A comparison of survival curves was performed according to BMI and NRS. There were no statistically significant differences (Table 7, Figures 2 and 3).

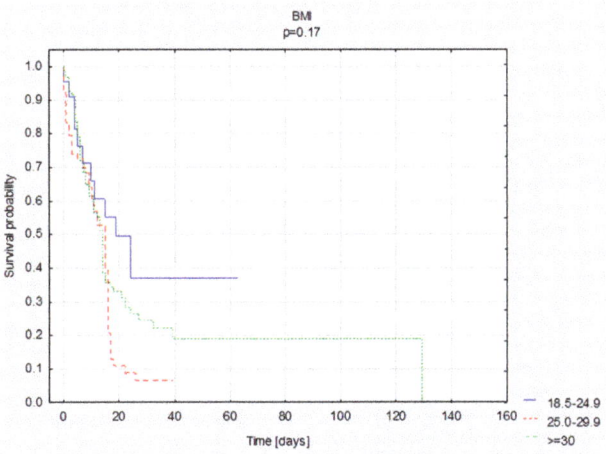

Figure 2. Comparison of survival curves according to BMI scores.

Table 7. Descriptive statistics for survival time, number of deaths and survival according to BMI and NRS scores.

		Descriptive Statistics				
		Me	x̄	SD	n—Death	n—Survivors
BMI	<18.5	-	-	-	-	-
	18.5–24.9	13.0	18.0	17.8	11	11
	25.0–29.9	11.5	10.8	8.2	63	15
	≥30	11.0	14.7	16.6	63	31
NRS	<3	10.0	13.2	14.8	19	9
	≥3	11.0	14.4	14.3	175	83

Abbreviations: n, number of participants; Me, median; x̄, mean; SD, standard deviation; BMI, body mass index; NRS, nutritional risk screening.

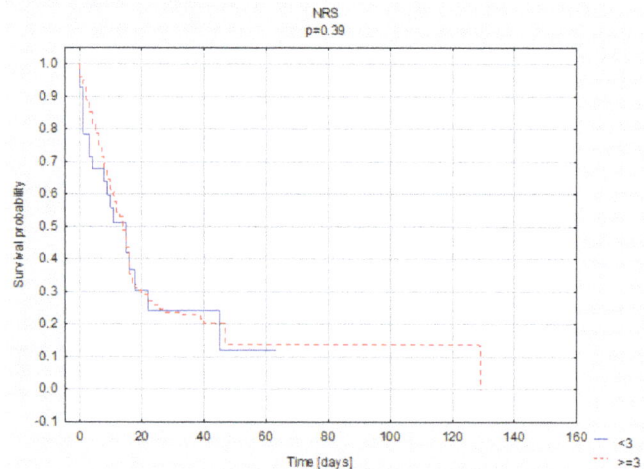

Figure 3. Comparison of survival curves according to NRS scores.

Assessment of the influence of selected variables on mortality is shown in Table 8 (Cox proportional hazards regression). It was observed that the risk of death increased in the group with BMI in the range of 25.0–29.9 (HR = 2.18; p = 0.010). Taking the quantitative variables into account, the risk of death was lower in patients with higher levels of TC (HR = 0.996; p = 0.034) and sodium (HR = 0.97; p = 0.033). However, age (HR = 1.03; p < 0.001), NRS (HR = 1.18; p = 0.019), high potassium (HR = 1.34; p = 0.002) and PCT (HR = 1.04; p < 0.001) also affected mortality.

Table 8. Assessment of the influence of variables on mortality: the Cox proportional hazards regression model, a single model.

		p-Value	HR	95% CI HR (Lower)	95% CI HR (Upper)
Sex (n = 286)	M	0.451	1.13	0.82	1.56
BMI (n = 194)	18.5–24.9		Ref.		
	25.0–29.9	0.010	2.18	1.14	4.16
	≥30	0.662	1.62	0.85	3.07
NRS (n = 286)	<3		Ref.		
	≥3	0.661	0.90	0.56	1.44

Table 8. *Cont.*

		p-Value	HR	95% CI HR (Lower)	95% CI HR (Upper)
HF (*n* = 286)	Yes	0.281	1.32	0.79	2.21
HT (*n* = 286)	Yes	0.733	1.05	0.79	1.40
DM (*n* = 286)	No	0.344	1.15	0.86	1.55
CVD (*n* = 286)	Yes	0.941	1.01	0.75	1.36
CRD (*n* = 286)	Yes	0.080	1.55	0.95	2.52
CKD (*n* = 286)	Yes	0.641	1.20	0.56	2.55
TGs (*n* = 251)	>150	0.671	1.08	0.77	1.51
TC (*n* = 232)	>190	0.184	0.76	0.51	1.14
Variables					
Age (*n* = 286)		0.000	1.03	1.02	1.04
NRS (*n* = 286)		0.019	1.18	1.03	1.35
BMI (*n* = 194)		0.522	0.99	0.96	1.02
Height [cm] (*n* = 193)		0.762	1.00	0.98	1.02
Body Mass [kg] (*n* = 194)		0.733	1.00	0.99	1.01
TGs [mg/dL] (*n* = 251)		0.844	1.00	1.00	1.00
TC [mg/dL] (*n* = 232)		0.034	1.00	0.99	1.00
Albumins [g/dL] (*n* = 276)		0.844	1.04	0.74	1.44
Lymphocytes [%] (*n* = 271)		0.011	1.00	0.99	1.02
Potassium [mmol/L] (*n* = 280)		0.002	1.34	1.11	1.61
Sodium [mmol/L] (*n* = 280)		0.033	0.97	0.95	1.00
CRP [mg/L] (*n* = 281)		0.283	1.00	1.00	1.00
PCT [ng/mL] (*n* = 280)		0.000	1.04	1.03	1.05

Abbreviations: *n*, number of participants; M, males; HR, hazard ratio; CI, confidence interval; *p*, level of significance; BMI, body mass index; NRS, nutritional risk screening; HF, heart failure; HT, arterial hypertension; DM, diabetes mellitus; CVD, cardiovascular disease; CRD, chronic respiratory disease; CKD, chronic kidney disease; TGs, triglycerides; TC, total cholesterol; CRP, C-reactive protein; PCT, procalcitonin.

Variables were included in the multivariate model in accordance with the adopted criteria. The criteria included the outcome of $p < 0.30$ in a univariate model, a lack of correlation of variables, and clinical recommendations. The following variables were included in the model: BMI (categories), HF, TC (quantitatively), age, NRS (quantitatively), potassium, sodium, CKD, CRP and PCT (Table 9).

The multivariate analysis showed that age (HR = 1.03, $p \leq 0.001$), potassium (HR = 1.40, $p = 0.023$), PCT (HR = 0.10, $p < 0.001$) and BMI 25.00–29.99 correlated with mortality (HR = 2.13, $p = 0.038$). Table 9 shows statistically significant variables.

Table 9. Assessment of the influence of variables on mortality: the Cox proportional hazards regression model, a multivariate model.

n = 153		Beta	Standard Error	Chi-Square	p-Value	HR	95% CI HR (Lower)	95% CI HR (Upper)
Age		0.03	0.01	11.2	0.001	1.03	1.01	1.05
Potassium [mmol/L]		0.34	0.15	5.2	0.023	1.40	1.05	1.88
PCT [ng/mL]		0.09	0.02	23.5	<0.001	1.10	1.06	1.14
BMI	25.0–29.9	0.33	0.16	4.3	0.038	2.13	1.03	4.40
	≥30	0.09	0.16	0.3	0.561	1.68	0.81	3.47

Abbreviations: n, number of participants; M, males; HR, hazard ratio; CI, confidence interval; p, level of significance; BMI, body mass index; TC, total cholesterol, PCT, procalcitonin.

4. Discussion

The nutritional status of COVID-19 patients is undoubtedly related to complications, and increased risk of death during in-patient treatment. The present study showed that patients with COVID-19 who died in the ICU were statistically significantly more likely to have comorbidities such as HF (p = 0.037) or HT (p = 0029). Nearly 68% of patients did not survive to discharge. Men died statistically significantly more often (p = 0.005). Other authors report between 20 and 62% of deaths during hospitalisation in the ICU and in the case of mechanically (either noninvasively or invasively) ventilated patients, from 50% to as much as 97% [15–17].

In the study group, the risk of death more than doubled (HR = 2.18) in patients who were overweight. The reasons for this may be that overweight patient are often not aware of their health condition because they do not have symptoms (e.g., metabolic disorders such as hypertension, insulin resistance, dyslipidemia or prediabetes, which frequently occur in overweight patients); therefore, they are less likely to undergo health examinations to diagnose their diseases, and comorbidities can lead to an increasingly severe course of, and consequent death from, COVID-19. It is widely known that both being overweight and obesity are risk factors for developing many comorbidities (including hypertension, CVD, DM2, obstructive sleep apnea) considered as risk factors for severe complications of COVID-19 [18–20]. In addition, being overweight and obesity alone may cause, e.g., chronic inflammation, which may lead to lowered immunity and lung function impairment. Jingzhou et.al. showed that being overweight was significantly associated with COVID-19 mortality at a global level [21].

Excessive body fat impedes respiratory gas exchange. Subcutaneous adipose tissue in the frontal part of the chest and at its sides increases its resistance during respiration, and, as a consequence, the patient might require higher positive pressure during mechanical ventilation [22]. It is also worth emphasising that abnormal body weight could be a problem during patient extubation. In such cases, especially in patients with obesity, there is a higher probability of upper airway obstruction and re-intubation [23]. According to Kompaniyets et al., in the United States from March to December 2020, among 34,899 patients hospitalised in the ICU for COVID-19, almost 28% were overweight and 50% were obese. The risk of death increased with increasing BMI [24]. In Europe (England), Gao et al. revealed in their prospective study that among 1601 patients in the ICU, 31% were overweight, and 50% were obese [25]. The results of the current study are similar. Among all inpatients, more than 40% were overweight, and nearly 50% were obese. Similar results were reported in France, where being overweight and obesity concerned 41.4% and 43.4% of ICU in-patients, respectively. In the cited study, the death rate was lower and amounted to 18.5%. Interestingly, multifactorial analysis indicated a paradoxical relationship between the category of BMI and mortality. Patients whose BMI was ≤29 kg/m^2 (OR = 3.64) and those whose BMI was >39 kg/m^2 (OR = 10.45) were more at risk of death compared to those with a BMI of 29–39 kg/m^2 [26]. Researchers point out that the risk of a severe COVID-19 disease course and invasive ventilation in the ICU is higher in patients being overweight or with obesity [27,28]. On the other hand, they also demonstrated that obesity is not a predictor of a higher risk of death in the ICU. A study by Zhaozhong et al. confirmed that there were more patients with obesity admitted to the ICU compared to those with a BMI < 30 kg/m^2 but, at the same time, obesity did not affect survival in these hospital units [29]. In another study, severe obesity classified as a BMI > 35 kg/m^2, and male sex, were independently related to the need for patient intubation and death [30]. Some studies, in this case, refer to the so-called "obesity paradox". Ironically, in patients with CVD, despite increased health risks associated with obesity, treatment outcomes were often better than in slimmer patients [31]. This can be observed, for example, in patients with HF. One of the possible explanations for this phenomenon is that the disease frequently develops in patients with obesity at a younger age, and intensive therapy, which might result in reduced mortality in this group, is provided earlier. In our study there was no significant difference regarding the age of obese and nonobese patients, but in some studies people with obesity were up to 10 years younger than individuals with normal body mass [32]. In these patients, their adipose tissue could serve as a nutrient when metabolism declines [33,34]. BMI itself is not a good indicator of obesity because it does not consider exact body composition, i.e., amount of muscle, fat distribution or water retention. However, due to its ease of use and availability, it is an integral part of the evaluation of patients with other diseases as well [35]. The index does not distinguish well between obesity phenotypes; thus, the same patient with a high BMI may be an individual with an athletic physique or sarcopenic obesity. In a recently published literature review, Dalamaga et al. confirmed that obesity and increased visceral fat were significant risk factors for poor outcomes related to COVID-19. Even though the presented study did not find any relation between obesity and the risk of death, its presence should still be considered a potential risk factor for severe complications and death.

In this study, univariate analysis revealed that the risk of death increased with the risk of malnutrition according to NRS2002 (HR = 1.18). Osuna-Padilla et al. showed that nutritional risk in mechanically ventilated ICU patients was related to an increased risk of death (OR = 2.4, and was found in 66% of patients [36]. A similar result was reported by Zhang et al., where nutritional risk was found in more than 60% of hospitalised patients. The mortality rate was statistically significantly higher in that group. Moreover, those patients suffered from more comorbidities [37]. In both studies, the nutritional risk was analysed using the NUTRIC score. In this study, the risk of malnutrition occurred in 90% of patients and the screening assessment of nutritional status was performed using the validated NRS2002 questionnaire. Studies by other authors show that it is a good tool to assess the nutritional status of COVID-19 patients [38]. Retrospective and review studies show a high percentage of patients who are not only critically ill are also affected by malnutrition. This number is as high as 70%. These studies also show that malnutrition risk is strongly associated with mortality [39–41]. Malnutrition results in decreased body weight, muscle weakness, impaired immunity, decreased protein levels and oxygen utilisation [42], which affects the course of the disease.

In the multivariate analysis, in addition to being overweight, increases in plasma potassium levels (HR = 1.40) and procalcitonin levels (HR = 1.10) were associated with higher mortality risk. Abnormal plasma potassium levels may be one of the symptoms of acid-base imbalance that occurs in patients with acute respiratory failure. It may also cause cardiac arrhythmia, bradyarrhythmia, complete heart block and circulatory arrest [43,44]. In a study concerning critically ill COVID-19 patients, Shengcong et al. found a significant increase in mortality rate in patients with potassium levels ≥5.0 mmol/L [45]. On the other hand, according to Perez, hypokalemia is associated with longer hospital and ICU stay but does not affect mortality [46]. Research shows that an increase in procalcitonin levels is one of the indicators of disease severity in COVID-19 patients, and is a risk factor of mortality [47,48]. The results of this study seem to be consistent with those published so far and indicate an association between the value of this inflammatory marker and the increased risk of in-hospital mortality (in multivariate analysis: HR = 1.10; $p < 0.001$) [49,50]. In the study by Fenk et al., the risk of death increased up to fivefold (OR = 5.65; $p < 0.001$) in patients with high procalcitonin levels, indicating that this marker may be useful to reflect the degree of lung involvement during SARS-CoV-2 infection [51]. Leoni et al., who studied 242 COVID-19 patients hospitalised in the ICU, also found that predictors of increased mortality rate in the ICU include, among others, age, obesity and higher procalcitonin levels (HR = 1.03, p = 0.04). These predictors were independently associated with 28-day mortality [52].

Study Limitations

This study has some limitations. As it involved critically ill and mechanically ventilated (using invasive methods) patients, complete data concerning their medical history and medications could not always be obtained due to the serious nature of the situation.

Besides, we obtained statistical significance according to our classification, although other classifications could have been done. In our study, the data with no statistical significance must be taken with caution, and cannot be excluded.

The inference analysis should be interpreted with the variables we selected, and considering the whole study. We also do not have information about the time between the first symptoms of COVID-19 and hospital admission to the ICU. In some cases, NRS and BMI scores were not included in medical records. Regarding to the high proportion (90%) of individuals with a NRS $\geq$ 3, this can interfere with the results. Moreover, body composition analysis was not conducted in patients, and BMI scores may not be a reliable indicator for assessing overweight and obesity. Patients did not have their waist-to-hip ratio (WHR) measured, and data concerning central obesity based on waist circumference was not reported either. Finally, the long-term survival of COVID-19 patients could not be assessed due to restrictions on access to personal data because of the anonymity of medical records.

5. Conclusions

Being overweight in critically ill COVID-19 patients requiring invasive mechanical ventilation increases their risk of death significantly. Additional factors indicating a higher risk of death include the patient's age, high PCT and potassium levels measured at the time of admission to the ICU. Even though the presented study did not find any association between obesity and the risk of death, obesity should still be considered a potential risk factor for severe complications and death. The lack of confirmation of this association in this study should not be interpreted as providing a potential protective effect. The risk of malnutrition at the time of ICU admission also increases the risk of in-hospital death. Undoubtedly, studies concerning the nutritional status of COVID-19 patients hospitalised in the ICU need further investigation.

Author Contributions: Conceptualisation, M.C. and R.J.-V.; methodology, M.C. and R.J.-V.; software, M.C., S.Z.; validation, M.C., R.J.-V.; formal analysis, M.C.; investigation, M.C.; resources, M.C.; data curation, M.C.; writing—original draft preparation, M.C.; writing—review and editing, M.C., R.J.-V., S.Z., V.G.-C.; supervision, M.Z.; project administration, M.C.; funding acquisition, M.C. and M.Z., S.Z. All authors have read and agreed to the published version of the manuscript.

Funding: The study was funded by the Ministry of Science and Higher Education of Poland under the statutory grant of the Wroclaw Medical University (SUB.E140.21.108).

Institutional Review Board Statement: The study was conducted according to the guidelines of the Declaration of Helsinki and approved by the Independent Bioethics Committee of the Wroclaw Medical University (decision No. KB-229/2021).

Informed Consent Statement: Not applicable.

Data Availability Statement: The data are available by contacting the corresponding author.

Acknowledgments: There were no other contributors to the article than the authors. Certified English language services were provided.

Conflicts of Interest: The authors declare no conflict of interest.

References

1. WHO Coronavirus (COVID-19) Dashboard. Available online: https://covid19.who.int (accessed on 30 August 2021).
2. Singer, P.; Blaser, A.R.; Berger, M.M.; Alhazzani, W.; Calder, P.C.; Casaer, M.P.; Hiesmayr, M.; Mayer, K.; Montejo, J.C.; Pichard, C.; et al. ESPEN Guideline on Clinical Nutrition in the Intensive Care Unit. *Clin. Nutr.* **2019**, *38*, 48–79. [CrossRef] [PubMed]
3. Wang, D.; Hu, B.; Hu, C.; Zhu, F.; Liu, X.; Zhang, J.; Wang, B.; Xiang, H.; Cheng, Z.; Xiong, Y.; et al. Clinical Characteristics of 138 Hospitalized Patients With 2019 Novel Coronavirus-Infected Pneumonia in Wuhan, China. *JAMA* **2020**, *323*, 1061–1069. [CrossRef] [PubMed]
4. Beck, M.A.; Levander, O.A. Host Nutritional Status and Its Effect on a Viral Pathogen. *J. Infect. Dis.* **2000**, *182* (Suppl. S1), S93–S96. [CrossRef] [PubMed]
5. James, P.T.; Ali, Z.; E Armitage, A.; Bonell, A.; Cerami, C.; Drakesmith, H.; Jobe, M.; Jones, K.S.; Liew, Z.; E Moore, S.; et al. The Role of Nutrition in COVID-19 Susceptibility and Severity of Disease: A Systematic Review. *J. Nutr.* **2021**, *151*, 1854–1878. [CrossRef] [PubMed]
6. Wei, C.; Liu, Y.; Li, Y.; Zhang, Y.; Zhong, M.; Meng, X. Evaluation of the Nutritional Status in Patients with COVID-19. *J. Clin. Biochem. Nutr.* **2020**, *67*, 116–121. [CrossRef]
7. Pironi, L.; Sasdelli, A.S.; Ravaioli, F.; Baracco, B.; Battaiola, C.; Bocedi, G.; Brodosi, L.; Leoni, L.; Mari, G.A.; Musio, A. Malnutrition and Nutritional Therapy in Patients with SARS-CoV-2 Disease. *Clin. Nutr.* **2021**, *40*, 1330–1337. [CrossRef]
8. Bedock, D.; Couffignal, J.; Lassen, P.B.; Soares, L.; Mathian, A.; Fadlallah, J.; Amoura, Z.; Oppert, J.-M.; Faucher, P. Evolution of Nutritional Status after Early Nutritional Management in COVID-19 Hospitalized Patients. *Nutrients* **2021**, *13*, 2276. [CrossRef]
9. Wolf, M.; Alladina, J.; Navarrete-Welton, A.; Shoults, B.; Brait, K.; Ziehr, D.; Malhotra, A.; Corey Hardin, C.; Hibbert, K.A. Obesity and Critical Illness in COVID-19: Respiratory Pathophysiology. *Obesity* **2021**, *29*, 870–878. [CrossRef]
10. Zhang, L.; Liu, Y. Potential Interventions for Novel Coronavirus in China: A Systematic Review. *J. Med Virol.* **2020**, *92*, 479–490. [CrossRef]
11. Cederholm, T.; Jensen, G.L.; Correia, M.I.T.D.; Gonzalez, M.C.; Fukushima, R.; Higashiguchi, T.; Baptista, G.; Barazzoni, R.; Blaauw, R.; Coats, A.J.; et al. GLIM Criteria for the Diagnosis of Malnutrition—A Consensus Report from the Global Clinical Nutrition Community. *Clin. Nutr.* **2019**, *38*, 207–217. [CrossRef]
12. Lewandowicz-Umyszkiewicz, M.; Wieczorowska-Tobis, K. Nowe kryteria diagnozowania niedożywienia. *GERIATRIA* **2019**, *13*, 101–105.
13. Barazzoni, R.; Bischoff, S.C.; Breda, J.; Wickramasinghe, K.; Krznaric, Z.; Nitzan, D.; Pirlich, M.; Singer, P. ESPEN Expert Statements and Practical Guidance for Nutritional Management of Individuals with SARS-CoV-2 Infection. *Clin. Nutr.* **2020**, *39*, 1631–1638, endorsed by the ESPEN Council. [CrossRef] [PubMed]
14. Kondrup, J.; Allison, S.P.; Elia, M.; Vellas, B.; Plauth, M. ESPEN Guidelines for Nutrition Screening 2002. *Clin. Nutr.* **2003**, *22*, 415–421. [CrossRef]
15. Myers, L.C.; Parodi, S.M.; Escobar, G.J.; Liu, V.C. Characteristics of Hospitalized Adults With COVID-19 in an Integrated Health Care System in California. *JAMA* **2020**, *323*, 2195–2198. [CrossRef] [PubMed]
16. Arentz, M.; Yim, E.; Klaff, L.; Lokhandwala, S.; Riedo, F.X.; Chong, M.; Lee, M. Characteristics and Outcomes of 21 Critically Ill Patients With COVID-19 in Washington State. *JAMA* **2020**, *323*, 1612–1614. [CrossRef]
17. Wang, Y.; Lu, X.; Li, Y.; Chen, H.; Chen, T.; Su, N.; Huang, F.; Zhou, J.; Zhang, B.; Yan, F.; et al. Clinical Course and Outcomes of 344 Intensive Care Patients with COVID-19. *Am. J. Respir. Crit. Care Med.* **2020**, *201*, 1430–1434. [CrossRef] [PubMed]
18. Dixon, A.E.; Peters, U. The Effect of Obesity on Lung Function. *Expert Rev. Respir. Med.* **2018**, *12*, 755–767. [CrossRef]
19. Cercato, C.; Fonseca, F.A. Cardiovascular Risk and Obesity. *Diabetol. Metab. Syndr.* **2019**, *11*, 74. [CrossRef]
20. Sanchis-Gomar, F.; Lavie, C.J.; Mehra, M.R.; Henry, B.M.; Lippi, G. Obesity and Outcomes in COVID-19: When an Epidemic and Pandemic Collide. *Mayo Clin. Proc.* **2020**, *95*, 1445–1453. [CrossRef]
21. Wang, J.; Sato, T.; Sakuraba, A. Worldwide Association of Lifestyle-Related Factors and COVID-19 Mortality. *Ann. Med.* **2021**, *53*, 1528–1533. [CrossRef]
22. Pelosi, P.; Croci, M.; Ravagnan, I.; Vicardi, P.; Gattinoni, L. Total Respiratory System, Lung, and Chest Wall Mechanics in Sedated-Paralyzed Postoperative Morbidly Obese Patients. *Chest* **1996**, *109*, 144–151. [CrossRef] [PubMed]
23. Hibbert, K.; Rice, M.; Malhotra, A. Obesity and ARDS. *Chest* **2012**, *142*, 785–790. [CrossRef] [PubMed]
24. Kompaniyets, L.; Goodman, A.B.; Belay, B.; Freedman, D.S.; Sucosky, M.S.; Lange, S.J.; Gundlapalli, A.V.; Boehmer, T.K.; Blanck, H.M. Body Mass Index and Risk for COVID-19–Related Hospitalization, Intensive Care Unit Admission, Invasive Mechanical Ventilation, and Death—United States, March–December 2020. *MMWR. Morb. Mortal. Wkly. Rep.* **2021**, *70*, 355–361. [CrossRef] [PubMed]
25. Gao, M.; Piernas, C.; Astbury, N.M.; Hippisley-Cox, J.; O'Rahilly, S.; Aveyard, P.; A Jebb, S. Associations between Body-Mass Index and COVID-19 Severity in 6·9 Million People in England: A Prospective, Community-Based, Cohort Study. *Lancet Diabetes Endocrinol.* **2021**, *9*, 350–359. [CrossRef]
26. Dana, R.; Bannay, A.; Bourst, P.; Ziegler, C.; Losser, M.-R.; Gibot, S.; Levy, B.; Audibert, G.; Ziegler, O. Obesity and Mortality in Critically Ill COVID-19 Patients with Respiratory Failure. *Int. J. Obes.* **2021**, *45*, 2028–2037. [CrossRef]
27. Zhu, Z.; Hasegawa, K.; Ma, B.; Fujiogi, M.; Camargo, C.A.; Liang, L. Association of Obesity and Its Genetic Predisposition with the Risk of Severe COVID-19: Analysis of Population-Based Cohort Data. *Metabolism* **2020**, *112*, 154345. [CrossRef]

28. Rottoli, M.; Bernante, P.; Belvedere, A.; Balsamo, F.; Garelli, S.; Giannella, M.; Cascavilla, A.; Tedeschi, S.; Ianniruberto, S.; Del Turco, E.R.; et al. How Important Is Obesity as a Risk Factor for Respiratory Failure, Intensive Care Admission and Death in Hospitalised COVID-19 Patients? Results from a Single Italian Centre. *Eur. J. Endocrinol.* **2020**, *183*, 389–397. [CrossRef]
29. Biscarini, S.; Colaneri, M.; Ludovisi, S.; Seminari, E.; Pieri, T.C.; Valsecchi, P.; Gallazzi, I.; Giusti, E.; Cammà, C.; Zuccaro, V.; et al. The Obesity Paradox: Analysis from the SMAtteo COvid-19 REgistry (SMACORE) Cohort. *Nutr.Metab. Cardiovasc. Dis.* **2020**, *30*, 1920–1925. [CrossRef]
30. Palaiodimos, L.; Kokkinidis, D.G.; Li, W.; Karamanis, D.; Ognibene, J.; Arora, S.; Southern, W.N.; Mantzoros, C.S. Severe Obesity, Increasing Age and Male Sex Are Independently Associated with Worse in-Hospital Outcomes, and Higher in-Hospital Mortality, in a Cohort of Patients with COVID-19 in the Bronx, New York. *Metab. Clin. Exp.* **2020**, *108*, 154262. [CrossRef]
31. Elagizi, A.; Carbone, S.; Lavie, C.J.; Mehra, M.R.; Ventura, H.O. Implications of Obesity across the Heart Failure Continuum. *Prog. Cardiovasc. Dis.* **2020**, *63*, 561–569. [CrossRef]
32. Niedziela, J.; Hudzik, B.; Niedziela, N.; Gąsior, M.; Gierlotka, M.; Wasilewski, J.; Myrda, K.; Lekston, A.; Poloński, L.; Rozentryt, P. The Obesity Paradox in Acute Coronary Syndrome: A Meta-Analysis. *Eur. J. Epidemiol.* **2014**, *29*, 801–812. [CrossRef] [PubMed]
33. Bucholz, E.M.; Beckman, A.L.; Krumholz, H.A.; Krumholz, H.M.; Beckman, A.L.; Krumholz, H.A.; Krumholz, H.M. Excess Weight and Life Expectancy after Acute Myocardial Infarction: The Obesity Paradox Reexamined. *Am. Heart J.* **2016**, *172*, 173–181. [CrossRef] [PubMed]
34. Karampela, I.; Chrysanthopoulou, E.; Christodoulatos, G.S.; Dalamaga, M. Is There an Obesity Paradox in Critical Illness? Epidemiologic and Metabolic Considerations. *Curr. Obes. Rep.* **2020**, *9*, 231–244. [CrossRef]
35. Yousufuddin, M.; Takahashi, P.Y.; Major, B.; Ahmmad, E.; Al-Zubi, H.; Peters, J.; Doyle, T.; Jensen, K.; Al Ward, R.Y.; Sharma, U.; et al. Association between Hyperlipidemia and Mortality after Incident Acute Myocardial Infarction or Acute Decompensated Heart Failure: A Propensity Score Matched Cohort Study and a Meta-Analysis. *BMJ Open* **2019**, *9*, e028638. [CrossRef] [PubMed]
36. Osuna-Padilla, I.A.; Rodríguez-Moguel, N.C.; Aguilar-Vargas, A.; Rodríguez-Llamazares, S. High Nutritional Risk Using NUTRIC-Score Is Associated with Worse Outcomes in COVID-19 Critically Ill Patients. *Nutr. Hosp.* **2021**, *38*, 540–544. [CrossRef]
37. Zhang, P.; He, Z.; Yu, G.; Peng, D.; Feng, Y.; Ling, J.; Wang, Y.; Li, S.; Bian, Y. The Modified NUTRIC Score Can Be Used for Nutritional Risk Assessment as Well as Prognosis Prediction in Critically Ill COVID-19 Patients. *Clin. Nutr.* **2021**, *40*, 534–541. [CrossRef]
38. Ali, A.; Kunugi, H. Approaches to Nutritional Screening in Patients with Coronavirus Disease 2019 (COVID-19). *Int. J. Environ. Res. Public Health* **2021**, *18*, 2772. [CrossRef]
39. Lechien, J.R.; Chiesa-Estomba, C.M.; De Siati, D.R.; Horoi, M.; Le Bon, S.D.; Rodrigues, A.; Dequanter, D.; Blecic, S.; El Afia, F.; Distinguin, L.; et al. Olfactory and Gustatory Dysfunctions as a Clinical Presentation of Mild-to-Moderate Forms of the Coronavirus Disease (COVID-19): A Multicenter European Study. *Eur. Arch. Oto-Rhino-Laryngol.* **2020**, *277*, 2251–2261. [CrossRef]
40. Lechien, J.R.; Chiesa-Estomba, C.M.; Place, S.; Van Laethem, Y.; Cabaraux, P.; Mat, Q.; Huet, K.; Plzak, J.; Horoi, M.; Hans, S.; et al. Clinical and Epidemiological Characteristics of 1420 European Patients with Mild-to-Moderate Coronavirus Disease 2019. *J. Intern. Med.* **2020**, *288*, 335–344. [CrossRef]
41. Li, G.; Zhou, C.-L.; Ba, Y.-M.; Wang, Y.-M.; Song, B.; Cheng, X.-B.; Dong, Q.-F.; Wang, L.-L.; You, S.-S. Nutritional Risk and Therapy for Severe and Critical COVID-19 Patients: A Multicenter Retrospective Observational Study. *Clin. Nutr.* **2021**, *40*, 2154–2161. [CrossRef]
42. Ljungqvist, O.; van Gossum, A.; Sanz, M.L.; de Man, F. The European Fight against Malnutrition. *Clin. Nutr.* **2010**, *29*, 149–150. [CrossRef]
43. Romano, T.G.; Correia, M.D.T.; Mendes, P.V.; Zampieri, F.G.; Maciel, A.T.; Park, M. Metabolic Acid-Base Adaptation Triggered by Acute Persistent Hypercapnia in Mechanically Ventilated Patients with Acute Respiratory Distress Syndrome. *Rev. Bras. De Ter. Intensiv.* **2016**, *28*, 19–26. [CrossRef] [PubMed]
44. McMahon, G.; Mendu, M.L.; Gibbons, F.K.; Christopher, K.B. Association between Hyperkalemia at Critical Care Initiation and Mortality. *Intensiv. Care Med.* **2012**, *38*, 1834–1842. [CrossRef] [PubMed]
45. Liu, S.; Zhang, L.; Weng, H.; Yang, F.; Jin, H.; Fan, F.; Zheng, X.; Yang, H.; Li, H.; Zhang, Y.; et al. Association Between Average Plasma Potassium Levels and 30-Day Mortality During Hospitalization in Patients with COVID-19 in Wuhan, China. *Int. J. Med. Sci.* **2021**, *18*, 736–743. [CrossRef] [PubMed]
46. Moreno-Pérez, O.; Leon-Ramirez, J.-M.; Fuertes-Kenneally, L.; Perdiguero, M.; Andres, M.; Garcia-Navarro, M.; Ruiz-Torregrosa, P.; Boix, V.; Gil, J.; Merino, E.; et al. Hypokalemia as a Sensitive Biomarker of Disease Severity and the Requirement for Invasive Mechanical Ventilation Requirement in COVID-19 Pneumonia: A Case Series of 306 Mediterranean Patients. *Int. J. Infect. Dis.* **2020**, *100*, 449–454. [CrossRef]
47. Hu, R.; Han, C.; Pei, S.; Yin, M.; Chen, X. Procalcitonin Levels in COVID-19 Patients. *Int. J. Antimicrob. Agents* **2020**, *56*, 106051. [CrossRef]
48. Liu, Z.-M.; Li, J.-P.; Wang, S.-P.; Chen, D.-Y.; Zeng, W.; Chen, S.-C.; Huang, Y.-H.; Huang, J.-L.; Long, W.; Li, M.; et al. Association of Procalcitonin Levels with the Progression and Prognosis of Hospitalized Patients with COVID-19. *Int. J. Med. Sci.* **2020**, *17*, 2468. [CrossRef]
49. Lippi, G.; Plebani, M. Procalcitonin in Patients with Severe Coronavirus Disease 2019 (COVID-19): A Meta-Analysis. *Clin. Chim. Acta Int. J. Clin. Chem.* **2020**, *505*, 190–191. [CrossRef]

50. Zhou, F.; Yu, T.; Du, R.; Fan, G.; Liu, Y.; Liu, Z.; Xiang, J.; Wang, Y.; Song, B.; Gu, X.; et al. Clinical Course and Risk Factors for Mortality of Adult Inpatients with COVID-19 in Wuhan, China: A Retrospective Cohort Study. *Lancet* **2020**, *395*, 1054–1062. [CrossRef]
51. Feng, T.; James, A.; Doumlele, K.; White, S.; Twardzik, W.; Zahid, K.; Sattar, Z.; Foronjy, R.; Nakeshbandi, M.; Chow, L. Procalcitonin Levels in COVID-19 Patients Are Strongly Associated with Mortality and ICU Acceptance in an Underserved, Inner City Population. In Proceedings of the American Thoracic Society International Conference, San Francisco, CA, USA, 14–19 May 2021.
52. Leoni, M.L.G.; Lombardelli, L.; Colombi, D.; Bignami, E.G.; Pergolotti, B.; Repetti, F.; Villani, M.; Bellini, V.; Rossi, T.; Halasz, G.; et al. Prediction of 28-Day Mortality in Critically Ill Patients with COVID-19: Development and Internal Validation of a Clinical Prediction Model. *PLoS ONE* **2021**, *16*, e0254550. [CrossRef]

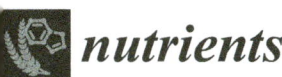

Article

Energy Achievement Rate Is an Independent Factor Associated with Intensive Care Unit Mortality in High-Nutritional-Risk Patients with Acute Respiratory Distress Syndrome Requiring Prolonged Prone Positioning Therapy

Pin-Kuei Fu [1,2,3,4,*,†], Chen-Yu Wang [1,5,†], Wei-Ning Wang [6], Chiann-Yi Hsu [7], Shih-Pin Lin [8] and Chen-Tsung Kuo [9]

1 Department of Critical Care Medicine, Taichung Veterans General Hospital, Taichung 407219, Taiwan; chestmen@gmail.com
2 Ph.D. Program in Translational Medicine, National Chung Hsing University, Taichung 402010, Taiwan
3 College of Human Science and Social Innovation, Hungkuang University, Taichung 433304, Taiwan
4 Department of Computer Science, Tunghai University, Taichung 407224, Taiwan
5 Department of Nursing, Hungkuang University, Taichung 43302, Taiwan
6 Department of Food and Nutrition, Taichung Veterans General Hospital, Taichung 40705, Taiwan; sherry@vghtc.gov.tw
7 Biostatistics Task Force of Taichung Veterans General Hospital, Taichung 407219, Taiwan; chiann@vghtc.gov.tw
8 Department of Information Engineering and Computer Science, Feng Chia University, Taichung 407802, Taiwan; yalebin.lin@gmail.com
9 Computer & Communications Center, Taipei Veterans General Hospital, Taipei 11217, Taiwan; jmskuo@gmail.com
* Correspondence: yetquen@gmail.com; Tel.: +886-4-23592525 (ext. 6536)
† These authors contributed equally to this work.

Abstract: Early enteral nutrition (EN) and a nutrition target >60% are recommended for patients in the intensive care unit (ICU), even for those with acute respiratory distress syndrome (ARDS). Prolonged prone positioning (PP) therapy (>48 h) is the rescue therapy of ARDS, but it may worsen the feeding status because it requires the heavy sedation and total paralysis of patients. Our previous studies demonstrated that energy achievement rate (EAR) >65% was a good prognostic factor in ICU. However, its impact on the mortality of patients with ARDS requiring prolonged PP therapy remains unclear. We retrospectively analyzed 79 patients with high nutritional risk (modified nutrition risk in the critically ill; mNUTRIC score ≥5); and identified factors associated with ICU mortality by using a Cox regression model. Through univariate analysis, mNUTRIC score, comorbid with malignancy, actual energy intake, and EAR (%) were associated with ICU mortality. By multivariate analysis, EAR (%) was a strong predictive factor of ICU mortality (HR: 0.19, 95% CI: 0.07–0.56). EAR >65% was associated with lower 14-day, 28-day, and ICU mortality after adjustment for confounding factors. We suggest early EN and increase EAR >65% may benefit patients with ARDS who required prolonged PP therapy.

Keywords: acute respiratory distress syndrome; energy achievement rate; high nutritional risk; mortality; modified nutrition risk in the critically ill; prolonged prone positioning

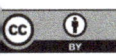

1. Introduction

Early enteral nutrition (EN) initiated within 48 h is recommended for all critically ill patients treated with invasive mechanical ventilation in the intensive care unit (ICU) [1–4]. According to current guidelines, a systemic survey of nutritional risk within 24 h of admission is recommended, accompanied by early EN [2–4] to reduce the risk of infectious complications and organ failure in critically ill patients [4,5]. The modified nutrition risk in the critically ill (mNUTRIC) score is a powerful screening tool that uses a cutoff value of ≥5 to identify patients with high nutritional risk [6] and even critically ill patients with COVID-19 infection [7]. After the identification of higher-risk groups, the second step is the achievement of feeding goals [1]. The ideal energy achievement rate (EAR) for the first week in the ICU is 60–70% of the nutritional target according to the 2016 American Society for Parenteral and Enteral Nutrition (ASPEN) and Society of Critical Care Medicine (SCCM) guidelines and the 2019 European Society for Clinical Nutrition and Metabolism (ESPN) guidelines [1,3,4]. Our previous studies have also demonstrated that an EAR of >65% was associated with lower mortality risk in medical ICUs [8–11]. However, the impact of EAR on the mortality of patients with high nutritional risk and acute respiratory distress syndrome (ARDS) requiring prolonged prone positioning (PP) therapy remains unclear.

The most severe condition for patients in medical ICUs is ARDS secondary to pneumonia or sepsis because the mortality rate can vary from 34.9% for mild ARDS to 46.1% for severe ARDS [12,13]. Prolonged PP therapy for at least 16 h per day is the standard of care for moderate to severe ARDS because a landmark study revealed that it reduced mortality [14,15]. PP therapy is an effective strategy to improve oxygenation and secretion clearance in cases of severe COVID-19-associated ARDS (CARDS) [16,17]. However, PP therapy may affect the achievement of feeding goals [18] because of the elevated intra-abdominal pressure and decreased gastrointestinal mobility caused by the heavy sedation induced by midazolam or propofol and the total paralysis caused by neuromuscular blocking agents [19]. One study discovered that EN was stopped more frequently for patients in the prone position than for those in the supine position [20]. Vomiting episodes were also more frequent for patients with ARDS receiving PP therapy [21]. Because prolonged PP therapy has become the standard of care for moderate to severe ARDS and CARDS, the aim of the current study investigated the association between EAR and ICU mortality in patients with high nutritional risk and ARDS receiving prolonged PP therapy.

2. Materials and Methods
2.1. Study Design and Patient Enrollment

This retrospective cohort study investigated the respiratory intensive care unit (RICU) of Taichung Veterans General Hospital (TCVGH), a tertiary referral center in Taiwan, from January 2014 to June 2018. We enrolled patients with high nutritional risk and a diagnosis of moderate to severe ARDS requiring mechanical ventilation and prolonged PP therapy for at least 48 h in the first week of ICU admission. High nutritional risk was defined as an mNUTRIC score of ≥5 in the first ICU stay or a feeding volume of <750 mL/day within 48 h of ICU admission, as in our previous publications [8,10]. Moderate to severe ARDS was defined as partial pressure of oxygen/fraction concentration of inspired oxygen ratio (PaO_2/FiO_2 ratio) of <150 mm Hg in accordance with the Berlin definition of ARDS [8,10,22,23]. The following patients were excluded: those requiring surgical intervention for acute abdominal infection or extracorporeal membrane oxygenation support within 48 h of admission because of failed PP therapy; those with comorbid poor cardiac function; those with active cancer in the terminal stage and a do not resuscitate order; and those who did not receive continuous PP therapy for more than 48 h (Figure 1). The demographic data, comorbidities, severity scores, daily feeding status, and clinical outcomes were extracted from electronic medical records. The study protocol was reviewed and approved by the Institutional Review Board of TCVGH (IRB number, CE20308B; date of approval, 16 September 2020). The study was conducted in accordance with the Declaration of Helsinki and relevant guidelines and regulations. The requirement for informed consent was waived because of the retrospective nature of the study, and the patients' personal information was deidentified prior to analysis.

2.2. Protocol of Prone Positioning Therapy

The RICU is a 24-bed medical ICU that services adult patients with diagnoses of sepsis, acute respiratory failure, and ARDS requiring mechanical ventilation. For patients diagnosed as having moderate to severe ARDS, the standard of care in the RICU is to follow a lung protective strategy to maintain plateau pressure at less than 30 cm H_2O by using low-tidal-volume ventilation (4–6 mL/kg) [14,24]. PP therapy is the first choice for rescue therapy in our RICU [25] when patients with moderate to severe ARDS experience refractory hypoxemia less than 24 h, a standard modified from that of landmark studies [14,15,26,27]. Since 2007, the protocol for PP therapy in our RICU was at least 48 h of continuous therapy [25,28]. Once the patients' hypoxemia improves and their clinical condition stabilizes (i.e., when peripheral capillary oxygen saturation >90% and FiO_2 <60% for >24 h after at least 48 h of PP therapy), patients are turned to the supine position. For prolonged PP therapy, patients require heavy sedation with medications such as midazolam or propofol and total paralysis through neuromuscular blocking agents to achieve a Richmond Agitation Sedation Scale score of less than −4. During PP therapy, patients are alternately turned right and left every 2 h to reduce the risk of pressure sore formation in the facial area, as described in our previous studies [25].

2.3. Protocol of Nutritional Risk Evaluation and Treatment

The evaluation of nutritional risk and suggestions for personalized nutritional prescriptions have been supported by a registered dietitian in our RICU since 2016. The mNUTRIC score and EAR were recorded, and nutritional prescriptions were suggested by the dietitian, as in our previous studies [8–11,29]. Early EN, the standard of care, was provided through a nasogastric tube on the first day of RICU admission for each patient, even for those requiring PP therapy [25]. The target energy requirement was 25–30 kcal/kg/day, and the target protein intake was 1.2 g/kg/day in accordance with the guidelines [3,4]. For patients who could not tolerate the standard feeding target, trophic feeding was provided to achieve a target of approximately 600 kcal/day, and 8–10 kcal/kg/day was also allowed during PP therapy [9].

2.4. Data Collection, Assessment, and Outcome Measures

Data on age, gender, body mass index (BMI), severity of illness score (Sequential Organ Failure Assessment [SOFA], Acute Physiology and Chronic Health Evaluation [APACHE] II, and mNUTRIC scores), major comorbidities, and PaO_2/FiO_2 ratio were extracted from the electronic medical records. The index date was the day of initiating PP therapy for ARDS. Daily EAR (%) was recorded on the index day and the seven days thereafter. The energy intake and energy intake achievement rate (%) of each day were calculated as follows: (actual energy intake/estimated energy requirement) × 100 [8–11]. The primary outcome was the correlation between energy intake achievement rate and ICU mortality. We identified an EAR of <65% in the first week of ICU admission as a poor prognostic factor for patients with high nutritional risk in our previous study [8,11], and this study was conducted to confirm the power of this predictor of ICU mortality.

2.5. Statistical Analysis

SPSS (version 22.0; International Business Machines Corp, Armonk, NY, USA) was used to perform the statistical analysis. The categorical variables are presented as frequencies and percentages. A chi-squared test was performed to determine significance. For nonparametric data distributions, a Mann–Whitney U test was performed to identify the differences between groups, and the results are presented as medians and interquartile ranges (IQRs). Cox regression analysis was performed to identify the factors associated with mortality. The strength of associations is presented with hazard ratios (HRs) and 95% confidence intervals (CIs). The survival curves were constructed through Kaplan–Meier analysis. A log-rank test was performed to identify significant differences in survival outcome between groups. All tests were two sided, with $p < 0.05$ considered significant.

3. Results

3.1. Patients' Clinical and Demographic Characteristics

A total of 79 patients with moderate to severe ARDS receiving prolonged PP therapy (>48 h) were enrolled in this study (Figure 1). The median mNUTRIC score of this cohort was 7 (IQR: 5–8), indicating that the enrollees had high nutrition risk and required additional energy intake to reduce mortality [3,4]. The median APACHE II and SOFA scores were 31 (IQR: 27–33) and 10 (IQR: 8–14), respectively, and the median PaO_2/FiO_2 was 92.5 (IQR: 70.1–114.3), indicating high clinical severity, severe hypoxemia, and a higher probability of mortality. The overall mortality rate in the ICU was 48.1%. The average EAR (%) was higher during the post–PP therapy period than during PP therapy (64.5% and 42%). However, the median EAR (55.5%, IQR: 33.1–81.8%) was lower than 65% in the first seven days after the index date (Table 1).

Table 1. Demographic characteristics, severity scores, comorbidities, and clinical outcomes of patients with moderate to severe ARDS receiving prolonged PP therapy in the ICU.

Characteristics	Median (IQR) or n (%) (n = 79)
Demographic data	
Age (y/o) (n, %)	61.5 (51.1–74)
Gender-Male (n, %)	48 (60.8%)
mNUTRIC score	7.0 (5–8)
APACHE II score	31.0 (27–33)
SOFA	10.0 (8–14)
Renal replacement therapy (n, %)	35 (44.30%)
Comorbidity	
CAD (n, %)	6 (7.59%)
COPD (n, %)	10 (12.66%)
Solid cancer (n, %)	11 (13.92%)
Hematologic malignancies (n, %)	5 (6.33%)
DM (n, %)	24 (30.38%)
CKD (n, %)	27 (34.18%)
Autoimmune disease (n, %)	12 (15.19%)
PaO_2/FiO_2 (PF ratio)	92.5 (70.1–114.3)
Actual energy intake (kcal/BW)	
During prolonged PP (d 1–d 3)	7.9 (4.6–13)
Post prolonged PP (d 4–d 7)	12.0 (7.3–18.8)
Average in the first 7 d	10.8 (6.6–15.2)
Energy achievement rate (%)	
During prolonged PP (d 1–d 3)	42.0 (23.8–64.9)
Post prolonged PP (d 4–d 7)	64.5 (36.4–91.8)
Average in the first 7 d	55.5 (33.1–81.8)
ICU mortality (n, %)	38 (48.10%)

Continuous data are expressed as medians and interquartile ranges (IQRs). Categorical data are expressed as numbers and percentages. APACH II: acute physiology and chronic health evaluation II; SOFA: Sequential Organ Failure Assessment; CAD: coronary artery disease; COPD: chronic obstructive pulmonary disease; DM: diabetes mellitus; CKD: chronic kidney disease. mNUTRIC: modified nutrition risk in the critically ill; PP: prone positioning; PF ratio: partial pressure of oxygen/fraction concentration of inspired oxygen ratio.

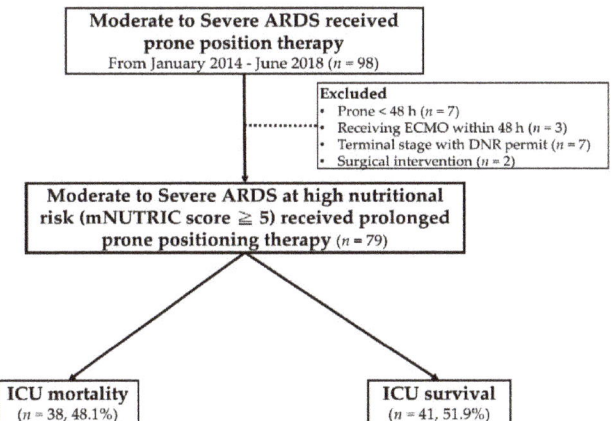

Figure 1. Study flowchart. ARDS: acute respiratory distress syndrome; ECMO: extracorporeal member oxygenation; DNR: do not resuscitate; ICU: intensive care unit.

3.2. Differences between Survival and Non-Survival Groups

Figure 2 presents a comparison of the EAR of the survival and non-survival groups in the first seven days of prolonged PP therapy. In the survival group, the EAR (%) significantly increased during the post–PP therapy period (days 4–7). However, only a minimal increase in EAR (%) was observed in the non-survival group. The survival group was significantly different from the non-survival group in terms of the distribution of the EAR (%) in the first seven days ($p = 0.004$; Figure 2).

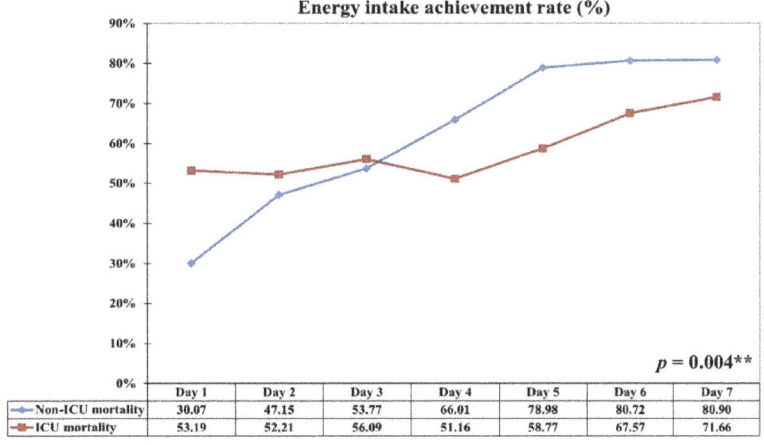

Figure 2. Comparison of energy achievement rate (EAR) during the first week of intensive care unit (ICU) admission between the survival and non-survival groups. ** $p < 0.01$.

The characteristics of the survival and non-survival groups were compared (Table 2). The non-survival group had a higher mNUTRIC score and lower EAR (%) in the post–PP therapy period (days 4–7). Significant differences were observed in age and number of patients who had renal replacement therapy (RRT) in the ICU and had comorbid active solid or hematologic malignancy between the survival and non-survival groups (all $p < 0.05$). For the survival group, the median EAR was 65% for days 4–7 (77.9%, IQR: 47.2–102.7%). In contrast, the median EAR (%) for the non-survival group was below 65% (51.1%, IQR: 26.6–87.4%), which was a significant difference ($p = 0.025$; Table 2). A significant difference was also observed on day 5 for the survival group compared with the non-survival group (73.8% and 47.0%, p = 0.033; Appendix A Table A1).

Table 2. Demographic characteristics, severity index, comorbidities, and EAR in survival and non-survival groups.

Characteristics	Survival (n = 41)	Non-Survival (n = 38)	p Value
Demographic data			
Age (y/o) (n, %)	56.8 (46–68.3)	63.8 (56.9–76.5)	0.036 *
Gender-Male (n, %)	27 (65.9%)	21 (55.3%)	0.464
mNUTRIC score	6.0 (4–7)	7.0 (6–8)	0.002 **
APACHE II score	31.0 (26.5–32.5)	31.0 (26.8–34.3)	0.470
SOFA	10.0 (8–14.5)	10.5 (8–14.3)	0.996
Renal replacement therapy (n, %)	13 (31.7%)	22 (57.9%)	0.034 *
Comorbidity			
CAD (n, %) [f]	3 (7.3%)	3 (7.9%)	1.000
COPD (n, %) [f]	6 (14.6%)	4 (10.5%)	0.739
Solid cancer (n, %)	1 (2.4%)	10 (26.3%)	0.006 **
Hematologic malignancies (n, %)	1 (2.4%)	4 (10.5%)	0.190
DM (n, %)	16 (39.0%)	8 (21.1%)	0.136
CKD (n, %)	12 (29.3%)	15 (39.5%)	0.473
Autoimmune disease (n, %)	5 (12.2%)	7 (18.4%)	0.648
PaO_2/FiO_2 (PF ratio)	96.5 (73.2–125.2)	88.7 (65.5–104.3)	0.133
Actual energy intake (kcal/BW)			
During prolonged PP (d 1–d 3)	6.5 (4–11.6)	9.2 (5.1–14.8)	0.133
Post prolonged PP (d 4–d 7)	12.8 (9–21.2)	10.2 (5.3–16.9)	0.049 *
Average in the first 7 d	10.5 (7.3–16.4)	10.9 (5.6–15.5)	0.638
Energy achievement rate (%)			
During prolonged PP (d 1–d 3)	39.3% (19.8–59.4%)	46.1% (29.2–76.0%)	0.192
Post prolonged PP (d 4–d 7)	77.9% (47.2–102.7%)	51.1% (26.6–87.4%)	0.025 *
Average in the first 7 d	57.4% (37.3–82.1%)	55.1% (28.2–82.1%)	0.498

Mann–Whitney U test. Chi-square test. [f] Fisher's exact test. * p < 0.05, ** p < 0.01. Continuous data are expressed as medians and IQRs. Categorical data are expressed as numbers and percentages. APACH II: acute physiology and chronic health evaluation II; SOFA: Sequential Organ Failure Assessment; CAD: coronary artery disease; COPD: chronic obstructive pulmonary disease; DM: diabetes mellitus; CKD: chronic kidney disease. mNUTRIC: modified nutrition risk in the critically ill; PP: prone positioning; PF ratio: partial pressure of oxygen/fraction concentration of inspired oxygen ratio.

3.3. Factors Associated with ICU Mortality for Patients with ARDS Who Received PP Therapy

Table 3 and Figure 3 present the results of the Cox regression analysis of the factors associated with mortality in the ICU. Univariate analysis revealed five factors associated with mortality in the ICU: mNUTRIC score (HR: 1.26; 95% CI: 1.01–1.58; p = 0.038), comorbid active solid cancer (HR: 2.68; 95% CI: 1.28–5.62; p = 0.009) and hematologic malignancy (HR: 2.90; 95% CI: 1.01–8.31; p = 0.47), average energy intake (kcal/body weight; HR: 0.94; 95% CI: 0.90–0.98; p = 0.007), and EAR (%) (HR: 0.21; 95% CI: 0.07–0.64; p = 0.006) in the post–PP therapy period (days 4–7). Multivariate analysis revealed that a higher EAR (%) for post-admission days 4–7 (HR: 0.19; 95% CI: 0.07–0.56) was a strong predictive factor in the survival and non-survival groups (Table 3 and Figure 2). The EAR (%) on the fifth day after the initiation of PP therapy was significantly different between the survival and non-survival groups (Appendix A Table A1). Therefore, we used an EAR of >65% on the fifth post–PP therapy day as the cutoff value to create the Kaplan–Meier survival curves and perform the log-rank test on the survival and non-survival groups. An EAR of >65% was associated with lower 14-day, 28-day, and ICU mortality (p = 0.021) after adjustment for age, sex, BMI, and APACHE II and SOFA scores (Figure 4).

Table 3. Univariate and multivariate analyses of factors associated with ICU mortality.

Characteristics	Univariate Analysis HR (95% CI)	p Value	Multivariate Analysis HR (95% CI)	p Value
Demographic data				
Age	1.02 (1.00–1.04)	0.062		
Sex (Female/Male)	0.76 (0.40–1.44)	0.401		
BMI (kg/m^2)	1.01 (0.94–1.08)	0.848		
mNUTRIC score	1.26 (1.01–1.58)	0.038 *	1.22 (0.95 0.56)	0.116
APACHE II score	1.04 (0.98–1.09)	0.182		
SOFA	1.03 (0.95–1.12)	0.510		
Renal replacement therapy (n, %)	1.31 (0.68–2.50)	0.422		
Comorbidity				
CAD (n, %) [f]	1.32 (0.40–4.32)	0.648		
COPD (n, %) [f]	0.65 (0.23–1.86)	0.426		
Solid cancer (n, %)	2.68 (1.28–5.62)	0.009 **	2.81 (1.25–6.33)	0.013 *
Hematologic malignancies (n, %)	2.90 (1.01–8.31)	0.047 *	2.74 (0.83–9.10)	0.099
DM (n, %)	1.03 (0.46–2.28)	0.945		
CKD (n, %)	1.15 (0.60–2.22)	0.668		
Autoimmune disease (n, %)	1.09 (0.48–2.48)	0.839		
PaO$_2$/FiO$_2$ (PF ratio)	0.99 (0.98–1.00)	0.084		
Actual energy intake (kcal/BW)				
During prolonged PP (d 1–d 3)	1.00 (0.96–1.04)	0.994		
Post prolonged PP (d 4–d 7)	0.94 (0.90–0.98)	0.007 **	0.93 (0.89–0.98)	0.006 **
Average in the first 7 d	0.97 (0.92–1.01)	0.144		
Energy achievement rate (%)				
During prolonged PP (d 1–d 3)	1.00 (0.38–2.59)	0.994		
Post prolonged PP (d 4–d 7)	0.21 (0.07–0.64)	0.006 **	0.19 (0.07–0.56)	0.002 **
Average in the first 7 d	0.42 (0.14–1.27)	0.124		

Cox regression. * $p < 0.05$, ** $p < 0.01$. APACH II: acute physiology and chronic health evaluation II; SOFA: Sequential Organ Failure Assessment; CAD: coronary artery disease; COPD: chronic obstructive pulmonary disease; DM: diabetes mellitus; CKD: chronic kidney disease. mNUTRIC: modified nutrition risk in the critically ill; PP: prone positioning; PF ratio: partial pressure of oxygen/fraction concentration of inspired oxygen ratio. [f] Fisher's exact test.

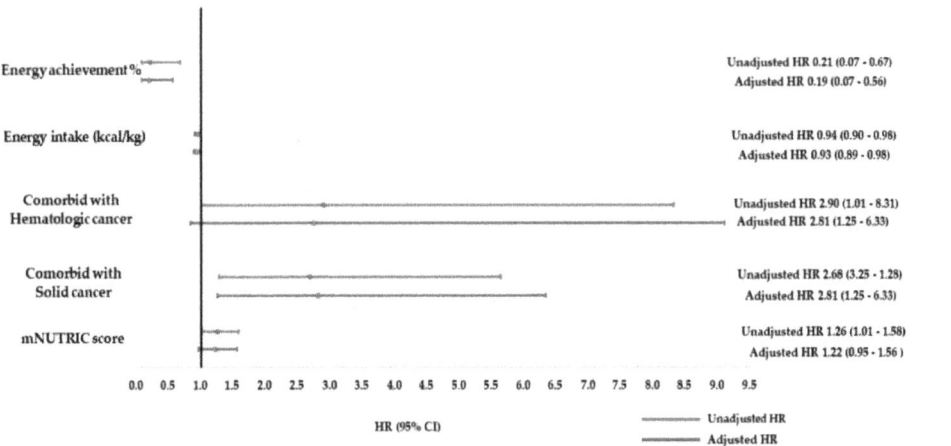

Figure 3. Hazard ratio (HR) of ICU mortality of critically ill patients with high nutritional risk and moderate to severe ARDS receiving prolong prone positioning (PP) therapy. mNUTRIC score: modified nutrition risk in the critically ill score.

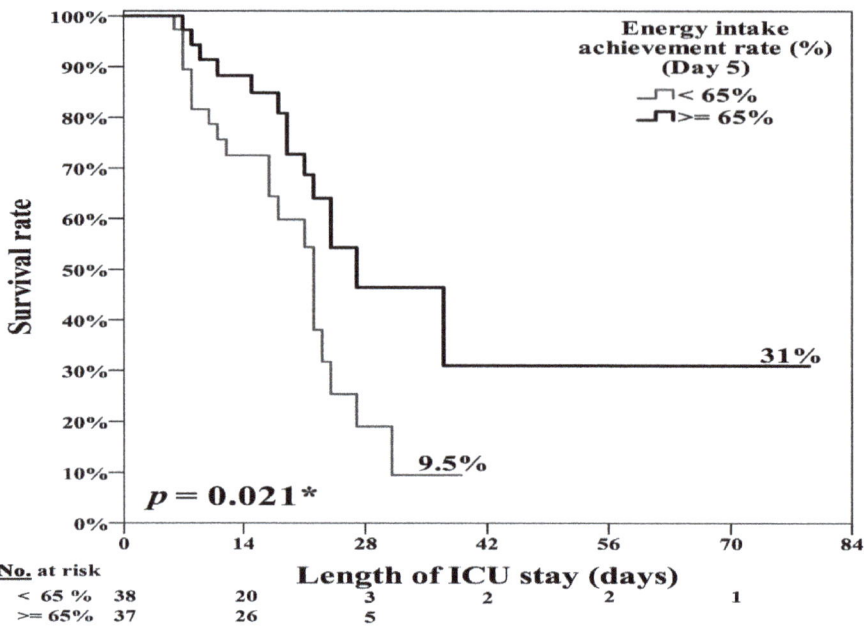

Figure 4. EAR >65% at the fifth ICU day was significantly associated with lower ICU mortality in patients with moderate to severe ARDS receiving prolonged PP therapy. * $p < 0.05$.

4. Discussion

This study yielded three major findings. First, ICU mortality was as high as 48.1% for patients with high nutritional risk and moderate to severe ARDS requiring prolonged PP therapy, even for those receiving EN within 24 h of admission. This high mortality may contribute to the severity of the disease and comorbidities, increase nutritional risk, and decrease EAR within seven days after initiating prolonged PP therapy. Second, although the average median EAR in the first seven days after PP therapy for the survival and non-survival groups was less than 65% (57.4% and 55.1%, respectively; $p = 0.498$), the EAR increased significantly in the survival group during PP therapy recovery (days 4–7). Third, an EAR of <65% on day 5 after prolonged PP therapy was an effective predictor of ICU mortality. To the best of our knowledge, this is the first study to evaluate the association between EAR and ICU mortality in patients with high nutritional risk and moderate to severe ARDS requiring prolonged PP therapy.

The prevalence of malnutrition and undernutrition is approximately 50–60% for critically ill patients admitted to the ICU. High nutritional risk is also correlated with morbidity and mortality in the ICU [30–32]. The standard to identify patients with malnourishment and high nutritional risk is uncertain in the current guidelines [1]. However, screening tools such as the Nutrition Risk Screening 2002 (NRS-2002), the nutrition risk in the critically ill (NUTRIC) and the mNUTRIC have been widely applied and recommended for use in the ICU [2–4]. The mNUTRIC score is a composite of five parameters: age, comorbidities, APACHE II score, SOFA score, and days in hospital before ICU admission [33]. Our previous study demonstrated that in critically ill patients, high nutritional risk (mNUTRIC score ≥ 5) was associated with higher ICU mortality [11]. Few studies have investigated the association between nutritional screening tools and clinical outcomes in critically ill patients with ARDS. One retrospective study conducted in South Korea proposed that the geriatric nutritional risk index (GNRI) is associated with 30-day mortality in elderly patients with ARDS [34]. However, another report noted the GNRI's low specificity (57.1%) compared with the specificity of other nutritional indexes such as NRS 2002 and Onodera's prognostic nutritional index for short-term outcomes in geriatric patients with respiratory failure [35]. In addition, the applicability of the GNRI may be limited because it is used to evaluate the geriatric population [36]. In our ICUs, the dietitian calculates the mNUTRIC score and feeding volume for all adult patients rather than only geriatric patients within 48 h to determine nutritional risk. Therefore, our study was the first to demonstrate that mNUTRIC score, rather than APACHE II or SOFA score, is significantly associated with ICU mortality for adult patients with ARDS requiring PP therapy. As our previous study also demonstrated [8–11], mNUTRIC score is a useful tool to evaluate nutritional risk in critically ill adult patients admitted to medical ICUs.

Several studies have proposed predictive factors associated with mortality in patients with ARDS requiring PP therapy [25,37,38]. However, few studies have addressed the effect of nutrition and the achievement of feeding goals on mortality. One retrospective study enrolled 43 patients who received PP therapy for ARDS and discovered three factors associated with mortality: APACHE II score, plateau pressure, and driving pressure in the lung mechanism [37]. Kao et al. retrospectively investigated factors associated with 60-day mortality in 65 patients with influenza-related ARDS who received PP therapy. The study identified higher pneumonia severity scores, increased driving pressure in the lung mechanism, and the comorbidity of requiring RRT [38]. Age, APACHE II score, malignant comorbidity, RRT requirement, and non-influenza-related ARDS were identified as predictive factors of ICU mortality in an investigation of 116 patients with severe ARDS requiring PP therapy [25]. However, the effects of nutritional support and the achievement of feeding goals in the first week of ICU admission on mortality in such patients were not considered. In the era of the COIVD-19 pandemic, PP therapy began to be widely recommended in treatment guidelines for patients with severe CARDS [16,17], and the crucial nature of nutrition support during PP therapy garnered attention [18,39,40]. This study identified two factors related to nutrition, namely mNUTRIC score (HR: 1.26; 95% CI: 1.01–1.58) and EAR (HR: 0.21; 95% CI, 0.07–0.64) on the fifth day after the initiation of PP therapy; this fills a gap in the research regarding the effect of nutritional support on ICU mortality for patients with ARDS requiring PP therapy.

This study demonstrated that even in patients with ARDS requiring a long period of PP therapy, an EAR >65% within the first week of ICU admission was associated with lower mortality risk in medical ICUs than that revealed in our previous studies [8,10,11]. The optimal EAR is 60–70% of the nutritional target in the first week in the ICU, as recommended by the 2016 ASPEN and SCCM guidelines and the 2019 ESPN guidelines [1,3,4]. PP therapy may be perceived as a barrier to providing early nutrition and achieving the energy target because of concerns regarding feasibility, safety, and tolerance. However, Reignier et al. revealed a significant improvement in feeding volume after a feeding protocol implementation in ARDS patients required PP therapy [41]. Because our RICU has evaluated nutritional risk and implemented the feeding protocol within 24 h of admission for all critically ill patients since 2016 [8–11], feeding targets are monitored and titrated to the maximum volume, even for patients requiring PP therapy. Therefore, our study also revealed that the difference in EAR on each day (Figure 2), rather than the average EAR in the first week of ICU admission, provides more information regarding mortality risk for patients receiving the feeding protocol. To the best of our knowledge, this study is the first to examine the EAR and its effect on ICU mortality in critically ill patients with moderate to severe ARDS requiring prolonged PP therapy.

This study had several limitations. First, the retrospective design limited the explanation of the results because of heterogeneity among the patients. Second, a single center, rather than multiple centers, was studied, which may have limited the generalizability of the results. Third, the enrollment of patients with moderate to severe ARDS may have confounded the ICU mortality risk. Because few studies have investigated the effect of nutritional support in patients with ARDS receiving PP therapy for at least 48 h, this study offers useful information for academic practice. Our RICU has practiced the standard protocol of lung protection, prolonged PP therapy [25], early EN within 24 h of admission, and feeding for all admitted critically ill patients with ARDS since 2007 [8–11]. Therefore, the limitations of the retrospective, single-center design should have been minimal. Although the severity of ARDS ranged from moderate to severe, the median PaO_2/FiO_2 ratio was less than 100 (median: 92.5; IQR: 70.1–114.3), and the difference in PaO_2/FiO_2 ratio was not significant in the univariate analysis of the Cox regression model. Therefore, the PaO_2/FiO_2 ratio was unlikely to be a confounding factor in the prediction of ICU mortality. Finally, our results may not be generalizable to critically ill patients in neurosurgical, surgical, cardiac, and pediatric ICUs because only adult patients admitted to a medical ICU were enrolled.

5. Conclusions

ICU mortality is high for adult patients with ARDS requiring PP therapy. The only score significantly associated with ICU mortality was mNUTRIC. An EAR of <50% was observed in both the survival and non-survival groups during PP therapy. However, only the survival group exhibited a significant increase in EAR during recovery from prolonged PP in the supine position (days 4–7 after initiation of PP therapy). The key factor in determining ICU mortality in this population was an EAR of <65% by day 5 after the initiation of prolonged PP therapy. For patients with high nutrition risk (mNUTRIC score ≥ 5) and moderate to severe ARDS requiring prolonged PP therapy, we suggest early EN and increasing the feeding volume to the goal of >65% during the first week of ICU admission. For patients with an EAR of <65% during the first week, nutrition support therapy with postpyloric tube placement or partial parenteral nutrition is required.

Author Contributions: Conceptualization, P.-K.F., C.-Y.W. and W.-N.W.; Data curation, P.-K.F.; Formal analysis, P.-K.F. and C.-Y.H.; Investigation, P.-K.F., C.-Y.W. and W.-N.W.; Methodology, P.-K.F., C.-Y.W. and W.-N.W.; Resources, P.-K.F.; Software, C.-Y.H., S.-P.L. and C.-T.K.; Validation, C.-Y.W.; Writing—original draft, P.-K.F. and W.-N.W.; Writing—review & editing, P.-K.F., C.-Y.W., W.-N.W., C.-Y.H., S.-P.L. and C.-T.K. All authors have read and agreed to the published version of the manuscript.

Funding: The authors sincerely appreciate the funding in part by the Department of Medical Research of Taichung Veterans General Hospital (TCVGH-1104401B) and the Ministry of Science and Technology (Taiwan) (MOST 110-2410-H-075A-001).

Institutional Review Board Statement: The study was conducted according to the guidelines of the Declaration of Helsinki and approved by the Institutional Review Board (or Ethics Committee) of Taichung Veterans General Hospital (CE20308B; date of approval, 16 September 2020).

Informed Consent Statement: Patient consent was waived due to the retrospective study design and anonymization and deidentification of patient data prior to analysis.

Data Availability Statement: The data presented in this study are available on request from the corresponding author. The data are not publicly available due to the regulation of Institutional Review Board of Taichung Veterans General Hospital in Taiwan.

Acknowledgments: This study was based in part on data from the Taichung Veterans General Hospital Research Database, which is managed by the Clinical Informatics Research & Development Center of Taichung Veterans General Hospital.

Conflicts of Interest: The authors declare no conflict of interest.

Appendix A

Table A1. Comparison of EAR between survival and non-survival groups during the first week of ICU admission.

Characteristics	Survival (n = 41)		Mortality (n = 38)		p Value
	%	IQR	%	IQR	
Energy achievement rate (%)					
day 1	18.3%	(7.3–46.8%)	50.1%	(17.0–79.8%)	0.010 *
day 2	46.8%	(19.1–71.3%)	47.4%	(22.4–77.1%)	0.603
day 3	49.9%	(23.4–74.5%)	46.6%	(28.4–76.0%)	0.791
day 4	69.9%	(40.7–86.1%)	39.3%	(25.5–73.6%)	0.052
day 5	73.8%	(44.0–112.4%)	47.0%	(30.7–83.0%)	0.033 *
day 6	73.1%	(45.6–115.5%)	65.2%	(24.6–98.5%)	0.185
day 7	72.3%	(52.1–105.3%)	76.0%	(24.0–101.2%)	0.388

Mann–Whitney U test. Chi-square test. * $p < 0.05$.

References

1. Singer, P.; Blaser, A.R.; Berger, M.M.; Alhazzani, W.; Calder, P.C.; Casaer, M.P.; Hiesmayr, M.; Mayer, K.; Montejo, J.C.; Pichard, C.; et al. ESPEN guideline on clinical nutrition in the intensive care unit. *Clin. Nutr.* **2019**, *38*, 48–79. [CrossRef] [PubMed]
2. Sioson, M.S.; Martindale, R.; Abayadeera, A.; Abouchaleh, N.; Aditianingsih, D.; Bhurayanontachai, R.; Chiou, W.C.; Higashibeppu, N.; Mat Nor, M.B.; Osland, E.; et al. Nutrition therapy for critically ill patients across the Asia-Pacific and Middle East regions: A consensus statement. *Clin. Nutr.* **2018**, *24*, 156–164. [CrossRef] [PubMed]
3. Taylor, B.E.; McClave, S.A.; Martindale, R.G.; Warren, M.M.; Johnson, D.R.; Braunschweig, C.; McCarthy, M.S.; Davanos, E.; Rice, T.W.; Cresci, G.A.; et al. Guidelines for the Provision and Assessment of Nutrition Support Therapy in the Adult Critically Ill Patient: Society of Critical Care Medicine (SCCM) and American Society for Parenteral and Enteral Nutrition (A.S.P.E.N.). *Crit. Care Med.* **2016**, *44*, 390–438. [CrossRef] [PubMed]
4. McClave, S.A.; Taylor, B.E.; Martindale, R.G.; Warren, M.M.; Johnson, D.R.; Braunschweig, C.; McCarthy, M.S.; Davanos, E.; Rice, T.W.; Cresci, G.A.; et al. Guidelines for the Provision and Assessment of Nutrition Support Therapy in the Adult Critically Ill Patient: Society of Critical Care Medicine (SCCM) and American Society for Parenteral and Enteral Nutrition (A.S.P.E.N.). *JPEN J. Parenter. Enteral. Nutr.* **2016**, *40*, 159–211. [CrossRef] [PubMed]
5. Li, P.F.; Wang, Y.L.; Fang, Y.L.; Nan, L.; Zhou, J.; Zhang, D. Effect of early enteral nutrition on outcomes of trauma patients requiring intensive care. *Chin. J. Traumatol.* **2020**, *23*, 163–167. [CrossRef] [PubMed]
6. Mukhopadhyay, A.; Henry, J.; Ong, V.; Leong, C.S.; Teh, A.L.; van Dam, R.M.; Kowitlawakul, Y. Association of modified NUTRIC score with 28-day mortality in critically ill patients. *Clin. Nutr.* **2017**, *36*, 1143–1148. [CrossRef] [PubMed]
7. Zhang, P.; He, Z.; Yu, G.; Peng, D.; Feng, Y.; Ling, J.; Wang, Y.; Li, S.; Bian, Y. The modified NUTRIC score can be used for nutritional risk assessment as well as prognosis prediction in critically ill COVID-19 patients. *Clin. Nutr.* **2021**, *40*, 534–541. [CrossRef]
8. Wang, W.N.; Wang, C.Y.; Hsu, C.Y.; Fu, P.K. Comparison of Feeding Efficiency and Hospital Mortality between Small Bowel and Nasogastric Tube Feeding in Critically Ill Patients at High Nutritional Risk. *Nutrients* **2020**, *12*, 2009. [CrossRef]
9. Wang, C.Y.; Fu, P.K.; Chao, W.C.; Wang, W.N.; Chen, C.H.; Huang, Y.C. Full Versus Trophic Feeds in Critically Ill Adults with High and Low Nutritional Risk Scores: A Randomized Controlled Trial. *Nutrients* **2020**, *12*, 3518. [CrossRef]
10. Wang, W.N.; Yang, M.F.; Wang, C.Y.; Hsu, C.Y.; Lee, B.J.; Fu, P.K. Optimal Time and Target for Evaluating Energy Delivery after Adjuvant Feeding with Small Bowel Enteral Nutrition in Critically Ill Patients at High Nutrition Risk. *Nutrients* **2019**, *11*, 645. [CrossRef] [PubMed]
11. Wang, C.Y.; Fu, P.K.; Huang, C.T.; Chen, C.H.; Lee, B.J.; Huang, Y.C. Targeted Energy Intake Is the Important Determinant of Clinical Outcomes in Medical Critically Ill Patients with High Nutrition Risk. *Nutrients* **2018**, *10*, 1731. [CrossRef]
12. Bellani, G.; Laffey, J.G.; Pham, T.; Fan, E.; Brochard, L.; Esteban, A.; Gattinoni, L.; van Haren, F.; Larsson, A.; McAuley, D.F.; et al. Epidemiology, Patterns of Care, and Mortality for Patients With Acute Respiratory Distress Syndrome in Intensive Care Units in 50 Countries. *JAMA* **2016**, *315*, 788–800. [CrossRef]
13. Hasan, S.S.; Capstick, T.; Ahmed, R.; Kow, C.S.; Mazhar, F.; Merchant, H.A.; Zaidi, S.T.R. Mortality in COVID-19 patients with acute respiratory distress syndrome and corticosteroids use: A systematic review and meta-analysis. *Expert Rev. Respir Med.* **2020**, *14*, 1149–1163. [CrossRef] [PubMed]
14. Griffiths, M.J.D.; McAuley, D.F.; Perkins, G.D.; Barrett, N.; Blackwood, B.; Boyle, A.; Chee, N.; Connolly, B.; Dark, P.; Finney, S.; et al. Guidelines on the management of acute respiratory distress syndrome. *BMJ Open Respir. Res.* **2019**, *6*, e000420. [CrossRef] [PubMed]
15. Guerin, C.; Reignier, J.; Richard, J.C.; Beuret, P.; Gacouin, A.; Boulain, T.; Mercier, E.; Badet, M.; Mercat, A.; Baudin, O.; et al. Prone positioning in severe acute respiratory distress syndrome. *N. Engl. J. Med.* **2013**, *368*, 2159–2168. [CrossRef]

16. Alhazzani, W.; Evans, L.; Alshamsi, F.; Moller, M.H.; Ostermann, M.; Prescott, H.C.; Arabi, Y.M.; Loeb, M.; Ng Gong, M.; Fan, E.; et al. Surviving Sepsis Campaign Guidelines on the Management of Adults With Coronavirus Disease 2019 (COVID-19) in the ICU: First Update. *Crit. Care Med.* **2021**, *49*, e219–e234. [CrossRef]
17. Coppo, A.; Bellani, G.; Winterton, D.; Di Pierro, M.; Soria, A.; Faverio, P.; Cairo, M.; Mori, S.; Messinesi, G.; Contro, E.; et al. Feasibility and physiological effects of prone positioning in non-intubated patients with acute respiratory failure due to COVID-19 (PRON-COVID): A prospective cohort study. *Lancet Respir. Med.* **2020**, *8*, 765–774. [CrossRef]
18. Behrens, S.; Kozeniecki, M.; Knapp, N.; Martindale, R.G. Nutrition Support During Prone Positioning: An Old Technique Reawakened by COVID-19. *Nutr. Clin. Pract.* **2021**, *36*, 105–109. [CrossRef]
19. Ohbe, H.; Jo, T.; Matsui, H.; Fushimi, K.; Yasunaga, H. Early Enteral Nutrition in Patients Undergoing Sustained Neuromuscular Blockade: A Propensity-Matched Analysis Using a Nationwide Inpatient Database. *Crit. Care Med.* **2019**, *47*, 1072–1080. [CrossRef]
20. Reignier, J.; Thenoz-Jost, N.; Fiancette, M.; Legendre, E.; Lebert, C.; Bontemps, F.; Clementi, E.; Martin-Lefevre, L. Early enteral nutrition in mechanically ventilated patients in the prone position. *Crit. Care Med.* **2004**, *32*, 94–99. [CrossRef]
21. Bruni, A.; Garofalo, E.; Grande, L.; Auletta, G.; Cubello, D.; Greco, M.; Lombardo, N.; Garieri, P.; Papaleo, A.; Doldo, P.; et al. Nursing issues in enteral nutrition during prone position in critically ill patients: A systematic review of the literature. *Intensive Crit. Care Nurs.* **2020**, *60*, 102899. [CrossRef]
22. Girard, R.; Baboi, L.; Ayzac, L.; Richard, J.C.; Guerin, C. The impact of patient positioning on pressure ulcers in patients with severe ARDS: Results from a multicentre randomised controlled trial on prone positioning. *Intensive Care Med.* **2014**, *40*, 397–403. [CrossRef] [PubMed]
23. Force, A.D.T.; Ranieri, V.M.; Rubenfeld, G.D.; Thompson, B.T.; Ferguson, N.D.; Caldwell, E.; Fan, E.; Camporota, L.; Slutsky, A.S. Acute respiratory distress syndrome: The Berlin Definition. *JAMA* **2012**, *307*, 2526–2533. [CrossRef]
24. Howell, M.D.; Davis, A.M. Management of ARDS in Adults. *JAMA* **2018**, *319*, 711–712. [CrossRef]
25. Lee, P.H.; Kuo, C.T.; Hsu, C.Y.; Lin, S.P.; Fu, P.K. Prognostic Factors to Predict ICU Mortality in Patients with Severe ARDS Who Received Early and Prolonged Prone Positioning Therapy. *J. Clin. Med.* **2021**, *10*, 2323. [CrossRef] [PubMed]
26. Hadaya, J.; Benharash, P. Prone Positioning for Acute Respiratory Distress Syndrome (ARDS). *JAMA* **2020**, *324*, 1361. [CrossRef]
27. Fan, E.; Del Sorbo, L.; Goligher, E.C.; Hodgson, C.L.; Munshi, L.; Walkey, A.J.; Adhikari, N.K.J.; Amato, M.B.P.; Branson, R.; Brower, R.G.; et al. An Official American Thoracic Society/European Society of Intensive Care Medicine/Society of Critical Care Medicine Clinical Practice Guideline: Mechanical Ventilation in Adult Patients with Acute Respiratory Distress Syndrome. *Am. J. Respir. Crit. Care Med.* **2017**, *195*, 1253–1263. [CrossRef]
28. Chan, M.C.; Hsu, J.Y.; Liu, H.H.; Lee, Y.L.; Pong, S.C.; Chang, L.Y.; Kuo, B.I.; Wu, C.L. Effects of prone position on inflammatory markers in patients with ARDS due to community-acquired pneumonia. *J. Formos. Med. Assoc.* **2007**, *106*, 708–716. [CrossRef]
29. Wang, Y.L.; Huang, C.T.; Chen, C.H.; Fu, P.K.; Wang, C.Y. Outcome of glycemic control in critically ill patients receiving enteral formulas. *Asia Pac. J. Clin. Nutr.* **2021**, *30*, 22–29. [CrossRef]
30. Weijs, P.J.M.; Mogensen, K.M.; Rawn, J.D.; Christopher, K.B. Protein Intake, Nutritional Status and Outcomes in ICU Survivors: A Single Center Cohort Study. *J. Clin. Med.* **2019**, *8*, 43. [CrossRef] [PubMed]
31. Kopp Lugli, A.; de Watteville, A.; Hollinger, A.; Goetz, N.; Heidegger, C. Medical Nutrition Therapy in Critically Ill Patients Treated on Intensive and Intermediate Care Units: A Literature Review. *J. Clin. Med.* **2019**, *8*, 1395. [CrossRef]
32. Havens, J.M.; Columbus, A.B.; Seshadri, A.J.; Olufajo, O.A.; Mogensen, K.M.; Rawn, J.D.; Salim, A.; Christopher, K.B. Malnutrition at Intensive Care Unit Admission Predicts Mortality in Emergency General Surgery Patients. *JPEN J. Parenter. Enteral. Nutr.* **2018**, *42*, 156–163. [CrossRef] [PubMed]
33. Rahman, A.; Hasan, R.M.; Agarwala, R.; Martin, C.; Day, A.G.; Heyland, D.K. Identifying critically-ill patients who will benefit most from nutritional therapy: Further validation of the "modified NUTRIC" nutritional risk assessment tool. *Clin. Nutr.* **2016**, *35*, 158–162. [CrossRef] [PubMed]
34. Yoo, J.W.; Ju, S.; Lee, S.J.; Cho, Y.J.; Lee, J.D.; Kim, H.C. Geriatric nutritional risk index is associated with 30-day mortality in patients with acute respiratory distress syndrome. *Medicine* **2020**, *99*, e20671. [CrossRef]
35. Yenibertiz, D.; Cirik, M.O. The comparison of GNRI and other nutritional indexes on short-term survival in geriatric patients treated for respiratory failure. *Aging Clin. Exp. Res.* **2021**, *33*, 611–617. [CrossRef]
36. Bouillanne, O.; Morineau, G.; Dupont, C.; Coulombel, I.; Vincent, J.P.; Nicolis, I.; Benazeth, S.; Cynober, L.; Aussel, C. Geriatric Nutritional Risk Index: A new index for evaluating at-risk elderly medical patients. *Am. J. Clin. Nutr.* **2005**, *82*, 777–783. [CrossRef]
37. Modrykamien, A.M.; Daoud, Y. Factors among patients receiving prone positioning for the acute respiratory distress syndrome found useful for predicting mortality in the intensive care unit. *Bayl. Univ. Med. Cent. Proc.* **2018**, *31*, 1–5. [CrossRef] [PubMed]
38. Kao, K.C.; Chang, K.W.; Chan, M.C.; Liang, S.J.; Chien, Y.C.; Hu, H.C.; Chiu, L.C.; Chen, W.C.; Fang, W.F.; Chen, Y.M.; et al. Predictors of survival in patients with influenza pneumonia-related severe acute respiratory distress syndrome treated with prone positioning. *Ann. Intensive Care* **2018**, *8*, 94. [CrossRef] [PubMed]
39. Savio, R.D.; Parasuraman, R.; Lovesly, D.; Shankar, B.; Ranganathan, L.; Ramakrishnan, N.; Venkataraman, R. Feasibility, tolerance and effectiveness of enteral feeding in critically ill patients in prone position. *J. Intensive Care Soc.* **2021**, *22*, 41–46. [CrossRef]

20. Machado, L.S.; Rizzi, P.; Silva, F.M. Administration of enteral nutrition in the prone position, gastric residual volume and other clinical outcomes in critically ill patients: A systematic review. *Rev. Bras. Ter. Intensiva* **2020**, *32*, 133–142. [CrossRef]
21. Reignier, J.; Dimet, J.; Martin-Lefevre, L.; Bontemps, F.; Fiancette, M.; Clementi, E.; Lebert, C.; Renard, B. Before-after study of a standardized ICU protocol for early enteral feeding in patients turned in the prone position. *Clin. Nutr.* **2010**, *29*, 210–216. [CrossRef] [PubMed]

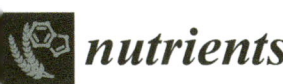

Article

Does Route of Full Feeding Affect Outcome among Ventilated Critically Ill COVID-19 Patients: A Prospective Observational Study

Dimitrios Karayiannis [1,*], Sotirios Kakavas [2], Aikaterini Sarri [3], Vassiliki Giannopoulou [3], Christina Liakopoulou [3], Edison Jahaj [3], Aggeliki Kanavou [3], Thodoris Pitsolis [3], Sotirios Malachias [3], George Adamos [3], Athina Mantelou [3], Avra Almperti [1], Konstantina Morogianni [1], Olga Kampouropoulou [3], Anastasia Kotanidou [3] and Zafeiria Mastora [3]

[1] Department of Clinical Nutrition, "Evangelismos" General Hospital of Athens, Ypsilantou 45-47, 10676 Athens, Greece; aalmperti@yahoo.gr (A.A.); konstantina.morogianni@gmail.com (K.M.)
[2] Intensive Care Unit, Center for Respiratory Failure, "Sotiria" General Hospital of Chest Diseases, 152 Mesogeion Avenue, 11527 Athens, Greece; sotikaka@yahoo.com
[3] First Department of Critical Care Medicine and Pulmonary Services, Evangelismos General Hospital, National and Kapodistrian University of Athens, 11527 Athens, Greece; katsarri5@hotmail.com (A.S.); vaso.giannop88@gmail.com (V.G.); chr1stieliak@gmail.com (C.L.); edison.jahaj@gmail.com (E.J.); agg_kan@hotmail.com (A.K.); theodorepitsolis@yahoo.com (T.P.); sotmalachias@gmail.com (S.M.); George.adamos1983@gmail.com (G.A.); athina.mantelou@gmail.com (A.M.); olgakampou@yahoo.com (O.K.); akotanid@gmail.com (A.K.); zafimast@yahoo.gr (Z.M.)
* Correspondence: dkarag@hua.gr; Tel.: +30-213-2045035; Fax: +30-213-2041385

Abstract: The outbreak of the new coronavirus strain SARS-CoV-2 (COVID-19) highlighted the need for appropriate feeding practices among critically ill patients admitted to the intensive care unit (ICU). This study aimed to describe feeding practices of intubated COVID-19 patients during their second week of hospitalization in the First Department of Critical Care Medicine, Evaggelismos General Hospital, and evaluate potential associations with all cause 30-day mortality, length of hospital stay, and duration of mechanical ventilation. We enrolled adult intubated COVID-19 patients admitted to the ICU between September 2020 and July 2021 and prospectively monitored until their hospital discharge. Of the 162 patients analyzed (52.8% men, 51.6% overweight/obese, mean age 63.2 ± 1.9 years), 27.2% of patients used parenteral nutrition, while the rest were fed enterally. By 30 days, 34.2% of the patients in the parenteral group had died compared to 32.7% of the patients in the enteral group (relative risk (RR) for the group receiving enteral nutrition = 0.97, 95% confidence interval = 0.88–1.06, $p = 0.120$). Those in the enteral group demonstrated a lower duration of hospital stay (RR = 0.91, 95% CI = 0.85–0.97, $p = 0.036$) as well as mechanical ventilation support (RR = 0.94, 95% CI = 0.89–0.99, $p = 0.043$). Enteral feeding during second week of ICU hospitalization may be associated with a shorter duration of hospitalization and stay in mechanical ventilation support among critically ill intubated patients with COVID-19.

Keywords: SARS-CoV-2 virus; energy target; enteral nutrition; parenteral nutrition; critical illness

Citation: Karayiannis, D.; Kakavas, S.; Sarri, A.; Giannopoulou, V.; Liakopoulou, C.; Jahaj, E.; Kanavou, A.; Pitsolis, T.; Malachias, S.; Adamos, G.; et al. Does Route of Full Feeding Affect Outcome among Ventilated Critically Ill COVID-19 Patients: A Prospective Observational Study. *Nutrients* 2022, 14, 153. https://doi.org/10.3390/nu14010153

Academic Editor: Arved Weimann

Received: 24 November 2021
Accepted: 26 December 2021
Published: 29 December 2021

Publisher's Note: MDPI stays neutral with regard to jurisdictional claims in published maps and institutional affiliations.

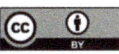

Copyright: © 2021 by the authors. Licensee MDPI, Basel, Switzerland. This article is an open access article distributed under the terms and conditions of the Creative Commons Attribution (CC BY) license (https://creativecommons.org/licenses/by/4.0/).

1. Introduction

The recent COVID-19 pandemic, which resulted from SARS-CoV-2 coronavirus infection, contributed to a rapid increment in hospital and intensive care unit (ICU) admissions [1]. Most patients exhibit mild to moderate symptoms, such as fever, cough, fatigue, respiratory failure, and multiple effects on the gastrointestinal tract, which appear especially in patients who are over 60 years old and those with concomitant diseases [2]. Approximately 5% of patients develop severe disease and require ICU admission, where the provision of adequate nutritional support is a challenge given the complex and fluctuating metabolic changes that accompany their nutritional status over time [3]. Critical illness, in general, is characterized by an inflammatory response that elicits a catabolic response and can be divided into different metabolic diseases: the early acute phase, which occurs in the first 48 h after entering the ICU, and the next, called the late acute phase, which usually lasts days after admission [4]. In severely ill patients with COVID-19, the acute phase presents with a prolonged severe inflammatory response, which is associated with a significant increase in resting energy expenditure [5,6], and current strategies for nutritional therapy seem to be unsuccessful in covering energy/protein needs [7]. In addition, COVID-19 patients spend extended periods in the ICU compared to the usual severely ill [8], and thus, metabolic phases of the disease are likely to be different and last longer.

Nutritional support is essential for all critically ill COVID-19 patients because acute illness carries an increased risk of malnutrition, muscle wasting, and increased mortality and requires a complex calculation of feeding route, time of onset, and amount and type of nutrients [4,9]. All the above may significantly affect patient's outcomes, such as length of hospital stay or duration of mechanical ventilation [10]. Recently, various guidelines from international societies were developed and published early in the pandemic without providing convincing answers to many critical questions [3,11,12]. One important question is route of nutritional support administration (enteral vs. parenteral), the effects of which on outcome remain unclear [13,14]. Up to the present moment, administration of energy needs via the enteral route is the preferred method of choice according to published guidelines [15,16] although it is affiliated with higher rates of gastrointestinal intolerance [17]. Parenteral feeding is more invasive, provides higher amounts of calories, and is associated with a higher risk of complications [18]. There are several published papers comparing different types of interventions regarding the route of feeding and ICU outcome but mainly among non COVID-19 patients during their first days of ICU stay [19].

Despite it being quoted in various guidelines, there is lack of data comparing enteral vs. parenteral feeding among critically ill patients with COVID-19 disease as well as the effect of full feeding (after 5–7 days of ICU stay) on clinical outcomes [20–23]. Therefore, the purpose of this study was to describe full feeding practices and highlight their long-term consequences among intubated patients with COVID-19 disease, who were treated within ICU at a reference hospital in Athens.

2. Methods
2.1. Participants

We conducted this single-center observational study from September 2020 to July 2021 in the first intensive care unit of Evaggelismos Athens General Hospital (tertiary hospital). Adult patients (aged > 18 years), requiring mechanical ventilation for >48 h, projected to receive nutritional support for at least 5 days, and with laboratory-confirmed COVID-19 by a positive reverse-transcriptase polymerase-chain-reaction (RT-PCR) assay of a nasopharyngeal swab specimen were eligible. The Institutional Review Board at Athens Evangelismos Hospital: 116/31-03-2021 approved data collection and waived the need for informed consent. Exclusion criteria were existence of metabolic diseases requiring a specific diet (for example phenylketonuria), history of gastrectomy or esophagectomy, initiation of nutrition support 5–7 days before ICU admission, ICU length of stay (LOS) shorter than 7 days, pregnancy, or patients that were expected to require no more than 48 h of invasive mechanical ventilation.

2.2. Study Design

Data were retrieved from patient electronic file and daily hospital sheet on the admission, 7th day, 14th day, and until discharge from hospital. During ICU hospitalization, anthropometric data, such as height (in cm) and weight (in kg), were collected, while body mass index (in kg/m^2) was determined. Besides patients' basic characteristics, the Acute Physiology and Chronic Health Evaluation (Apache) score was calculated 24 h after ICU admission. After the initiation of nutrition support, various data, such as pre-existing illness, initiation/duration of mechanical ventilation, resource to organ support (vasopressors and kidney replacement therapy), use of prone position, and laboratory markers, such as serum albumin and CRP levels, were also computed.

2.3. Feeding Practices

Nutritional support was initiated as soon as possible after admission to the ICU and no later than 48 h after intubation. Data on feeding practices and tolerance to feeding were collected every day by the Nutrition Support Team (NST), while nutrient delivery was based on ESPEN guidelines by the hospital NST [4]. Feeding practices included enteral and parenteral feeding, while nutritional parameters assessed included calorie (from nutrient and non-nutrient calorie sources such as propofol and dextrose) and protein intake Regarding caloric requirements, calculations were based on previously published indirect calorimetry measurements in a subset of patients [6]. In our ICU, we had established protocols for nutrition support from the first day of the COVID-19 pandemic, based on the ESPEN guidelines or local consensus. The NST made the decision on the nutrition regimen as well as the route of nutrition support in collaboration with the treating physician.

Patients in the enteral nutrition group were fed through a nasogastric or nasoduodenal catheter depending on tolerance and comorbidities. The aim was to meet the caloric requirements by the 7th day of hospitalization using isosmotic, isocaloric, high-protein, polymeric preparations, after which the decision was at the discretion of the bedside physician [9]. In all cases, nutrition support was administered continuously (mL per h). Malnourished patients (BMI < 17 or clinical diagnosis) were assigned to a parenteral nutrition protocol designed to reduce the risk of refeeding syndrome [11,16]. In the parenteral group (presence of uncontrolled shock, uncontrolled life-threatening hypoxemia, hypercapnia or acidosis, hemodynamic instability, or when energy intake was consistently <50% of targets over 5–7 days), all patients received only parenteral nutrition via a central venous catheter depending on the results of daily haemodynamic assessments and nonfunctional digestive tract. We excluded from the analysis patients using supplemental parenteral nutrition to achieve predefined calorie targets after day 8. Parenteral nutrition was stopped and replaced with enteral nutrition at the flow rate needed to achieve the pre-defined calorie target once the patient met pre-defined criteria for haemodynamic stability. Bedside physician provided extra water, electrolytes, vitamins, and trace elements using standard preparations.

2.4. Outcome

The primary outcome was death by day 30. Secondary outcomes included mortality up to day 60 of hospitalization, ICU mortality, length of hospital and ICU stay, days of mechanical ventilation support, days of renal replacement, and percentage of patients who received mechanical ventilation, vasopressors and renal replacement therapy.

2.5. Statistical Analysis

The categorical variables are expressed as frequencies while the continuous variables as means (with standard deviations) or medians (with interquartile ranges (IQRs)), according to the rejection/not rejection of null hypothesis by the Shapiro–Wilk test, and then compared using Students t-test or Mann–Whitney U test. Due to the lack of information regarding effect of the feeding route on COVID-19 patients at the time of study design, it was not possible to perform a sample size calculation prior to the beginning of the current study when we performed hypothesis testing. The comparison between the groups was made using the Wilcoxon rank sum tests for continuous variables, while a chi-square test of independence (χ^2) (Fisher exact tests where appropriate) was performed for categorical variables. We used generalized linear models to test associations between feeding groups (enteral vs. parenteral nutrition) and study final outcomes. A Poisson distribution with log-link function was used to test association of number of count data, while a Binomial distribution with logit link function was used for clinical endpoints. The results are presented as relative risk (RR) and 95% confidence intervals (CIs). Statistical tests were considered significant if $p < 0.05$. All statistical analyzes were conducted using SPSS version 21.0.

3. Results
3.1. Patients

From September 2020 to July 2021, 192 patients with a confirmed SARS-CoV-2 infection during the second and third wave of the COVID-19 pandemic were admitted to the Evangelismos intensive care unit (ICU). Of these, 16 patients were excluded from the study because they either died within the first 48 h after admission or were under nutritional support, while four had mechanical ventilation started more than 24 h earlier, resulting in 176 patients (Figure 1). Participants were intubated within 24 h of admission, and their mean age was 62.1 ± 10.9 years, while 51.2% were male. The demographic, baseline, and nutritional characteristics of the patients analyzed are presented in Table 1. There was no clear categorization of patients as malnourished or not at admission, as it was not possible to collect information on dietary intake, weight loss, and the usual body weight. Almost half of the participants had Nutric Score values >5, indicating a high nutritional risk upon admission to the ICU.

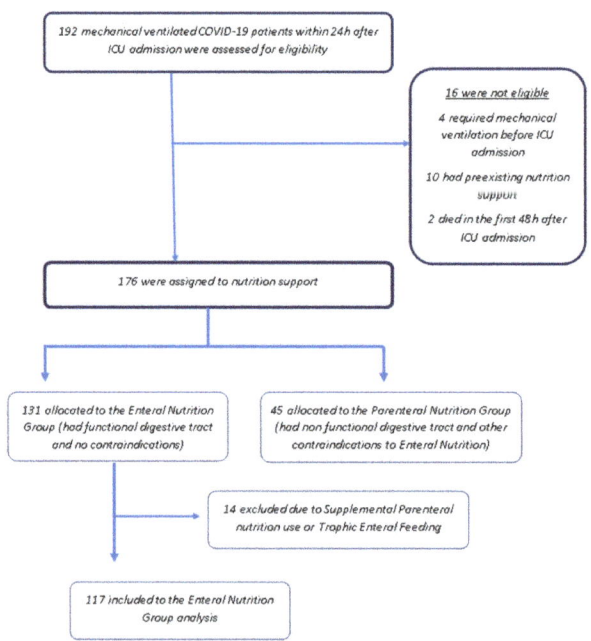

Figure 1. Patient recruitment flow chart.

Table 1. Baseline characteristics of the participants ($n = 162$).

Characteristics	Parenteral Nutrition Group $n = 45$ (27.7%)	Enteral Nutrition Group $n = 117$ (72.3%)	p-Value
Age (year)	62.7 ± 10.7	63.2 ± 11.9	0.181
Sex, male (n) %	21 (46.6)	62 (52.9)	0.093
Active Smoker (n)%	9 (20.0)	21 (17.8)	0.233
Comorbidities, (n) %			0.112
Hypertension	23 (51.1)	62 (52.9)	

Table 1. Cont.

Characteristics	Parenteral Nutrition Group n = 45 (27.7%)	Enteral Nutrition Group n = 117 (72.3%)	p-Value
Diabetes	21 (46.6)	52 (44.4)	
COPD	7 (15.5)	16 (13.6)	
Chronic Renal Failure	2 (4.4)	3 (2.5)	
Nutritional data			
BMI on admission, (kg/m^2), (n) %			0.233
Normal (18.5–24.9)	16 (36.2)	45 (38.5)	
Overweight (25–29.9)	12 (26.6)	31 (26.4)	
Obese ($\geq$30)	14 (31.1)	41 (35.0)	
NUTRIC Score on admission, (n) %			0.046 *
Low risk (0–4 points)	21 (46.7)	15 (59.7)	
High risk (5–9 points)	24 (53.3)	57 (40.3)	
Fluid balance (mL/day)	1250 ± 215	1015 ± 188	
Coverage of energy need during 7–14th day of ICU stay (n) %	89.1	86.5	0.076
Protein delivered during ICU (g/kg ideal body weight/day)	1.09 ± 0.61	1.17 ± 0.68	0.122
Time from ICU admission to start nutrition (IQR)—h	17.8 (13.4–27.2)	22.3 (15.2–31.2)	0.041 *
Calories administered—kcal/kg of body weight/day	27.8 ± 7.8	26.3 ± 6.9	0.098
Clinical Data			
APACHE II score on admission	18.3 ± 6.8	17.1 ± 6.2	0.249
Use of prone positioning, n (%)	26 (58.4)	67 (57.2)	0.135
PaO$_2$/FiO$_2$ ratio (mmHg)	126 (92-170)	128 (96–171)	0.338
Serum albumin g/L	3.16 ± 0.80	3.05 ± 0.96	0.224
Vasopressor therapy, n (%)	33 (73.3)	83 (70.9)	0.336
Side effects, n (%)			0.039 *
Electrolyte disturbances	2 (4.4)	1 (0.8%)	
Vomiting	10 (22.1)	37 (31.6%)	
Diarrhea	13 (29.2)	43 (36.7%)	
Hypoglycemia	-	-	
Other (cholestasis, pneumothorax)	1 (1.2)	-	

Values represent median (IQR) or means (+SD) or number of subjects (n, %). * Denotes statistically significant different between groups at <0.05 level, p = p value for Students t-test or Mann-Whitney U test or Chi square test. Abbreviations: APACHE, Acute Physiology and Chronic Health Evaluation; COPD, chronic obstructive pulmonary disease; BMI, body mass index; PEEP, positive end expiratory pressure; Nutric Score, Nutrition Risk in the Critically Ill; Fi02, fraction of inspired oxygen; NMBAs, neuromuscular blocking agents.

3.2. Outcomes

Data on feeding practices are presented in Table 1. A total of 117 individuals were fed enterally, while the rest were fed through the parenteral route. Of those belonging to the parenteral nutrition group, 5.6% experienced side effects, such as electrolyte disturbances, pneumothorax, hypoglycemia, and cholestasis, while in those receiving enteral nutrition, vomiting (32.3%) was the most common side effect.

Fifteen of 45 patients (33.3%) in the parenteral group and 38 of 117 patients (34.2%) in the enteral group died, with no significant between-group difference by day 30 even after adjusting for various baseline factors, such as age, sex, and race, APACHE score, Nutric

Score (as a dichotomous variable), BMI, diabetes, and chronic kidney disease (relative risk in the enteral group, 0.97; 95% confidence interval (CI), 0.88 to 1.06, Table 2). There were significant reductions in the enteral group as compared with the parenteral group for in-hospital length of stay (RR = 0.92; 95% CI, 0.86 to 0.98; p = 0.039), ventilator days (RR = 0.94; 95% CI, 0.89 to 0.99; p = 0.043), and elevated liver enzymes ((RR = 0.91; 95% CI, 0.85 to 0.97; p = 0.039); p = 0.022). However, there were also significant differences regarding the rates of adverse gastrointestinal events between the parenteral group and the enteral group (32.3% vs. 22.1% for vomiting and 37.2% vs. 29.2% for diarrhea, p < 0.05). There was no significant difference in the duration of survival up to 60 days. Initiation of feeding was delayed in 37 patients in the parenteral nutrition group and in 41 patients in the enteral nutrition group, while caloric and protein intake are shown in Table 1. The energy target of 25–30 calories per kilogram of body weight per day was reached in the majority of patients in both groups, and the average caloric intake was almost identical in both groups.

Table 2. Patients primary and secondary outcomes (n = 162).

Outcome	Parenteral Nutrition Group (n = 45)	Enteral Nutrition Group (n = 117)	Relative Risk (95% CI) [#]	p-Value
Primary				
Death within 30 days, n (%)	15 (33.3)	38 (32.4)	0.97 (0.88–1.06)	0.120
Secondary				
Death, n (%)				
In-hospital mortality,	14 (31.1%)	36 (30.7%)	0.98 (0.86–1.10)	0.132
ICU mortality,	17 (37.9%)	43 (36.7%)	0.96 (0.85–1.08)	0.124
60-day mortality	16 (35.5%)	41 (35%)	0.97 (0.82–1.10)	0.233
Hospital length of stay (days)	35 (7–59)	30 (8–52)	0.92 (0.86–0.98)	0.039 *
ICU length of stay (days)	23 (6–51)	21 (7–49)	0.98 (0.90–1.06)	0.078
Ventilator days (30-day study period only)	21 (6–28)	17 (6–24)	0.94 (0.89–0.99)	0.043 *
Days on RRT (30-day study period only)	17 (5–28)	18 (6–29)	0.98 (0.89–1.07)	0.180
Kidney failure requiring RRT	13 (28.8%)	34 (29.1%)	0.95 (0.81–1.09)	0.337
Tracheostomy, n (%)	11 (24.4%)	29 (24.7%)	0.96 (0.83–1.09)	0.197
ICU acquired Infections, n (%)	7 (15.5%)	20 (17.1%)	0.89 (0.72–1.06)	0.221
Septic shock, n (%)	30 (66.6%)	75 (64.1%)	0.94 (0.86–1.02)	0.063
Elevated liver enzymes	13 (28.8%)	17 (14.5%)	0.91 (0.85–0.97)	0.022 *

Values represent median (IQR) or means (+SD) or number of subjects (n, %). * Denotes statistically significant different between groups at <0.05 level [#] Covariates were selected a priori, incorporating demographic information (age, sex, and race). APACHE score, Nutric Score (dichotomous variable), BMI, diabetes, and chronic kidney disease. Abbreviations: ICU, intensive care unit; RRT, renal replacement therapy.

4. Discussion

This single-center prospective study evaluated the effect of the nutritional support administration route after the seventh day of hospitalization on outcome among critically ill intubated COVID-19 patients. Our data suggest that enteral feeding is superior to parenteral feeding in terms of length of hospital stay and mechanical ventilation, but these findings were not accompanied by a corresponding improvement in mortality both in-hospital and out-of-hospital at 60 days. These two groups also did not exhibit any differences regarding infections incidence, days on RRT, and septic shock prevalence.

Are there other data available to date on feeding practices and their effect on outcome among COVID-19 critically ill patients? Only a few studies so far have provided limited data about nutrition support. A USA cohort [24] revealed that more than half of the participants (56%) presented intolerance to enteral nutrition, which was associated with higher ICU stay and in-hospital mortality, whereas a similar study among intubated patients from Mexico revealed a lower prevalence of intolerance to enteral nutrition—about 32% [25]. A series of 176 critically ill patients with COVID-19 disease [26] managed to reach their energy and protein requirements during the first week of admission especially through the use of supplemental parenteral nutrition. Parenteral nutrition use was comparable to our study, as approximately 35% of patients were fed through the parenteral route compared with 27.7% of our patients. Reports from another study—the ISIIC point prevalence study—also suggest that there is a growing interest in the role of nutrition support, which resulted in providing COVID-19 patients with higher amounts of energy and protein compared to non-COVID-19 patients [27].

There is also lack of available data regarding the effect of feeding administration after the first week of ICU hospitalization when energy and protein targets are theoretically achieved [26]. All previous major studies tried to investigate the effect of either early administration (during the first 72 h following admission) of nutritional support [28] either up to the fifth day of hospitalization [19,29] or the first week of hospitalization [14] on outcome. The two largest multicenter clinical trials among critically ill patients assessing the effects of nutritional support route during first week of ICU stay suggest nonsignificant difference in all-cause mortality, frequency of infectious complications, ICU, and hospital length of stay (LOS) [14,19]. In our cohort, feeding practices were investigated during the second week of hospitalization and not the first. This was settled for two reasons: so far, most studies that explore the relationship between feeding practices during the first week of ICU and outcome have not provided any clear association [10,14,19,21]. The other reason is that in critically ill patients, energy metabolic demands usually peak within five to seven days before returning to normal (ebb/flow phases) [30]. Regarding COVID-19 disease, there is a stable hypermetabolic condition probably because of hyperinflammatory response, which persists during the second week of hospitalization and appears to stabilize after the 10th day of ICU stay, as recent studies have demonstrated [5,6].

The total length of hospital stay was lower in those patients receiving enteral nutrition although ICU length of stay (LOS) was not different. A systematic review and meta-analysis show that early enteral feeding is associated with a reduced postoperative length of stay among patients undergoing lower gastrointestinal surgery [31], while among critically ill patients, route of nutrition support during first week of hospitalization was not related to LOS although there was a trend for reduced ICU stay [14]. Harvey et al. revealed that there was no difference in both length of hospital and ICU stay among critically ill patients according to feeding rout e [19]. Another main finding of this study was that those receiving enteral feeding presented a shorter duration of mechanical ventilation support. As compared to earlier times, enteral feeding is no longer contraindicated in patients under mechanical ventilation and is the preferred route of feeding administration [32], while some data do not suggest that enteral feeding is superior [33]. On the other hand, parenteral feeding is well recognized for its higher caloric intake, leading to hyperglycemia and increased ventilator stay [34].

In addition to these findings, parenteral nutrition group was more likely to experience an increase in liver enzymes during hospitalization. Research on the effects of parenteral nutrition has focused on the possibility of liver dysfunction as well as an increase in liver enzymes [35]. This phenomenon is a potential result of cholestasis, which is caused by biliary obstruction or impaired secretion of bile [36]. On appearance, γ-glutamyl transpeptidase, alkaline phosphatase, and conjugated bilirubin levels are elevated. This is a clinical manifestation accompanying long-term parenteral nutrition therapy among pediatric patients or adults. Long-term PN therapy-induced cholestasis is a significant consequence that can progress to cirrhosis and liver failure [37].

The present study was not without limitations. First, our study had a relatively small sample size, which limits the generalizability to other ICUs and countries. Second, the prospective nature of this study does not define a causal relationship and reflects only associations between the implemented nutrition protocols and study outcomes. Moreover, we did not obtain data regarding energy expenditure by using indirect calorimetry in the whole sample because it was very time consuming to get such a large quantity of data. Our study was not a randomized evaluation of feeding practices; even if the indication for parenteral and enteral nutrition followed guidelines and local treatment protocols, a selection bias cannot be excluded. We should also point out that a higher proportion of patients belonging to the parenteral nutrition group exhibited high Nutric Score values, but we have controlled for this confounding factor in the multivariate models. Furthermore, it was not possible to assess all possible covariates among our patients, and future studies might lead to different results regarding the provision of nutrition therapy in critically ill patients.

5. Conclusions

There are scarce data on feeding practices among critically ill COVID-19 patients and their effects on outcome. Our study demonstrated that the majority of COVID-19 intubated patients were fed through the enteral route during their second week of ICU hospitalization. Enteral nutrition was not superior compared to parenteral feeding in relation to the main study outcome, which was 30-day mortality, but it was associated with reduced length of hospital stay, less demand for mechanical ventilation support, and a more favorable profile for liver enzyme levels.

Author Contributions: Conceptualization, D.K., Z.M. and A.K. (Anastasia Kotanidou); formal analysis, D.K. and A.A.; methodology, Z.M., A.A., K.M., D.K., E.J. and T.P.; project administration, D.K.; supervision, D.K. and Z.M.; writing—original draft, D.K.; writing—review and editing, A.K. (Aggeliki Kanavou), A.M., V.G., D.K., A.S., C.L., S.K., O.K., S.M., A.S. and G.A. All authors have read and agreed to the published version of the manuscript.

Funding: This research received no external funding.

Institutional Review Board Statement: The study was conducted in accordance with the Declaration of Helsinki, and approved by the Institutional Review Board at Athens Evangelismos Hospital: 116/31-03-2021.

Informed Consent Statement: The Institutional Review Board at Athens Evangelismos Hospital: 116/31-03-2021 approved data collection and waived the need for informed consent.

Acknowledgments: We are grateful to Athina Kardara and Emy Valavani for their assistance in data collection.

Conflicts of Interest: The authors declare no conflict of interest.

Abbreviations

APACHE	Acute Physiology And Chronic Health Evaluation
BMI	Body mass index
ICU	Intensive care unit
LOS	Length of stay
NST	Nutrition Support Team
Nutric Score	Nutrition Risk in the Critically Il
PEEP	Positive end expiratory pressure
RR	Relative risk

References

1. Zhou, F.; Yu, T.; Du, R.; Fan, G.; Liu, Y.; Liu, Z.; Xiang, J.; Wang, Y.; Song, B.; Gu, X.; et al. Clinical course and risk factors for mortality of adult inpatients with COVID-19 in Wuhan, China: A retrospective cohort study. *Lancet* **2020**, *395*, 1054–1062. [CrossRef]
2. Struyf, T.; Deeks, J.J.; Dinnes, J.; Takwoingi, Y.; Davenport, C.; Leeflang, M.M.; Spijker, R.; Hooft, L.; Emperador, D.; Dittrich, S.; et al. Signs and symptoms to determine if a patient presenting in primary care or hospital outpatient settings has COVID-19 disease. *Cochrane Database Syst. Rev.* **2020**, *7*, Cd013665. [CrossRef] [PubMed]

3. Barazzoni, R.; Bischoff, S.C.; Breda, J.; Wickramasinghe, K.; Krznaric, Z.; Nitzan, D.; Pirlich, M.; Singer, P. ESPEN expert statements and practical guidance for nutritional management of individuals with SARS-CoV-2 infection. *Clin. Nutr.* **2020**, *39*, 1631–1638. [CrossRef] [PubMed]
4. Singer, P.; Blaser, A.R.; Berger, M.M.; Alhazzani, W.; Calder, P.C.; Casaer, M.P.; Hiesmayr, M.; Mayer, K.; Montejo, J.C.; Pichard, C.; et al. ESPEN guideline on clinical nutrition in the intensive care unit. *Clin. Nutr.* **2019**, *38*, 48–79. [CrossRef]
5. Whittle, J.; Molinger, J.; MacLeod, D.; Haines, K.; Wischmeyer, P.E. Persistent hypermetabolism and longitudinal energy expenditure in critically ill patients with COVID-19. *Crit. Care* **2020**, *24*, 581. [CrossRef]
6. Karayiannis, D.; Maragkouti, A.; Mikropoulos, T.; Sarri, A.; Kanavou, A.; Katsagoni, C.; Jahaj, E.; Kotanidou, A.; Mastora, Z. Neuromuscular blockade administration is associated with altered energy expenditure in critically ill intubated patients with COVID-19. *Clin. Nutr.* **2021**. [CrossRef] [PubMed]
7. Suliman, S.; McClave, S.A.; Taylor, B.E.; Patel, J.; Omer, E.; Martindale, R.G. Barriers to nutrition therapy in the critically ill patient with COVID-19. *J. Parenter. Enteral Nutr.* **2021**. [CrossRef]
8. Vekaria, B.; Overton, C.; Wiśniowski, A.; Ahmad, S.; Aparicio-Castro, A.; Curran-Sebastian, J.; Eddleston, J.; Hanley, N.A.; House, T.; Kim, J.; et al. Hospital length of stay for COVID-19 patients: Data-driven methods for forward planning. *BMC Infect. Dis.* **2021**, *21*, 700. [CrossRef]
9. Achamrah, N.; Delsoglio, M.; De Waele, E.; Berger, M.M.; Pichard, C. Indirect calorimetry: The 6 main issues. *Clin. Nutr.* **2021**, *40*, 4–14. [CrossRef]
10. Doig, G.S.; Simpson, F.; Sweetman, E.A.; Finfer, S.R.; Cooper, D.J.; Heighes, P.T.; Davies, A.R.; O'Leary, M.; Solano, T.; Peake, S. Early parenteral nutrition in critically ill patients with short-term relative contraindications to early enteral nutrition: A randomized controlled trial. *JAMA* **2013**, *309*, 2130–2138. [CrossRef]
11. Martindale, R.; Patel, J.J.; Taylor, B.; Arabi, Y.M.; Warren, M.; McClave, S.A. Nutrition Therapy in Critically Ill Patients With Coronavirus Disease 2019. *J. Parenter. Enteral Nutr.* **2020**, *44*, 1174–1184. [CrossRef] [PubMed]
12. Chapple, L.S.; Fetterplace, K.; Asrani, V.; Burrell, A.; Cheng, A.C.; Collins, P.; Doola, R.; Ferrie, S.; Marshall, A.P.; Ridley, E.J. Nutrition management for critically and acutely unwell hospitalised patients with coronavirus disease 2019 (COVID-19) in Australia and New Zealand. *Aust. Crit. Care* **2020**, *33*, 399–406. [CrossRef]
13. Preiser, J.C.; van Zanten, A.R.; Berger, M.M.; Biolo, G.; Casaer, M.P.; Doig, G.S.; Griffiths, R.D.; Heyland, D.K.; Hiesmayr, M.; Iapichino, G.; et al. Metabolic and nutritional support of critically ill patients: Consensus and controversies. *Crit. Care* **2015**, *19*, 35. [CrossRef]
14. Reignier, J.; Boisramé-Helms, J.; Brisard, L.; Lascarrou, J.B.; Ait Hssain, A.; Anguel, N.; Argaud, L.; Asehnoune, K.; Asfar, P.; Bellec, F.; et al. Enteral versus parenteral early nutrition in ventilated adults with shock: A randomised, controlled, multicentre, open-label, parallel-group study (NUTRIREA-2). *Lancet* **2018**, *391*, 133–143. [CrossRef]
15. Jeejeebhoy, K.N. Enteral nutrition versus parenteral nutrition—the risks and benefits. *Nat. Clin. Pract. Gastroenterol. Hepatol.* **2007**, *4*, 260–265. [CrossRef] [PubMed]
16. Chapple, L.S.; Tatucu-Babet, O.A.; Lambell, K.J.; Fetterplace, K.; Ridley, E.J. Nutrition guidelines for critically ill adults admitted with COVID-19: Is there consensus? *Clin. Nutr. ESPEN* **2021**, *44*, 69–77. [CrossRef] [PubMed]
17. Lewis, S.R.; Schofield-Robinson, O.J.; Alderson, P.; Smith, A.F. Enteral versus parenteral nutrition and enteral versus a combination of enteral and parenteral nutrition for adults in the intensive care unit. *Cochrane Database Syst. Rev.* **2018**, *6*, Cd012276. [CrossRef]
18. Hill, A.; Elke, G.; Weimann, A. Nutrition in the Intensive Care Unit-A Narrative Review. *Nutrients* **2021**, *13*, 2851. [CrossRef] [PubMed]
19. Harvey, S.E.; Parrott, F.; Harrison, D.A.; Bear, D.E.; Segaran, E.; Beale, R.; Bellingan, G.; Leonard, R.; Mythen, M.G.; Rowan, K.M. Trial of the route of early nutritional support in critically ill adults. *N. Engl. J. Med.* **2014**, *371*, 1673–1684. [CrossRef]
20. Rives-Lange, C.; Zimmer, A.; Merazka, A.; Carette, C.; Martins-Bexinga, A.; Hauw-Berlemont, C.; Guerot, E.; Jannot, A.S.; Diehl, J.L.; Czernichow, S.; et al. Evolution of the nutritional status of COVID-19 critically-ill patients: A prospective observational study from ICU admission to three months after ICU discharge. *Clin. Nutr.* **2021**. [CrossRef]
21. Lakenman, P.L.M.; van der Hoven, B.; Schuijs, J.M.; Eveleens, R.D.; van Bommel, J.; Olieman, J.F.; Joosten, K.F.M. Energy expenditure and feeding practices and tolerance during the acute and late phase of critically ill COVID-19 patients. *Clin. Nutr. ESPEN* **2021**, *43*, 383–389. [CrossRef] [PubMed]
22. Alves, T.; Guimarães, R.S.; Souza, S.F.; Brandão, N.A.; Daltro, C.; Conceição-Machado, M.E.P.; Oliveira, L.P.M.; Cunha, C.M. Influence of nutritional assistance on mortality by COVID-19 in critically ill patients. *Clin. Nutr. ESPEN* **2021**, *44*, 469–471. [CrossRef] [PubMed]
23. Lin, J.; Ke, L.; Doig, G.S.; Ye, B.; Jiang, Z.; Liu, Z.; Guo, F.; Yin, J.; Yu, W.; Sun, J.; et al. Nutritional practice in critically ill COVID-19 patients: A multicenter ambidirectional cohort study in Wuhan and Jingzhou. *Asia Pac. J. Clin. Nutr.* **2021**, *30*, 15–21. [CrossRef]
24. Liu, R.; Paz, M.; Siraj, L.; Boyd, T.; Salamone, S.; Lite, T.V.; Leung, K.M.; Chirinos, J.D.; Shang, H.H.; Townsend, M.J.; et al. Feeding intolerance in critically ill patients with COVID-19. *Clin. Nutr.* **2021**. [CrossRef]
25. Osuna-Padilla, I.; Rodríguez-Moguel, N.C.; Aguilar-Vargas, A.; Rodríguez-Llamazares, S. Safety and tolerance of enteral nutrition in COVID-19 critically ill patients, a retrospective study. *Clin. Nutr. ESPEN* **2021**, *43*, 495–500. [CrossRef] [PubMed]
26. Miguélez, M.; Velasco, C.; Camblor, M.; Cedeño, J.; Serrano, C.; Bretón, I.; Arhip, L.; Motilla, M.; Carrascal, M.L.; Morales, A.; et al. Nutritional management and clinical outcome of critically ill patients with COVID-19: A retrospective study in a tertiary hospital. *Clin. Nutr.* **2021**. [CrossRef]

27. Nakamura, K.; Liu, K.; Katsukawa, H.; Nydahl, P.; Ely, E.W.; Kudchadkar, S.R.; Inoue, S.; Lefor, A.K.; Nishida, O. Nutrition therapy in the intensive care unit during the COVID-19 pandemic: Findings from the ISIIC point prevalence study. *Clin. Nutr.* **2021**. [CrossRef] [PubMed]
28. Sim, J.; Hong, J.; Na, E.M.; Doo, S.; Jung, Y.T. Early supplemental parenteral nutrition is associated with reduced mortality in critically ill surgical patients with high nutritional risk. *Clin. Nutr.* **2021**, *40*, 5678–5683. [CrossRef] [PubMed]
29. Hise, M.E.; Halterman, K.; Gajewski, B.J.; Parkhurst, M.; Moncure, M.; Brown, J.C. Feeding practices of severely ill intensive care unit patients: An evaluation of energy sources and clinical outcomes. *J. Am. Diet. Assoc.* **2007**, *107*, 458–465. [CrossRef]
30. Stahel, P.F.; Flierl, M.A.; Moore, E.E. "Metabolic staging" after major trauma—A guide for clinical decision making? *Scand J. Trauma Resusc. Emerg. Med.* **2010**, *18*, 34. [CrossRef]
31. Herbert, G.; Perry, R.; Andersen, H.K.; Atkinson, C.; Penfold, C.; Lewis, S.J.; Ness, A.R.; Thomas, S. Early enteral nutrition within 24 hours of lower gastrointestinal surgery versus later commencement for length of hospital stay and postoperative complications. *Cochrane Database Syst. Rev.* **2018**, *10*, Cd004080. [CrossRef]
32. Allen, K.; Hoffman, L. Enteral Nutrition in the Mechanically Ventilated Patient. *Nutr. Clin. Pract.* **2019**, *34*, 540–557. [CrossRef] [PubMed]
33. Altintas, N.D.; Aydin, K.; Türkoğlu, M.A.; Abbasoğlu, O.; Topeli, A. Effect of enteral versus parenteral nutrition on outcome of medical patients requiring mechanical ventilation. *Nutr. Clin. Pract.* **2011**, *26*, 322–329. [CrossRef] [PubMed]
34. Reid, C. Frequency of under- and overfeeding in mechanically ventilated ICU patients: Causes and possible consequences. *J. Hum. Nutr. Diet.* **2006**, *19*, 13–22. [CrossRef] [PubMed]
35. Nowak, K. Parenteral Nutrition-Associated Liver Disease. *Clin. Liver Dis.* **2020**, *15*, 59–62. [CrossRef] [PubMed]
36. Żalikowska-Gardocka, M.; Przybyłkowski, A. Review of parenteral nutrition-associated liver disease. *Clin. Exp. Hepatol.* **2020**, *6*, 65–73. [CrossRef] [PubMed]
37. Kumpf, V.J.; Gervasio, J. Complications of parenteral nutrition. In *The ASPEN Adult Nutrition Support Core Curriculum*, 3rd ed.; Mueller, C.M., Ed.; American Society of Parenteral and Enteral Nutrition: Silver Spring, MD, USA, 2017; pp. 352–355.

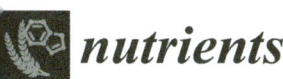

Article

Stress Hyperglycemia and Osteocalcin in COVID-19 Critically Ill Patients on Artificial Nutrition

Francisco Arrieta [1,2], Victoria Martinez-Vaello [1], Nuria Bengoa [1], Marta Rosillo [3], Angélica de Pablo [4], Cristina Voguel [4], Rosario Pintor [5], Amaya Belanger-Quintana [6], Raquel Mateo-Lobo [1], Angel Candela [4] and José I. Botella-Carretero [1,2,*]

1. Department of Endocrinology and Nutrition, Hospital Universitario Ramón y Cajal, 28034 Madrid, Spain; arri68@hotmail.com (F.A.); vmartinezvaello@gmail.com (V.M.-V.); nuria.bengoa@salud.madrid.org (N.B.); raquel.mateo@salud.madrid.org (R.M.-L.)
2. Centro de Investigación Biomédica en Red Fisiopatología de la Obesidad y Nutrición (CIBERobn) & Instituto Ramón y Cajal de Investigación Sanitaria (IRyCIS), 28034 Madrid, Spain
3. Department of Biochemistry, Hospital Universitario Ramón y Cajal, 28034 Madrid, Spain; marta.rosillo@salud.madrid.org
4. Department of Anesthesiology, Hospital Universitario Ramón y Cajal, 28034 Madrid, Spain; angelicadepabl@hotmail.com (A.d.P.); crivomed@gmail.com (C.V.); angel.candela@salud.madrid.org (A.C.)
5. Department of Pharmacy, Hospital Universitario Ramón y Cajal, 28034 Madrid, Spain; mariarosario.pintor@salud.madrid.org
6. Department of Pediatrics, Hospital Universitario Ramón y Cajal, 28034 Madrid, Spain; amaya.belanger@salud.madrid.org
* Correspondence: joseignacio.botella@salud.madrid.org; Tel.: +34-913368383

Abstract: We aimed to study the possible association of stress hyperglycemia in COVID-19 critically ill patients with prognosis, artificial nutrition, circulating osteocalcin, and other serum markers of inflammation and compare them with non-COVID-19 patients. Fifty-two critical patients at the intensive care unit (ICU), 26 with COVID-19 and 26 non-COVID-19, were included. Glycemic control, delivery of artificial nutrition, serum osteocalcin, total and ICU stays, and mortality were recorded. Patients with COVID-19 had higher ICU stays, were on artificial nutrition for longer ($p = 0.004$), and needed more frequently insulin infusion therapy ($p = 0.022$) to control stress hyperglycemia. The need for insulin infusion therapy was associated with higher energy ($p = 0.001$) and glucose delivered through artificial nutrition ($p = 0.040$). Those patients with stress hyperglycemia showed higher ICU stays (23 ± 17 vs. 11 ± 13 days, $p = 0.007$). Serum osteocalcin was a good marker for hyperglycemia, as it inversely correlated with glycemia at admission in the ICU ($r = -0.476$, $p = 0.001$) and at days 2 ($r = -0.409$, $p = 0.007$) and 3 ($r = -0.351$, $p = 0.049$). In conclusion, hyperglycemia in critically ill COVID-19 patients was associated with longer ICU stays. Low circulating osteocalcin was a good marker for stress hyperglycemia.

Keywords: COVID-19; hyperglycemia; parenteral nutrition; enteral nutrition; osteocalcin

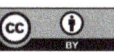

1. Introduction

Severe acute respiratory syndrome coronavirus 2 (SARS-CoV-2) is the cause of the coronavirus disease 2019 (COVID-19) pandemic, which has affected more than two hundred million individuals and is the cause of more than four million deaths worldwide as of this writing (https://coronavirus.jhu.edu/map.html, last accessed on 24 August 2021). Hyperglycemia is a risk factor for a more severe course of the disease, as hospitalized COVID-19 patients with diabetes show longer hospital stays than patients without diabetes [1]. They suffer disproportionately from acute COVID-19, with higher rates of serious complications and death [2]. Chronic inflammation, increased coagulation activity, immune response impairment, and potential direct pancreatic damage by SARS-CoV-2 might be among the underlying mechanisms for this association [3]. Furthermore, an important proportion of COVID-19 patients need admission to an intensive care unit (ICU) and may develop stress hyperglycemia—whether or not having a previous history of diabetes mellitus—which has been shown to be a prognostic factor [4,5].

Among the factors associated with stress hyperglycemia, the need for parenteral nutrition (PN)—which is normally part of the nutritional therapy together with enteral nutrition (EN) in critically ill patients [6]—might be one of them, especially in older individuals [7]. Besides, several interactions between some counter-regulatory hormones, adipokines, and inflammatory cytokines produce excessive production of glucose by the liver and insulin resistance at the peripheral tissues [8]. The resultant hyperglycemia further exacerbates the inflammatory and oxidative stress response, potentially setting up a vicious cycle whereby hyperglycemia leads to further hyperglycemia [9].

In the last few years, circulating osteocalcin, an osteoblast-specific protein, has shown extraskeletal metabolic activity, such as promoting insulin secretion and increasing peripheral insulin sensitivity [10]. Reduced circulating osteocalcin was found in patients with type 2 diabetes mellitus and also associated with insulin sensitivity [11,12].

Therefore, given this previous knowledge, we aimed to study the possible association of stress hyperglycemia in COVID-19 critically ill patients with a worse prognosis compared to non-COVID-19 patients. We also aimed to explore the possible associations of hyperglycemia with circulating osteocalcin concentrations, the composition of artificial nutrition, and serum markers of inflammation.

2. Materials and Methods

2.1. Subjects and Measurements

Fifty-two patients were included in this study: 26 consecutive patients with severe COVID-19 requiring admission to the ICU and 26 non-COVID-19 critically ill postsurgical patients. The latter were historical controls before the COVID-19 pandemic occurred and had the following procedures: 7 cardiovascular surgery, 12 renal/urological surgery, 6 pelvic surgery, and 1 surgery for traumatic hemothorax. Patients with COVID-19 were diagnosed by the presence of SARS-CoV-2 in respiratory specimens by real-time polymerase chain reaction (RT-PCR) in pharyngeal swabs. All COVID-19 patients were critically-ill and on mechanical ventilation. They received our standard treatment protocol, including low molecular-weight heparin, glucocorticoids, and tocilizumab. Non-COVID-19 patients were all complicated postsurgical ones in need of mechanical ventilation and vasoactive drugs. Patients under 18 y were excluded as well as those with active cancer, pregnancy, or with end-stage renal or liver disease before the diagnosis of COVID-19.

Patients in both groups were categorized as with or without diabetes mellitus based on a previous diagnosis. Stress hyperglycemia was defined as a plasma glucose level of ≥ 140 mg/dl. Continuous insulin infusion (50 IU of Actrapid in 50 mL of 0.9% saline using an IV pump) was started when blood glucose was ≥ 180 mg/dl and adjusted for a glycemic range of 140–179 mg/dl [13]. Capillary glycemia was measured every one or two hours to adjust the infusion rate. When blood glucose fell to <140 mg/dl, insulin infusion was stopped and subcutaneous insulin started. Capillary glycemia was then measured every six hours. ICU stay and total hospital stay were recorded as well as mortality.

The type of composition of artificial nutrition administered to the included patients were recorded. PN was delivered through a central line as soon as the patient was hemodynamically stable. Individualized formulae or standardized commercial bags were prepared by the hospital pharmacy. We aimed at 20–25 kcal/Kg/day, with a proportion of 3–6 g/Kg/day for glucose, 1.0 g/Kg/day for amino-acids, and less than 1 g/Kg/day for lipids, with 7–10 g/day of essential fatty acids. Vitamins and trace elements were also added by the hospital pharmacy. For those patients with ICU stays above 7 days, and whenever possible, EN was started with a standard, fiber-free formulation and PN gradually tapered as EN was tolerated and increased.

2.2. Ethics

The study protocol was approved by the Institutional Ethics Committee of our center (study code 147/20) and performed according to the Declaration of Helsinki. Written or verbal informed consent was obtained from all patients.

2.3. Analytical Assays

Serum concentrations of glucose and other biochemical variables were measured with an Architect c16000/i2000-analyzer (Abbot Diagnostics, Maidenhead, UK) and HbA1c by high-performance liquid chromatography (A. Menarini Diagnostics, Bagno a Ripoli, Italy). Immunoanalysis was employed for the measurement of C-reactive protein (CRP), procalcitonin (Abbott, Illinois, IL, USA) and D-dimer (Siemens, Münich, Germany), and interleukins 6 (IL-6) and 12 (IL-12) by enzyme-linked immunosorbent assay (Invitrogen, Waltham, MA, USA) at ICU admission. Serum osteocalcin was measured by electrochemi-luminescence Cobas-e601 (Roche Diagnostics, Rotkreuz ZG, Switzerland), with normal range of 15.0–45.0 µg/L also at ICU admission. The intra- and inter-assay coefficients of variation were below 10%.

2.4. Statistical Analysis

We used GRANMO 7.12 [14] for sample size analysis. The primary outcome was to study the possible association of stress hyperglycemia in COVID-19 critically ill patients with a worse prognosis compared to non-COVID-19 patients. In order to find a mean difference of 10 days in ICU stay with a SD of 10, we needed a sample size of at least 16 individuals in each group for a two-tail estimates setting α at 0.05 and β at 0.20. Secondary outcomes were the possible associations of hyperglycemia with circulating osteocalcin concentrations, the composition of artificial nutrition, and serum markers of inflammation. Based on our previous results [12], in order to find a mean difference of 7.6 µg/L in osteocalcin concentrations with a SD of 8.8, we needed a sample size of at least 21 individuals in each group for a two-tail estimates setting α at 0.05 and β at 0.20. Sample size analyses for the composition of artificial nutrition and inflammatory markers were not performed.

Results are expressed as means ± SD unless otherwise stated. The Kolmogorov–Smirnov statistic was applied to continuous variables. Logarithmic or square root transformations were used as needed to ensure normal distribution of the variables. To compare discontinuous variables, we used the χ^2 test and Fisher's exact test as appropriate. Unpaired t-tests or Mann–Whitney U tests were used to compare the central tendencies of the different groups as appropriate. Bivariate correlation was employed to study the association between two continuous variables using Pearson or Spearman's tests as appropriate. Two-way ANOVA was employed to analyze the effect of both COVID-19 and stress hyperglycemia on the studied continuous prognostic variables and corrected χ^2 test for categorical ones. Finally a multivariate linear regression analysis was also performed with a backwards strategy. Analyses were performed using SPSS 17 (SPSS Inc, Chicago, IL, USA). $p < 0.05$ was considered statistically significant.

3. Results

3.1. Baseline Characteristics of Patients

Of the 52 initially included patients, the results of 49 patients were finally analyzed, as three patients with COVID-19 had undetectable levels of osteocalcin (Table 1). Patients with COVID-19 were younger, with a higher proportion of males. Previous diagnosis of diabetes mellitus was similar in both groups as well as their HbA1c.

Table 1. Characteristics of the critically ill included patients.

	Patients with COVID-19 (n = 23)	Non-COVID-19 Patients (n = 26)	p
Male sex (n, %)	19 (83)	14 (54)	0.039
Age (y)	64 ± 9	71 ± 8	0.005
Time to ICU admission (days)	8.1 ± 12.2	4.0 ± 6.7	0.158
Glucose metabolism			
Previous diabetes mellitus (n, %)	6 (23)	6 (26)	0.806
HbA1c (%)	6.0 ± 0.9	6.0 ± 0.8	0.977
Glycemia at ICU admission (mg/dl)	148 ± 62	129 ± 41	0.207
Mean glycemia 1 week at ICU (mg/dl)	136 ± 37	128 ± 39	0.523
Patients with stress hyperglycemia (n, %) *	10 (48)	12 (46)	0.920
Patients with insulin infusion therapy (n, %)	14 (61)	7 (27)	0.022
Artificial nutrition			
Time on TPN (days)	15.7 ± 9.6	7.2 ± 10.1	0.004
Time on EN (days)	10.0 ± 12.9	2.1 ± 4.3	0.010
Mean energy delivered (kcal/day)	1222 ± 180	900 ± 329	<0.001
Mean glucose delivered (g/day)	141 ± 15	137 ± 29	0.600
Metabolic and inflammatory markers			
Osteocalcin (μg/L)	7.0 ± 3.5	12.9 ± 7.0	<0.001
Creatinine (mg/dl)	1.0 ± 0.6	1.3 ± 1.3	0.309
CRP (mg/L)	181 ± 129	161 ± 105	0.652
Procalcitonin (ng/mL)	1.0 ± 2.2	2.4 ± 3.5	0.156
D-dimer (μg/mL)	3791 ± 5403	-	-
IL-6 (pg/mL)	280 ± 400	-	-
IL-12 (pg/mL)	0.8 ± 1.1	-	-
Prognostic parameters			
ICU stay (days)	24 ± 16	9 ± 13	<0.001
Total hospital stay (days)	46 ± 19	32 ± 39	0.138
Mortality (n, %)	8 (35)	7 (27)	0.551

Data are means ± SD unless otherwise stated. TPN, total parenteral nutrition; EN, enteral nutrition; CRP, C-reactive protein; IL, interleukin; ICU, intensive care unit. * Stress hyperglycemia was defined as glycemia ≥ 140 mg/dl.

We did not find a difference in glycemia at ICU admission in the proportion of patients with stress hyperglycemia or in mean glycemia at ICU. However, patients with COVID-19 more frequently needed insulin infusion therapy for glycemic control and showed lower osteocalcin concentrations. Patients with COVID-19 were also on artificial nutrition for longer (both PN and EN) and received higher energy per day than non-COVID-19 ones but with similar amounts of delivered glucose per day. Serum CRP and procalcitonin at ICU admission were similar in both groups (Table 1).

Mortality did not differ between groups. Non-COVID-19 patients died as a result of cardiac arrest (n = 3), pulmonary embolism (n = 1), and multiorgan failure after septic shock (n = 3). COVID-19 patients died as a result of respiratory distress syndrome (n = 6) and pulmonary embolism (n = 2). The possibility of stroke and or any other CNS complications as the cause of death could not be accurately assessed due to profound sedation in these patients (Table 1).

3.2. Impact of Stress Hyperglycemia

When both patients with and without COVID-19 were considered together and classified according to the presence of stress hyperglycemia, the latter group showed a higher proportion of previous diagnosis of type 2 diabetes mellitus and higher HbA1c levels

(Table 2). They were on PN for longer, received higher amounts of energy and glucose from artificial nutrition, and showed higher ICU stays.

Table 2. Characteristics of patients with and without stress hyperglycemia *.

	Patients with Stress Hyperglycemia (n = 22)	Patients without Stress Hyperglycemia (n = 27)	p
COVID-19 diagnosis (n, %)	10 (46)	13 (48)	0.851
Male sex (n, %)	14 (64)	19 (70)	0.617
Age (y)	69 ± 9	67 ± 10	0.574
Glucose metabolism			
Previous diabetes mellitus (n, %)	9 (41)	3 (11)	0.022
HbA1c (%)	6.4 ± 0.9	5.7 ± 0.7	0.013
Glycemia at ICU admission (mg/dl)	162 ± 44	118 ± 42	0.003
Mean glycemia 1-week at ICU (mg/dl)	161 ± 29	112 ± 26	<0.001
Artificial nutrition			
Time on TPN (days)	14.7 ± 11.8	8.3 ± 8.9	0.035
Time on EN (days)	8.6 ± 12.6	3.5 ± 6.8	0.075
Mean energy delivered (kcal/day)	1185 ± 296	941 ± 287	0.006
Mean glucose delivered (g/day)	147 ± 24	132 ± 20	0.026
Metabolic and inflammatory markers			
Osteocalcin (µg/L)	8.2 ± 5.3	12.3 ± 7.0	0.034
CRP (mg/L)	170 ± 102	180 ± 144	0.808
Procalcitonin (ng/mL)	1.8 ± 3.2	0.8 ± 1.5	0.314
Prognostic parameters			
ICU stay (days)	23 ± 17	11 ± 13	0.007
Total hospital stay (days)	47 ± 39	31 ± 23	0.090
Mortality (n, %)	5 (19)	10 (45)	0.085

Data are means ± SD unless otherwise stated. TPN, total parenteral nutrition; EN, enteral nutrition; CRP, C-reactive protein; ICU, intensive care unit. * Stress hyperglycemia was defined as glycemia ≥ 140 mg/dl.

Total hospital stay did not correlate with glucose control, but ICU stay correlated with glycemia at admission in ICU ($r = 0.337$, $p = 0.018$) and at day 2 ($r = 0.427$, $p = 0.015$). Those patients with stress hyperglycemia showed higher ICU stays. As expected, those patients with longer ICU stays needed more days on artificial nutrition for both PN ($r = 0.741$, $p < 0.001$) and EN ($r = 0.829$, $p < 0.001$).

3.3. Circulating Osteocalcin as a Marker for Hyperglycemia and Prognosis

Circulating osteocalcin was lower in patients with COVID-19 (Table 1). It was lower in patients with stress hyperglycemia (Table 2) and in those in need for insulin infusion therapy (7.0 ± 4.7 vs. 12.3 ± 7.0 µg/L for subcutaneous insulin, $t = 3.672$, $p = 0.001$).

Circulating osteocalcin concentrations inversely correlated with glycemia at the day of admission in the ICU ($r = -0.476$, $p = 0.001$) and at days 2 ($r = -0.409$, $p = 0.007$) and 3 ($r = -0.351$, $p = 0.049$) (Figure 1). Osteocalcin did not correlate with HbA1c ($r = -0.207$, $p = 0.225$) or age ($r = 0.145$, $p = 0.319$), and their levels were similar in men and women ($t = 0.482$, $p = 0.632$).

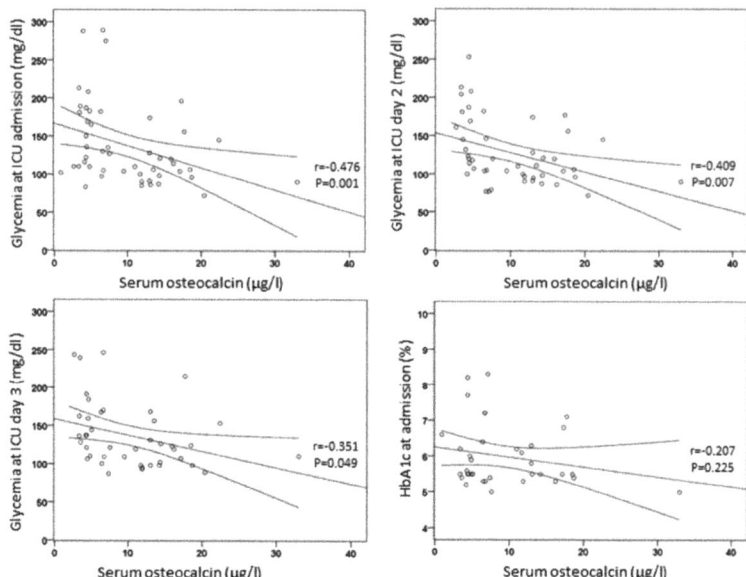

Figure 1. Correlations of circulating osteocalcin with glycemia and HbA1c.

3.4. Impact of the Composition of Artificial Nutrition

The amount of energy delivered through PN did not correlate with glycemia at the day of admission in the ICU ($r = 0.245$, $p = 0.097$), at day 2 ($r = 0.211$, $p = 0.245$), or 3 ($r = 0.069$, $p = 0.750$). Conversely, the amount of glucose delivered through PN was positively correlated with glycemia at the day of admission in the ICU ($r = 0.395$, $p = 0.006$). In addition, mean glucose and energy delivered through artificial nutrition correlated with mean glycemia during ICU stay ($r = 0.399$, $p = 0.007$ and $r = 0.291$, $p = 0.048$, respectively) (Figure 2).

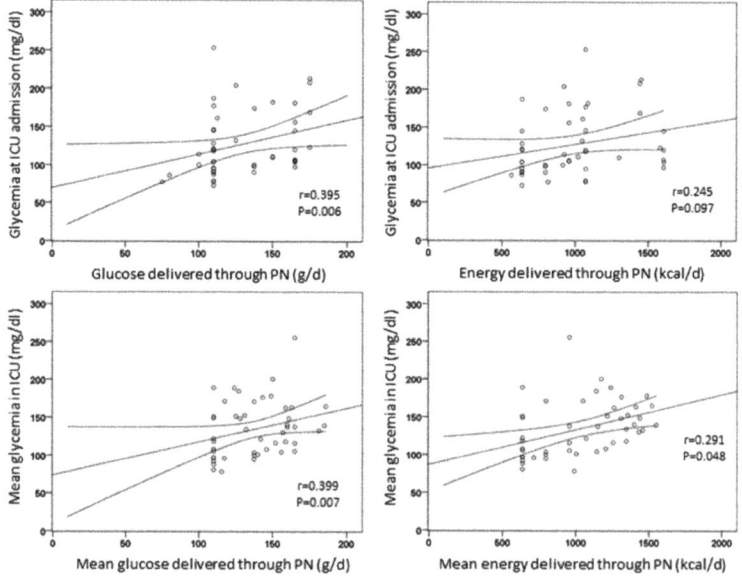

Figure 2. Correlations of energy and glucose delivered through artificial nutrition with glycemia.

Those patients in need of insulin infusion therapy compared with those on subcutaneous insulin received higher energy (1221 ± 256 vs. 923 ± 294 kcal/day, respectively, $t = 3.709$, $p = 0.001$) and glucose delivered through artificial nutrition (146 ± 22 vs. 133 ± 22 g/day, respectively, $t = 2.112$, $p = 0.040$).

3.5. Circulating Inflammatory Markers

Glycemia at the day of admission in the ICU was positively correlated with IL-12 ($r = 0.454$, $p = 0.038$) but not with CRP ($r = 0.065$, $p = 0.722$), procalcitonin ($r = 0.145$, $p = 0.446$), IL-6 ($r = 0.138$, $p = 0.551$), or D-dimer ($r = 0.232$, $p = 0.312$) (Figure 3).

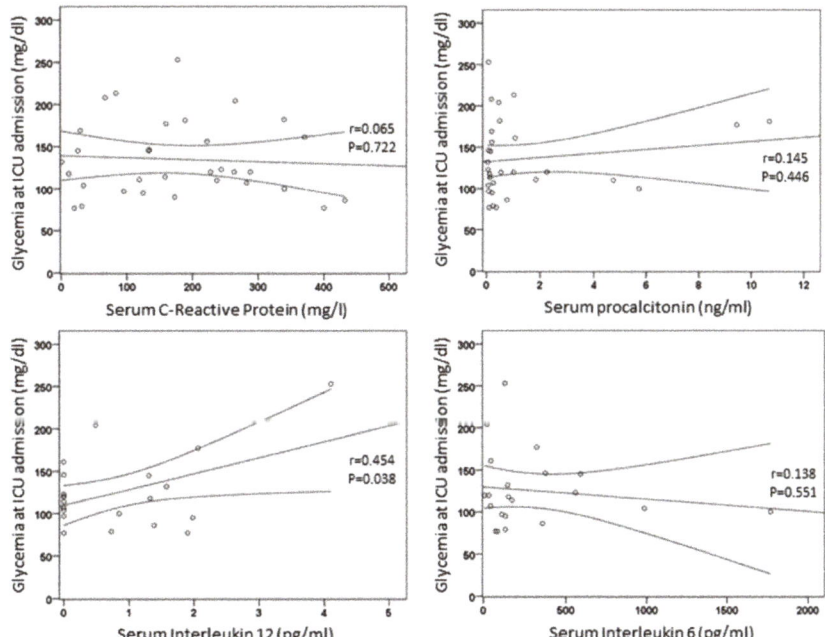

Figure 3. Correlations of serum inflammatory markers with glycemia.

Patients with stress hyperglycemia had more similar inflammatory markers at ICU admission than those without it (Table 2). The same occurred between those patients in need for insulin infusion therapy compared with those on subcutaneous insulin ($p > 0.05$ for IL-12, CRP, procalcitonin, D-dimer, and IL-6).

3.6. Ancillary Analyses

In order to correct for the effects of both the presence of COVID-19 and stress hyperglycemia in prognostic parameters and osteocalcin, we performed a two-way analysis of variance for continuous variables and corrected χ^2 test for categorical ones. Separated data in four groups are shown in Table 3.

Table 3. Prognosis and serum markers of patients with and without COVID-19 and with or without stress hyperglycemia *,†.

	COVID-19 with Stress Hyperglycemia (n = 10)	COVID-19 without Stress Hyperglycemia (n = 13)	Non-COVID-19 with Stress Hyperglycemia (n = 12)	Non-COVID-19 without Stress Hyperglycemia (n = 14)	p for COVID-19 Effect	p for Hyperglycemia	p for Interaction
Male sex (n, %)	9 (90)	10 (77)	5 (42)	9 (64)	0.031	0.678	
Age (y)	65 ± 8	63 ± 10	72 ± 9	71 ± 8	0.006	0.595	0.878
ICU stay (days)	30 ± 17	20 ± 14	17 ± 15	2 ± 2	<0.001	0.002	0.172
Total hospital stay (days)	47 ± 20	46 ± 19	47 ± 52	20 ± 20	0.263	0.110	0.255
Mortality (n, %)	5 (50)	3 (23)	5 (42)	2 (14)	0.391	0.120	
Osteocalcin (μg/L)	6.2 ± 4.2	6.9 ± 4.3	9.8 ± 6.3	15.7 ± 6.2	0.001	0.027	0.172
CRP (mg/L)	192 ± 98	173 ± 153	146 ± 108	230 ± 82	0.926	0.560	0.354
Procalcitonin (ng/mL)	1.2 ± 2.9	0.7 ± 1.5	2.4 ± 3.7	1.3 ± 0.7	0.373	0.816	0.904
Patients with insulin infusion (n, %)	8 (80)	6 (46)	7 (58)	0 (0)	0.040	0.041	
Time on TPN (days)	16.4 ± 11.5	15.2 ± 8.4	13.3 ± 12.5	2.0 ± 1.3	0.003	0.020	0.060
Time on EN (days)	13.5 ± 17.0	7.2 ± 8.3	4.6 ± 5.5	1.0 ± 0.5	0.004	0.045	0.750
Mean energy delivered (kcal/day)	1274 ± 135	1182 ± 205	1109 ± 373	717 ± 121	<0.001	0.001	0.029
Mean glucose delivered (g/day)	140 ± 16	141 ± 15	153 ± 29	124 ± 21	0.721	0.029	0.015

Data are means ± SD unless otherwise stated. ICU, intensive care unit; CRP, C-reactive protein. * Stress hyperglycemia was defined as glycemia ≥ 140 mg/dl. †, p show the results of two-way ANOVA except for categorical variables that were analyzed by corrected χ^2 tests.

ICU stay was higher with both COVID-19 diagnosis and the presence of stress hyperglycemia, indicating these two were independent prognostic factors. Conversely total hospital stay and mortality were not associated with either COVID-19 diagnosis or the presence of stress hyperglycemia. Circulating osteocalcin was lower in both COVID-19 patients and with the presence of stress hyperglycemia, but CRP and procalcitonin showed no associations (Table 3).

Insulin infusion was more frequent for both COVID-19 diagnosis and the presence of stress hyperglycemia. The time on artificial nutrition, both on TPN and EN, was longer in those patients with COVID-19 and with stress hyperglycemia. The amount of energy and glucose delivered by artificial nutrition were also associated with both the presence of COVID-19 and stress hyperglycemia and with their interaction (Table 3).

Finally, a multivariate linear regression analysis was also performed with a backwards strategy, introducing COVID-19 diagnosis, the presence of stress hyperglycemia, the need for insulin infusion, age, and sex as independent variables and ICU stay as the dependent variable. Both COVID-19 diagnosis (β = 0.488, p < 0.001) and the presence of stress hyperglycemia (β = 0.394, p = 0.001) were retained by the model (R^2 = 0.383, F = 14.297, p < 0.001). When osteocalcin was introduced as the dependent variable, both COVID-19 diagnosis (β = −0.375, p = 0.005) and the presence of stress hyperglycemia (β = −0.344, p = 0.009) were retained by the model (R^2 = 0.347, F = 12.224, p < 0.001).

Another multivariate regression analysis model was performed as to take into account the artificial nutrition characteristics on ICU stay, which was introduced as the dependent variable. The independent variables in this model were the days on artificial nutrition, both TPN and EN, the amount of energy and glucose delivered by artificial nutrition, and the need for insulin infusion. The presence of COVID-19 and stress hyperglycemia could not be introduced in the model, as they showed collinearity with the variables of artificial nutrition. The variables retained by the model ($R^2 = 0.965$, $F = 438.5$, $p < 0.001$) were the days on both TPN ($\beta = 0.535$, $p < 0.001$) and EN ($\beta = 0.652$, $p < 0.001$) and the need for insulin infusion ($\beta = 0.066$, $p = 0.031$).

4. Discussion

In the present study, we have shown that hyperglycemia in critically ill COVID-19 patients was associated with longer ICU stays and higher amounts of glucose delivered through artificial nutrition. Low circulating osteocalcin was lower in COVID-19 patients, in those with stress hyperglycemia, and in those in need for insulin infusion therapy. Therefore, osteocalcin could be considered a useful marker for stress hyperglycemia and prognosis at ICU.

Osteocalcin, while playing important roles in bone remodeling, also contributes to glucose metabolism by affecting both insulin secretion and insulin sensitivity [15]. In vitro, co-cultures of pancreatic islets and wild-type osteoblasts stimulated insulin secretion, whereas knockout osteocalcin osteoblasts did not [15]. Furthermore, the link between bone and glucose metabolism is supported by clinical observations indicating that patients with diabetes show an increased risk of fractures because of osteopenia or osteoporosis [16,17] and similarly in animal models [10].

Circulating osteocalcin was reduced in patients with severe COVID-19, in accordance with a recent report in which 40 patients were compared with 57 non-COVID-19 controls in a cross-sectional design [18]. We further analyzed the serum osteocalcin association with glycemia in COVID-19 patients, as we and other authors reported in the past this relationship in other type of patients [12,19]. We found that circulating osteocalcin was inversely correlated with glycemia: it was lower in those with stress hyperglycemia, those in need for insulin infusion therapy, and also associated with longer ICU stays. To our knowledge, this is the first time that this association is reported in critically ill patients.

Diabetes mellitus has shown to be a risk factor for a worse prognosis in patients with COVID-19 [20,21] as well as those who develop stress hyperglycemia [4]. Furthermore, the severity of COVID-19 illness increases progressively in relation to glucose abnormalities at admission [22], and this has also been shown to happen in patients without a previous diagnosis of diabetes [23]. Conversely, a recent report has shown no difference in mortality based on the diabetes status, previous control, or complications [1]. Therefore, glycemic control may be important to all COVID-19 patients even if they have no pre-existing diabetes, as most COVID-19 patients are prone to glucose metabolic disorders as a result of stress hyperglycemia and probably the adverse effects of several treatments.

Among the factors that may influence the appearance of stress hyperglycemia in critically ill patients, the release of inflammatory mediators might be one of the physiopathological pathways. Inflammatory cytokines excessively produce glucose by the liver and insulin resistance at the peripheral tissues [8], and the resultant hyperglycemia further exacerbates the inflammatory and oxidative stress response [9]. The modulation of the immune response in patients receiving insulin treatment may partially explain a reduction in morbidity and mortality [24]. In agreement, we have shown that circulating IL-12 concentrations correlated with hyperglycemia at ICU admission and that those patients with stress hyperglycemia showed higher ICU stays.

The amount or glucose delivered through artificial nutrition might be another associated factor with stress hyperglycemia. It has been shown that among the metabolic complications of parenteral nutrition, hyperglycemia is one of them, and this may be especially important in older individuals [7]. Therefore, nutrition-support regimens need to minimize stress hyperglycemia and assist glucose management [25]. Recent recommendations from the European Society of Clinical Nutrition and Metabolism (ESPEN) state that in critically COVID-19 patients who do not tolerate full-dose EN during the first week in the ICU, initiating PN should be weighed on a case-by-case basis [14]. Conversely, in the last two decades, evidence-based recommendations suggest PN use in patients in whom EN cannot be initiated within 24 h of ICU admission or injury [26–28], as it produces similar outcomes as EN alone. Even a combination of PN and EN in critically ill patients has been recently recommended as a better approach [29].

However, there is still a paucity of data in critically ill COVID-19 patients regarding the recommendation of the type of artificial nutrition and also its composition. Our results showed that the amount of glucose delivered by artificial nutrition did not differ between COVID-19 and non-COVID-19 patients. It is true that the former needed higher rates of insulin infusion, but this could be related to the use of glucocorticoids as part of their treatment. In the present study, we have also shown that the amount of glucose delivered through parenteral nutrition was associated with higher glycemia at ICU independently of COVID-19 diagnosis.

An important limitation of our study is that it was enabled to find differences in ICU stay and serum osteocalcin but not in the composition of artificial nutrition. In this regard, we showed after performing a multivariate analysis that both ICU stay and osteocalcin were independently associated with COVID-19 diagnosis and the presence of stress hyperglycemia. However, the latter were also associated with longer artificial nutrition support and higher energy needs, so the design of our study precludes us from reaching valid, nonbiased associations regarding artificial nutrition. Therefore, future studies are needed to address the role of the type and composition of artificial nutrition in critically ill COVID-19 patients.

5. Conclusions

Hyperglycemia in critically ill COVID-19 patients was associated with longer ICU stays and with higher amounts of glucose delivered through artificial nutrition in both COVID-19 and non-COVID-19 patients. Low circulating osteocalcin was a good marker for stress hyperglycemia.

Author Contributions: J.I.B.-C. and F.A. equally contributed to the conception and design of the research; A.C. contributed to the design of the research; N.B., V.M.-V., M.R., A.d.P., C.V., R.P., A.B.-Q. and R.M.-L. contributed to the acquisition and analysis of the data; J.I.B.-C., A.C. and F.A. contributed to the interpretation of the data; and J.I.B.-C. and F.A. drafted the manuscript. All authors critically revised the manuscript, agree to be fully accountable for ensuring the integrity and accuracy of the work, and read and approved the final manuscript. All authors have read and agreed to the published version of the manuscript.

Funding: This research was funded by Vegenat Healthcare, grant for partly support study 147/20.

Institutional Review Board Statement: The study was conducted according to the guidelines of the Declaration of Helsinki and approved by the Ethics Committee of Hospital Universitario Ramón y Cajal (study code 147/20).

Informed Consent Statement: Written or verbal informed consent was obtained from all patients.

Data Availability Statement: Restrictions apply to the availability of data generated or analyzed during this study to preserve patient confidentiality or because they were used under license. The corresponding author will on request detail the restrictions and any conditions under which access to some data may be provided.

Acknowledgments: CIBERobn is an initiative of Instituto de Salud Carlos III (ISCIII).

Conflicts of Interest: The authors declare no conflict of interest. The funders had no role in the design of the study; in the collection, analyses, or interpretation of data; in the writing of the manuscript, or in the decision to publish the results.

References

1. Alkundi, A.; Mahmoud, I.; Musa, A.; Naveed, S.; Alshawwaf, M. Clinical characteristics and outcomes of COVID-19 hospitalized patients with diabetes in the United Kingdom: A retrospective single centre study. *Diabetes Res. Clin. Pract.* **2020**, *165*, 108263. [CrossRef]
2. Wake, D.J.; Gibb, F.W.; Kar, P.; Kennon, B.; Klonoff, D.C.; Rayman, G.; Rutter, M.K.; Sainsbury, C.; Semple, R.K. Endocrinology in the time of COVID-19: Remodelling diabetes services and emerging innovation. *Eur. J. Endocrinol.* **2020**, *183*, G67–G77. [CrossRef] [PubMed]
3. Hussain, A.; Bhowmik, B.; do Vale Moreira, N.C. COVID-19 and diabetes: Knowledge in progress. *Diabetes Res. Clin. Pract.* **2020**, *162*, 108142. [CrossRef] [PubMed]
4. Sardu, C.; D'Onofrio, N.; Balestrieri, M.L.; Barbieri, M.; Rizzo, M.R.; Messina, V.; Maggi, P.; Coppola, N.; Paolisso, G.; Marfella, R. Outcomes in Patients With Hyperglycemia Affected by COVID-19: Can We Do More on Glycemic Control? *Diabetes Care* **2020**, *43*, 1408–1415. [CrossRef]
5. Mantovani, A.; Byrne, C.D.; Zheng, M.H.; Targher, G. Diabetes as a risk factor for greater COVID-19 severity and in-hospital death: A meta-analysis of observational studies. *Nutr. Metab. Cardiovasc. Dis.* **2020**, *30*, 1236–1248. [CrossRef]
6. Singer, P.; Blaser, A.R.; Berger, M.M.; Alhazzani, W.; Calder, P.C.; Casaer, M.P.; Hiesmayr, M.; Mayer, K.; Montejo, J.C.; Pichard, C.; et al. ESPEN guideline on clinical nutrition in the intensive care unit. *Clin. Nutr.* **2019**, *38*, 48–79. [CrossRef] [PubMed]
7. Solomon, D.M.; Hollands, J.M.; Pontiggia, L.; Delic, J.J.; Bingham, A.L. Metabolic Complications Occur More Frequently in Older Patients Receiving Parenteral Nutrition. *Nutr. Clin. Pract.* **2020**, *35*, 627–633. [CrossRef]
8. Dungan, K.M.; Braithwaite, S.S.; Preiser, J.C. Stress hyperglycaemia. *Lancet* **2009**, *373*, 1798–1807. [CrossRef]
9. Lheureux, O.; Prevedello, D.; Preiser, J.C. Update on glucose in critical care. *Nutrition* **2019**, *59*, 14–20. [CrossRef]
10. Bilotta, F.L.; Arcidiacono, B.; Messineo, S.; Greco, M.; Chiefari, E.; Britti, D.; Nakanishi, T.; Foti, D.P.; Brunetti, A. Insulin and osteocalcin: Further evidence for a mutual cross-talk. *Endocrine* **2018**, *59*, 622–632. [CrossRef]
11. Gower, B.A.; Pollock, N.K.; Casazza, K.; Clemens, T.L.; Goree, L.L.; Granger, W.M. Associations of total and undercarboxylated osteocalcin with peripheral and hepatic insulin sensitivity and beta-cell function in overweight adults. *J. Clin. Endocrinol. Metab.* **2013**, *98*, E1173–E1180. [CrossRef]
12. Iglesias, P.; Arrieta, F.; Pinera, M.; Botella-Carretero, J.I.; Balsa, J.A.; Zamarrón, I.; Menacho, M.; Díez, J.J.; Muñoz, T.; Vázquez, C. Serum concentrations of osteocalcin, procollagen type 1 N-terminal propeptide and beta-CrossLaps in obese subjects with varying degrees of glucose tolerance. *Clin. Endocrinol.* **2011**, *75*, 104–188. [CrossRef]
13. American Diabetes Association. 15. Diabetes Care in the Hospital: Standards of Medical Care in Diabetes-2019. *Diabetes Care* **2019**, *42*, S173–S181. [CrossRef]
14. Barazzoni, R.; Bischoff, S.C.; Breda, J.; Wickramasinghe, K.; Krznarić, Z.; Nitzan, D.; Pirlich, M.; Singer, P. ESPEN expert statements and practical guidance for nutritional management of individuals with SARS-CoV-2 infection. *Clin. Nutr.* **2020**, *39*, 1631–1638. [CrossRef]
15. Zoch, M.L.; Clemens, T.L.; Riddle, R.C. New insights into the biology of osteocalcin. *Bone* **2016**, *82*, 42–49. [CrossRef] [PubMed]
16. Janghorbani, M.; Feskanich, D.; Willett, W.C.; Hu, F. Prospective study of diabetes and risk of hip fracture: The Nurses' Health Study. *Diabetes Care* **2006**, *29*, 1573–1578. [CrossRef]
17. Starup-Linde, J.; Frost, M.; Vestergaard, P.; Abrahamsen, B. Epidemiology of Fractures in Diabetes. *Calcif. Tissue Int.* **2017**, *100*, 109–121. [CrossRef] [PubMed]
18. Li, T.; Wang, L.; Wang, H.; Gao, Y.; Hu, X.; Li, X.; Zhang, S.; Xu, Y.; Wei, W. Characteristics of laboratory indexes in COVID-19 patients with non-severe symptoms in Hefei City, China: Diagnostic value in organ injuries. *Eur. J. Clin. Microbiol. Infect. Dis.* **2020**, *39*, 2447–2455. [CrossRef]
19. Liu, D.-M.; Guo, X.-Z.; Tong, H.-J.; Tao, B.; Sun, L.-H.; Zhao, H.-Y.; Ning, G.; Liu, J.-M. Association between osteocalcin and glucose metabolism: A meta-analysis. *Osteoporos. Int.* **2015**, *26*, 2823–2833. [CrossRef] [PubMed]
20. Riddle, M.C.; Buse, J.B.; Franks, P.W.; Knowler, W.C.; Ratner, R.E.; Selvin, E.; Wexler, D.J.; Kahn, S.E. COVID-19 in People with Diabetes: Urgently Needed Lessons From Early Reports. *Diabetes Care* **2020**, *43*, 1378–1381. [CrossRef]
21. Hartmann-Boyce, J.; Morris, E.; Goyder, C.; Kinton, J.; Perring, J.; Nunan, D.; Mahtani, K.; Buse, J.B.; Del Prato, S.; Ji, L.; et al. Diabetes and COVID-19: Risks, Management, and Learnings from Other National Disasters. *Diabetes Care* **2020**, *43*, 1695–1703. [CrossRef]
22. Targher, G.; Mantovani, A.; Wang, X.-B.; Yan, H.-D.; Sun, Q.-F.; Pan, K.-H.; Byrne, C.D.; Zheng, K.I.; Chen, Y.-P.; Eslam, M.; et al. Patients with diabetes are at higher risk for severe illness from COVID-19. *Diabetes Metab.* **2020**, *46*, 335–337. [CrossRef]
23. Wang, S.; Ma, P.; Zhang, S.; Song, S.; Wang, Z.; Ma, Y.; Xu, J.; Wu, F.; Duan, L.; Yin, Z.; et al. Fasting blood glucose at admission is an independent predictor for 28-day mortality in patients with COVID-19 without previous diagnosis of diabetes: A multi-centre retrospective study. *Diabetologia* **2020**, *63*, 2102–2111. [CrossRef] [PubMed]
24. Xiu, F.; Stanojcic, M.; Diao, L.; Jeschke, M.G. Stress hyperglycemia, insulin treatment, and innate immune cells. *Int. J. Endocrinol.* **2014**, *2014*, 486403. [CrossRef]
25. Krenitsky, J. Glucose control in the intensive care unit: A nutrition support perspective. *Nutr. Clin. Pract.* **2011**, *26*, 31–43. [CrossRef]
26. Simpson, F.; Doig, G.S. Parenteral vs. enteral nutrition in the critically ill patient: A meta-analysis of trials using the intention to treat principle. *Intensive Care Med.* **2005**, *31*, 12–23. [CrossRef]

27. Doig, G.S.; Simpson, F. CALORIES trial offers confirmatory evidence that parenteral nutrition does not cause infectious complications in critically ill patients. *Evid. Based Med.* **2015**, *20*, 60. [CrossRef] [PubMed]
28. Reignier, J.; Boisrame-Helms, J.; Brisard, L.; Lascarrou, J.-B.; Hssain, A.A.; Anguel, N.; Argaud, L.; Asehnoune, K.; Asfar, P.; Bellec, F.; et al. Enteral versus parenteral early nutrition in ventilated adults with shock: A randomised, controlled, multicentre, open-label, parallel-group study (NUTRIREA-2). *Lancet* **2018**, *391*, 133–143. [CrossRef]
29. Heidegger, C.P.; Darmon, P.; Pichard, C. Enteral vs. parenteral nutrition for the critically ill patient: A combined support should be preferred. *Curr. Opin. Crit. Care* **2008**, *14*, 408–414. [CrossRef] [PubMed]

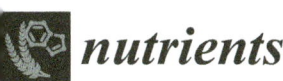

Article

Bad Prognosis in Critical Ill Patients with COVID-19 during Short-Term ICU Stay regarding Vitamin D Levels

Lourdes Herrera-Quintana [1], Yenifer Gamarra-Morales [1], Héctor Vázquez-Lorente [1], Jorge Molina-López [2,*], José Castaño-Pérez [3], Juan Francisco Machado-Casas [3], Ramón Coca-Zúñiga [3], José Miguel Pérez-Villares [3] and Elena Planells [1,*]

[1] Department of Physiology, Institute of Nutrition and Food Technology "Jose Mataix", School of Pharmacy, University of Granada, 18071 Granada, Spain; lourdesherrera@ugr.es (L.H.-Q.); jennifer_gamo@hotmail.com (Y.G.-M.); hectorvazquez@ugr.es (H.V.-L.)
[2] Faculty of Education, Psychology and Sports Sciences, University of Huelva, 21007 Huelva, Spain
[3] Intensive Care Unit, Virgen de las Nieves Hospital, Fuerzas Armadas Avenue, 18014 Granada, Spain; jcastaoperez@yahoo.com (J.C.-P.); jmachc2@hotmail.com (J.F.M.-C.); ramon.coca.sspa@juntadeandalucia.es (R.C.-Z.); josem.perez.villares.sspa@juntadeandalucia.es (J.M.P.-V.)
* Correspondence: jorge.molina@ddi.uhu.es (J.M.-L.); elenamp@ugr.es (E.P.)

Abstract: Background and aims: Vitamin D inadequacy may be involved in the mechanisms of SARS-CoV-2 infection and in potential risk factors for disease propagation or control of coronavirus disease 2019 (COVID-19). This study assessed a short-term evolution of vitamin D status and its influence upon different clinical parameters in critically ill patients with COVID-19. Methods: A prospective analytical study in which 37 critically ill volunteers between 41 and 71 years of age with COVID-19 were evaluated at baseline and three days of intensive care unit (ICU) stay. 25-OH-D$_3$ and 25-OH-D$_2$ were analyzed by liquid chromatography–tandem mass spectrometry and total 25-OH-D levels were calculated as the sum of both. Results: All patients presented low 25-OH-D levels at baseline, decreasing total 25-OH-D ($p = 0.011$) mainly through 25-OH-D$_2$ ($p = 0.006$) levels during ICU stay. 25-OH-D$_2$ levels decreased a mean of 41.6% ± 89.6% versus 7.0% ± 23.4% for the 25-OH-D$_3$ form during the ICU stay. Patients who did not need invasive mechanical ventilation presented higher levels of 25-OH-D$_2$ at baseline and follow-up. Lower 25-OH-D and 25-OH-D$_3$ levels were associated with higher D-dimer at baseline ($p = 0.003$; $p = 0.001$) and at follow up ($p = 0.029$), higher procalcitonin levels ($p = 0.002$; $p = 0.018$) at follow up, and lower percentage lymphocyte counts ($p = 0.044$; $p = 0.040$) during ICU stay. Conclusions: Deficient vitamin D status in critical patients was established at the admission and further worsened after three days of stay. Lower vitamin D levels were related to key altered clinical and biochemical parameters on patients with SARS-CoV-2 infection. Given the different response of the 25-OH-D$_3$ and 25-OH-D$_2$ forms, it would be useful to monitor them on the evolution of the critically ill patient.

Keywords: coronavirus disease 2019; SARS-CoV-2; Vitamin D; critical care; intensive care patient

1. Introduction

The global public health crisis caused by the SARS-CoV-2 virus has created the need for urgent actions in order to reduce the risk of infection, progression, and the severity of coronavirus disease 2019 (COVID-19) [1], which triggers an acute inflammatory process and uncontrolled oxidative stress [2]. This in turn results in severe acute respiratory distress syndrome (ARDS) characterized by a cytokine storm, mainly in critical cases [3], which may lead to multiple organ damage [4] and further complicate the patient's critical condition previously described during their ICU stay [5,6].

There is currently great concern regarding the clinical management and intensive care of patients with critical stages of the disease and who are at a higher risk of death [7]. The implementation of prompt and appropriate nutritional assessment in COVID-19 must be

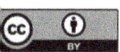

considered, [8,9] because possible modulation of the status of key micronutrients appears to be a relevant factor influencing the development of this disease [10]. No information about nutritional monitoring in critical patients with COVID-19 is available to date [11], and this lack of data precludes the definition of firm micronutrient recommendations in this particular risk population [12].

Certain micronutrients are essential for adequate immunocompetence and antioxidant defense, which are related to inflammatory response, such as vitamin D [13]. 25-Hydroxyvitamin D (25-OH-D) is the metabolite used to assess vitamin D status, due to its long half-life in plasma or serum (one month) [14], and is characterized by synergic action of its two main forms: 25-hydroxyvitamin D_2 (25-OH-D_2), which is obtained from plant sources, and 25-hydroxyvitamin D_3 (25-OH-D_3), which comes from animal products and endogenous synthesis in skin through exposure to sunlight [15], both of them can be supplemented with commercial products [16]. Recently, vitamin D has generated particular interest because of its role in reducing the risk of pneumonia and viral upper respiratory tract infections at a physical barrier and cellular natural and adaptive immunity level [17,18]. The underlying mechanisms can be grouped into two main actions: anti-inflammatory and anti-infective [19]. Vitamin D is associated with a decrease in proinflammatory cytokines, reducing the cytokine storm induced by the innate immune system, which is exacerbated in COVID-19 [17,20]. Moreover, it must be noted that serum 25-OH-D is considered as a negative acute phase reactant [21] and low vitamin D status in critical ill patients may be related to a decrease of binding protein concentration [22]. On the other hand, vitamin D is able to reduce viral infection and replication rates by inducing transcription of proteins with antimicrobial functions, enhancing autophagic encapsulation of viral particles, favoring lung epithelial cell barrier integrity, and ultimately regulating both innate and adaptive immunity [17–20,23,24].

Thus, vitamin D inadequacy has emerged as a factor that may be involved in the mechanisms of virus infection and in potential risk factors for disease propagation or control [24,25]. In fact, low vitamin D status in patients with COVID-19 has been reported [26–28], being associated with a poorer prognosis, infection risk, or unregulated inflammation. Thus, due to the lack of evidence on the importance of monitoring vitamin D status in critical patients with COVID-19, the present study was designed to assess the short-term evolution of the status of vitamin D and its influence upon different clinical parameters in critically ill patients with COVID-19 in the province of Granada, Spain.

2. Materials and Methods

2.1. Study Design and Subjects

A prospective analytical study was carried out of patients monitored from the first day of admission to the intensive care unit (ICU) (baseline) until day three of stay (follow-up). Of a total of 43 initially recruited patients, 37 participants from the province of Granada (Spain), aged 41–74 years, were included in the period from 1 March to 1 June 2020, after been informed about the study protocol. Six patients died during the study and were excluded. All eligible participants enrolled in the study were critical patients aged 18 years or older and hospitalized for more than 48 h, who agreed to participate in the study or for whom approval of participation was obtained from the family. All patients had a diagnosis of critical active SARS-CoV-2 infection according to the Chinese Clinical Guideline for the classification of COVID-19 [29] (analyzed by real-time reverse transcriptase–PCR (RT-PCR) testing of nasal and pharyngeal swab samples) and had an ICU stay of at least three days and did not receive vitamin D support. The present study was conducted in accordance with the principles of the Declaration of Helsinki, following the International Conference on Harmonization/Good Clinical Practice standards, and was approved by the Ethics Committee of the University of Granada (Ref. 149/CEIH/2016).

2.2. Data Collection

Data including age, sex, body mass index (BMI), smoking habits, comorbidities, respiratory and clinical parameters, ICU length of stay, length of hospitalization, and 28-day mortality were retrieved from the hospital electronic database system and recorded for each study participant at ICU admission (baseline) and after three days (follow-up). The Acute Physiology and Chronic Health Evaluation II (APACHE-II) score and Sequential Organ Failure Assessment (SOFA) score were obtained by intensivists at baseline and follow-up.

Patient clinical outcomes were recorded both at admission and during the ICU stay: heart rate (beats per minute); respiratory rate (breaths per minute); mean blood pressure (mmHg); positive end-expiratory pressure (PEEP); fraction of inspired oxygen (FiO_2); partial oxygen arterial pressure/fraction of inspired oxygen (PaO_2/FiO_2); ARDS; invasive mechanical ventilation (IMV).

2.3. Blood Sampling and Biochemical Parameters

Two measurements were performed (baseline and follow-up). Blood sampling was carried out in the morning under fasting conditions, followed by centrifugation (4 °C for 15 min at 3500 rpm) to separate the plasma. The samples were frozen at −80 °C until analysis of the different parameters. All samples were measured in one run, in the same assay batch, and blinded quality control samples were included in the same assay batches to determine laboratory error in the measurements.

The recorded biochemical parameters were total proteins, albumin, prealbumin, ferritin, transferrin, glucose, total cholesterol, glutamic oxaloacetic transaminase or aspartate transaminase (GOT or AST), glutamic pyruvic transaminase or alanine transaminase (GPT or ALT), lactate dehydrogenase (LDH), C-reactive protein (CRP), procalcitonin (PCT), hemoglobin, leukocytes, neutrophils, lymphocytes, platelets, D-dimer, fibrinogen, calcium (Ca), phosphorous (P), and magnesium (Mg), using routine hospital analytical assays (ECLIA, Elecsys 2010 and Modular Analytics E170, Roche Diagnostics, Mannheim, Germany).

2.4. Analytical Determination of Vitamin D

Vitamin D was measured in plasma samples by liquid chromatography–tandem mass spectrometry (LC-MS/MS). Plasma sample treatment involved protein precipitation adding 500 μL of acetonitrile in an Eppendorf flask with 200 μL of plasma and 20 μL of 25-hydroxyvitamin D_3 and 25-hydroxyvitamin D_2 deuterated solutions as Internal Standard (IS) (Sigma Aldrich, St. Louis, MO, USA) (0.5 μg/mL). The samples were slightly shaken for 1 min on a plate shaker and centrifuged at 10,000 rpm for 15 min at 4 °C. The supernatant was collected in another Eppendorf flask and dried with N_2. The dry residue was vortexed for 30 s after the addition of 200 μL of ethyl acetate and 100 μL of deionized water and centrifuged at 3000 rpm for 5 min. The supernatant was again collected in another Eppendorf flask, and the previous steps were repeated with the remaining liquid phase, subsequently pooling the second supernatant with the first. The total supernatant was dried with N_2.

For samples derivatization, we prepared a solution of 4-phenyl-3H-1,2,4-triazole-3,5(4H)-dione (PTAD) (Sigma Aldrich, St. Louis, MO, USA) in acetonitrile (0.5 mg/mL), using 50 μL of this solution in standards and in each sample, with vortexing. All samples were placed on the plate shaker for 1 h at room temperature and covered with aluminum foil. Lastly, the samples were transferred to vials, diluted with 50 μL of deionized water and stored in freezer at −20 °C covered with aluminum foil until injection into the chromatograph. For the calibration line, increasing concentrations of 1, 2, 5, 10, 25, 50, and 100 ppb of the standards 25-OH-D_3 and 25-OH-D_2 (Sigma Aldrich, St. Louis, MO, USA) with 20 μL of IS were used and dried with N_2 and derivatized at the same time as the samples. For sample measurements, use was made of a Waters Acquity UHPLC I-Class System chromatograph (Waters, London, UK), with the Acquity UHPLC BEH C18 column 2.1, 50 mm, 1.7 m at room temperature. The mobile phase of channel A was water with 50 mM of ammonium formate, while that of channel B was methanol. The injection volume of the sample was 10 µL and the flow rate was 0.4 mL/min. The detector was a Waters XEVO-TQ-XS Triple Quadrupole Low Resolution Spectrometer. Total 25-OH-D was calculated as the sum of the 25-OH-D_3 and 25-OH-D_2 forms. According to the Endocrine Society Practice Guidelines on Vitamin D, the threshold for biochemical 25-OH-D sufficiency values was considered to be >30 ng/mL, with deficiency being defined as 20–29 ng/mL and insufficiency as <20 ng/mL [28].

2.5. Statistical Analysis

Qualitative variables were presented as frequencies and percentages. Quantitative variables with normal distribution were expressed as the arithmetic mean and standard deviation (SD), and variables with non-normal distribution were expressed as the median and the interquartile range. Normal data distribution for continuous variables was tested using the Shapiro–Wilk test. The Wilcoxon signed-rank test for nonparametric samples was used for the comparative analyses at baseline and follow-up. The unpaired Student t-test for parametric samples was used for the comparative analysis based on clinical outcomes. The effect size (ES) was estimated and interpreted as follows: small = 0.01, moderate = 0.06, and large = 0.14 [30]. Correlation analyses and partial correlation coefficients were performed using the Spearman test. Statistical significance was considered for $p < 0.05$. The SPSS version 22.0 statistical package (IBM SPSS, Armonk, NY, USA) was used throughout.

3. Results

The demographic and clinical characteristics of the 37 patients enrolled in the study are shown in Table 1. The median age of the study population was 60 years, and the gender distribution of the sample was 26 males and 11 females. With regard to the anthropometric parameters, over a third of the patients were overweight, and more than half of them were obese. Most of the patients had one or more underlying diseases. With regard to the severity parameters, the mean APACHE-II and SOFA scores were 12.3 and 6.54, respectively, upon admission. A total of 26 of 37 patients (70.2%) had at least 1 infection, and 5 of them had 3 or more infections during their admission in ICU. The most frequent infection was bacteremia in 25 out of 48 total infections (52%), followed by respiratory infections 15 out of 48 total infections (31%), and finally urinary tract infections associated with urethral catheterization in 7 out of 48 total infections (14.5%). The most frequent germs causing these infections were Gram-positive (39%), followed by Gram-negative bacteria (33%) and fungi (20%). The mean length of hospitalization was 39.5 days. More than two-thirds of the patients presented ARDS on admission, requiring invasive mechanical ventilation with a mean duration of over 20 days. The mortality rate after 28 days of ICU stay was over two-thirds of the total study population.

The clinical and biochemical parameters of the study population at baseline and follow-up are shown in Table 2. Respiratory parameters were altered with significant changes in FiO_2 and PEEP after three days. Total proteins ($p = 0.012$), albumin ($p = 0.035$), prealbumin ($p = 0.017$), LDH ($p = 0.002$), CRP ($p = 0.001$), hemoglobin ($p = 0.001$), and fibrinogen ($p = 0.001$) were outside the reference values and decreased significantly after three days of ICU stay. Parameters such as ferritin, transaminases, or D-dimer were also outside the reference values although no changes were observed in their evolution during the ICU stay. The results showed the 25-OH-D, 25-OH-D_3, and 25-OH-D_2 levels to be lower at follow-up versus baseline—with statistical significance being reached for 25-OH-D ($p = 0.011$) and 25-OH-D_2 ($p = 0.006$).

Figure 1 shows the distribution of patient vitamin D status upon ICU admission and after three days of stay. In no case were the 25-OH-D levels > 25 ng/mL. Only 16.7% (6/37) of the patients had 25-OH-D > 20 ng/mL at baseline, versus 3.2% (1/37) at follow-up. Furthermore, 22.2% (8/37) presented 25-OH-D < 10 ng/mL—this percentage reaching 25.8% (10/37) after three days of stay.

Table 1. Demographic and clinical characteristics of the patients.

Baseline Characteristics (N = 37)	Mean ± SD	Min–Max	95% CI
Age (years)	60.0 ± 10.2	41.0–74.0	56.6–63.4
Sex (M/F, %)	26/11 (70.3/29.7)	-	-
BMI (kg/m^2)	30.77 ± 4.17	22.8–42.2	29.4–32.2
BMI < 25 kg/m^2 (n/N, %)	3/37 (8.10)	-	-
BMI 25–30 kg/m^2 (n/N, %)	14/37 (37.8)	-	-
BMI > 30 kg/m^2 (n/N, %)	20/37 (54.1)	-	-
Smoking habit (n/N, %)			
Smokers	3/37 (8.10)	-	-
Ex-smokers	12/37 (32.4)	-	-
Never smokers	22/37 (59.5)	-	-
Patients with comorbidity (n/N, %)	26/37 (70.3)	-	-
Diabetes	13/37 (35.1)	-	-
Hypertension	20/37 (54.1)	-	-
Dyslipidemia	11/37 (29.7)	-	-
Chronic kidney disease	2/37 (5.40)	-	-
COPD	10/37 (27.0)	-	-
Cardiovascular disease	6/37 (16.2)	-	-
APACHE-II score	12.3 ± 3.77	6.00–21.0	11.1–13.6
SOFA score	6.54 ± 2.60	2.00–13.0	5.67–7.41
Bacterial and fungal infection (n/N, %)	26/37 (70.3)	-	-
Sepsis (n/N, %)	7/36 (19.4)	-	-
PaO$_2$/FiO$_2$	212.9 ± 103.8	15.0–550.0	169.2–248.6
ARDS (PaO$_2$/FiO$_2$ < 300) (n/N, %)	26/37 (70.0)	-	-
Mild (300 < PaO$_2$/FiO$_2$ ≤ 200) (n/N, %)	12/37 (32.4)	-	-
Moderate (200 < PaO$_2$/FiO$_2$ ≤ 100) (n/N, %)	10/37 (27.0)	-	-
Severe (PaO$_2$/FiO$_2$ < 100) (n/N, %)	4/37 (10.8)	-	-
IMV (n/N, %)	30/37 (81.1)	-	-
Duration of IMV (days)	21.7 ± 14.6	1.00–73.0	16.0–27.4
ICU length of stay (days)	25.4 ± 22.6	6.00–104.0	17.8–32.9
Length of hospitalization (days)	39.5 ± 27.0	9.00–131.0	30.5–48.5
Patient 28-day mortality (n/N, %)	26/37 (70.3)	-	-

N = 37. Data expressed as mean ± standard deviation. Abbreviations: SD = standard deviation; Min–Max = minimum–maximum; CI = confidence interval; M/F = male/female; BMI = body mass index; COPD = chronic obstructive pulmonary disease; APACHE-II = Acute Physiology and Chronic Health Evaluation II; SOFA = Sequential Organ Failure Assessment; PaO$_2$/FiO$_2$ = partial oxygen arterial pressure/fraction of inspired oxygen; ARDS = acute respiratory distress syndrome; IMV = invasive mechanical ventilation; ICU = intensive care unit.

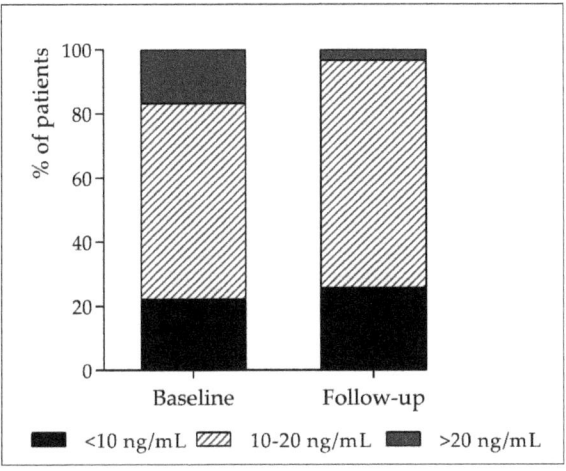

Figure 1. Vitamin D status in the study population at ICU admission (baseline) and after three days (follow-up).

Table 2. Clinical and biochemical parameters of the critical patients with COVID-19 at baseline and follow-up.

	Reference	Baseline Median (IQR) N = 37	Follow-Up Median (IQR) N = 37	Z	p-Value Initial–Final	ES
Clinical						
Heart rate (bpm)	60–100	80.0 (28.7)	64.0 (38.0)	−1.69	0.091	0.411
Respiratory rate (brpm)	15–20	30.0 (3.50)	22.0 (4.50)	−1.63	0.102	0.582
Mean blood pressure (mmHg)	70–105	93.5 (18.0)	91.5 (25.7)	−0.31	0.753	0.095
PEEP (cm H_2O)	2–5	14.0 (3.50)	12.0 (2.00)	−2.76	0.006	0.779
FiO_2	>68%	0.70 (0.25)	0.60 (0.15)	−3.81	0.001	0.825
PaO_2/FiO_2	200–300	200.0 (101.5)	222.0 (119.0)	−0.05	0.964	0.010
Biochemical						
Total Proteins (g/dL)	6.60–8.30	6.40 (0.90)	6.10 (1.13)	−2.51	0.012	0.513
Albumin (g/dL)	3.50–5.20	3.20 (0.65)	3.00 (0.60)	−2.11	0.035	0.444
Prealbumin (mg/dL)	16.0–42.0	9.00 (16.2)	25.0 (23.0)	−2.39	0.017	0.782
Ferritin (ng/mL)	20.0–275.0	1139.3 (1772.9)	1490.1 (1815.7)	−0.52	0.603	0.117
Transferrin (mg/dL)	200.0–360.0	132.0 (31.7)	136.0 (68.0)	−0.82	0.410	0.269
Glucose (mg/dL)	75.0–115.0	154.0 (81.0)	184.5 (113.5)	−1.62	0.106	0.328
Total Cholesterol (mg/dL)	140.0–200.0	138.5 (51.5)	159.0 (103.0)	−2.02	0.044	0.574
GOT or AST (U/L)	5.00–40.0	37.0 (32.5)	31.0 (32.0)	−1.76	0.078	0.351
GPT or ALT (U/L)	0.00–55.0	35.0 (40.0)	36.5 (46.5)	−1.21	0.228	0.248
LDH (U/L)	0.00–248.0	490.5 (183.0)	429.0 (138.0)	−3.05	0.002	0.590
CRP (mg/L)	0.00–5.00	153.7 (210.7)	35.4 (56.4)	−4.66	0.001	0.991
PCT (ng/dL)	0.02–0.50	0.22 (0.44)	0.11 (0.46)	−1.59	0.112	0.360
Hemoglobin (g/dL)	11.0–17.0	13.3 (2.80)	12.6 (3.93)	−4.06	0.001	0.789
Leukocytes ($*10^3/\mu L$)	3.50–10.5	9.67 (6.94)	9.45 (7.44)	−1.25	0.212	0.240
Neutrophils (%)	42.0–77.0	88.5 (8.15)	88.0 (6.82)	−0.34	0.737	0.067
Lymphocytes (%)	20.0–44.0	6.40 (5.68)	5.75 (4.13)	−0.28	0.777	0.056
Platelets ($*10^3/\mu L$)	120.0–450.0	212.0 (135.5)	266.0 (131.5)	−2.52	0.012	0.482
D-dimer (ng/dL)	0.00–500.0	1080.0 (1647.5)	1520.0 (3050.0)	−1.14	0.254	0.231
Fibrinogen (mg/dL)	200.0–350.0	750.5 (356.5)	556.0 (336.7)	−3.52	0.001	0.683
Ca (mg/dL)	8.80–10.6	8.40 (0.48)	8.10 (0.98)	−0.81	0.421	0.190
P (mg/dL)	2.30–4.50	3.55 (1.93)	3.15 (1.43)	−0.02	0.984	0.005
Mg (mg/dL)	1.60–2.60	2.23 (0.37)	2.20 (0.50)	−0.80	0.421	0.253
25–OH–D (ng/mL)	20.0–100.0	13.6 (9.02)	12.2 (6.01)	−2.53	0.011	0.600
25–OH–D_3 (ng/mL)	-	8.45 (6.38)	7.92 (5.85)	−1.35	0.176	0.520
25–OH–D_2 (ng/mL)	-	5.85 (2.95)	4.66 (2.02)	−2.74	0.006	0.278

N = 37. Data expressed as median (interquartile range, IQR). Abbreviations: SD = standard deviation; ES = effect size; bpm = beats per minute; brpm = breaths per minute; PEEP = positive end-expiratory pressure; PaO_2/FiO_2 = partial oxygen arterial pressure/fraction of inspired oxygen; GOT or AST = glutamic oxaloacetic transaminase or aspartate transaminase; GPT or ALT = glutamic pyruvic transaminase or alanine transaminase; LDH = lactate dehydrogenase; CRP = C-reactive protein; PCT = procalcitonin; Ca = calcium, P = phosphorous, Mg = magnesium, $*10^3$ = multiplied by 1000. The sixth column reports statistical significance after the Wilcoxon signed-rank test; evolution is shown after 3 days. ES effect size calculations were also made to determine the effect of ICU stay (ES: small ≤ 0.01, moderate = 0.06, and large ≤ 0.14) [28]. Statistical significance = $p < 0.05$.

Figure 2 corresponds to the comparative analysis of clinical parameters in relation to 25-OH-D, 25-OH-D_3, and 25-OH-D_2 levels upon ICU admission and after three days of stay. Based on the sepsis (Figure 2A) and infectious processes (Figure 2B), there was a trend toward statistical significance in the follow-up observing lower levels of 25-OH-D and 25-OH-D_3 for septic patients and lower levels of 25-OH-D_2 for infected patients. Patients who did not need invasive mechanical ventilation presented higher levels of 25-OH-D_2 at baseline and 25-OH-D and 25-OH-D_2 at follow-up (Figure 2C).

Table 3 shows the Spearman bivariate correlations between the 25-OH-D, 25-OH-D_3, and 25-OH-D_2 levels at baseline and follow-up and the clinical and biochemical parameters analyzed in our study. At baseline, the 25-OH-D levels were correlated to albumin ($p = 0.021$), hemoglobin ($p = 0.028$), D-dimer ($p = 0.003$), and fibrinogen ($p = 0.020$)— with albumin also being correlated to 25-OH-D_2 ($p = 0.037$); and D-dimer ($p = 0.001$) and fibrinogen to 25-OH-D_3 ($p = 0.029$). Respiratory rate was negatively correlated to 25-OH-D_2 ($p = 0.025$). At follow-up, 25-OH-D and 25-OH-D_3 were significantly correlated to PCT ($p = 0.002$; $p = 0.018$) and lymphocytes ($p = 0.044$; $p = 0.040$). In the case of D-dimer and Ca, an inverse correlation to 25-OH-D_3 was observed ($p = 0.029$ and $p = 0.006$, respectively). Finally, the 25-OH-D_2 levels showed a significant correlation to both the fibrinogen ($p = 0.003$) and Ca levels ($p = 0.030$). We did not find correlation between mortality rate after 28 days of ICU stay and 25-OH-D_3, 25-OH-D_2, and 25-OH-D levels.

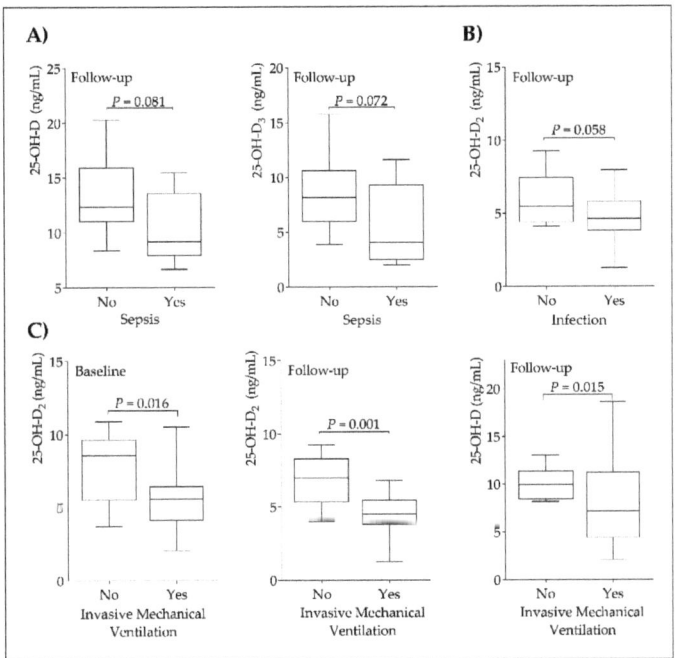

Figure 2. Comparative analysis of septic and non-septic patients with 25-OH-D and 25-OH-D_3 levels at follow-up (**A**); infection with 25-OH-D_2 levels at follow-up (**B**); invasive mechanical ventilation with 25-OH-D_2 levels at baseline and 25-OH-D_2 and 25-OH-D levels at follow-up (**C**). Statistical significance = $p < 0.05$.

Table 3. Matrix for correlation coefficients (rho) showing the simple linear relationship between clinical and biochemical parameters with 25-OH-D, 25-OH-D_2, and 25-OH-D_3 levels.

	Baseline			Follow-Up		
	25-OH-D (ng/mL)	25-OH-D_3 (ng/mL)	25-OH-D_2 (ng/mL)	25-OH-D (ng/mL)	25-OH-D_3 (ng/mL)	25-OH-D_2 (ng/mL)
Age (years)	−0.129	−0.132	−0.035	−0.089	−0.132	0.065
BMI (kg/m^2)	0.111	0.165	−0.026	0.091	0.261	−0.231
APACHE-II	−0.103	−0.066	−0.040	-	-	-
SOFA	−0.154	−0.053	−0.167	−0.133	0.008	−0.290
Respiratory rate (brpm)	−0.176	0.053	−0.456 [a]	−0.277	0.047	−0.374
Albumin (g/dL)	0.403 [a]	0.285	0.390 [a]	0.015	−0.097	0.234
PCT (ng/dL)	−0.270	−0.294	−0.026	−0.587 [b]	−0.458 [a]	−0.331
Hemoglobin (g/dL)	0.387 [a]	0.307	0.261	0.301	0.223	0.224
Lymphocytes (%)	−0.046	−0.059	0.084	0.364 [a]	0.371 [a]	0.034
D-dimer (ng/dL)	−0.521 [b]	−0.644 [b]	0.148	−0.264	−0.405 [a]	0.302
Fibrinogen (mg/dL)	0.350 [a]	0.370 [a]	0.128	0.116	0.335	−0.521 [b]
Ca (mg/dL)	0.285	0.180	0.306	−0.333	−0.527 [b]	0.426 [a]

Matrix correlations are presented as correlation coefficients (rho). Abbreviations: BMI = body mass index; APACHE-II = Acute Physiology and Chronic Health Evaluation II; SOFA = Sequential Organ Failure Assessment; FiO_2 = fraction of inspired oxygen; PCT = procalcitonin; Ca = calcium. Statistical significance [a] = $p < 0.05$; [b] = $p < 0.01$.

4. Discussion

The main finding of the present study was the low 25-OH-D levels in the patients upon admission (baseline), followed by a significant decrease after three days of ICU stay. The entire population was below the sufficiency reference values for 25-OH-D, and most of them presented insufficient 25-OH-D status. We also analyzed the 25-OH-D$_3$ and 25-OH-D$_2$ levels, both of which were seen to decrease after three days (though statistical significance was only reached in the case of 25-OH-D$_2$), thus influencing upon 25-OH-D decreased levels and presenting a worsening during their stay at 3 days. Moreover, vitamin D was associated with clinical parameters such as the need for mechanical ventilation or respiratory frequency and with biochemical parameters also associated with the severity of the critically ill patient such as albumin, hemoglobin, D-dimer, fibrinogen, PCT, and lymphocytes.

Previous evidence points to poorer COVID-19 outcomes associated with factors such as the male gender, older age, BMI > 35 kg/m^2, and the presence of certain comorbidities [31]. The demographic and clinical characteristics of our patients (Table 1) are consistent with this evidence. In effect, the population was fundamentally elderly, two-thirds were males, and there was a high prevalence of comorbidities and obesity. It should be noted that metabolically ill patients with obesity may have a high risk of suffering inflammatory processes [32], which could contribute to a greater probability of poorer outcomes.

Many of the clinical and biochemical parameters in our patients were altered (Table 2). In the case of PEEP and FiO$_2$, levels were above reference values and, they even decreased significantly in three days and remained altered in the most cases. It should be noted that ferritin, CRP, D-dimer, and fibrinogen were well above the reference values. Parameters related to inflammation (such as CRP) or coagulation (such as D-dimer) have been correlated to a poor prognosis and have been described as possible predictive biomarkers of COVID-19 [33].

Our results with reference to vitamin D status showed all patients to have insufficient levels (<30 ng/mL) both upon admission and during the study period—with the vitamin D status being seen to worsen in only three days. The great majority of patients presented vitamin D deficiency (<20 ng/mL), while extreme deficient values of <10 ng/mL were recorded in a quarter of the study sample. It is known that, compared to the general population, the prevalence of hypovitaminosis D is greater in the critically ill and may constitute a risk factor for adverse outcomes [34]. Moreover, these levels could be influenced by seasonality. In an observational study carried out in critical ill patients from Austria, significant differences were noted in the prevalence of vitamin D deficiency and in the mean 25-OH-D values between the winter and summer months [35]. Our study covered the period from March to June; we, therefore, could not demonstrate the influence of seasonality in our patients.

On the other hand, there is concern about the high prevalence of hypovitaminosis D in the general population—being regarded as a global health issue with important consequences [36]. Moreover, SARS-CoV-2 positivity has been strongly and inversely correlated to circulating 25-OH-D levels—a relationship that persists across latitudes, races/ethnicities, both genders, and age ranges [37], thereby evidencing that the COVID-19 fatality rates parallel the vitamin D deficiency rates [38]. These negative correlations between vitamin D deficiency and the number of COVID-19 cases and mortality have also been reported in another 20 European countries [39]. It could be expected that countries such as Spain have a better vitamin D status and therefore less severe consequences than other countries in northern Europe. However, our results reinforced the evidence of a possible widespread vitamin D deficiency in the Spanish population. Indeed, vitamin D deficiency in Italy and Spain (the countries presenting the highest age-specific case fatality ratio) [40] is more severe than elsewhere in Europe [41], particularly in the aging population [39].

On the other hand, Maghbooli et al. found 25-OH-D levels >30 ng/mL to reduce the risk of adverse clinical outcomes in patients with COVID-19 [42]. None of our critical patients with COVID-19 presented 25-OH-D levels >25 ng/mL, which is consistent with the findings of Maghbooli. Low 25-OH-D levels have been reported by many authors in hospitalized patients with COVID-19 [43], with such deficiency being associated with a greater mortality risk [26]. In fact, Vassiliou et al. found that low 25-OH-D levels in patients with COVID-19 at ICU admission could predispose to an increased 28-day mortality risk [44]. In the present study, although we did not observe an association between 25-OH-D levels with 28-day mortality risk, we found an association with clinical outcomes, reporting that higher 25-OH-D and 25-OH-D_2 levels were associated with those patients who did not require invasive mechanical ventilation. Moreover, lower 25-OH-D values, as a result of decreased 25-OH-D_3 and 25-OH-D_2 levels were observed with the presence of infection (bacterial/fungal) and sepsis (Figure 2). It should be noted that 25-OH-D_2 levels were in agreement with previous studies in the Spanish population [45], being also similar to those found in other studies performed in Belgian and Chinese populations [46,47]. Likewise, observational studies have also shown that higher 25-OH-D levels would be associated with better clinical outcomes in respiratory diseases [48]. Nevertheless, reference values are needed to have more contrastable evidence on 25-OH-D_2 levels.

In relation to infection, a high percentage of our patients (70.3%) showed bacteriological or fungal infection, which would support the idea that the daily risk rate of infection in COVID-critically-ill patients is increased during ICU stay [49]. Recent studies [50], consistent with the high prevalence of hypovitaminosis D observed in our study, suggest a possible role of low vitamin D in the increased risk of SARS-CoV-2 infection and subsequent hospitalization. Likewise, 25-OH-D levels were inversely associated with coagulation and sepsis, in addition to major comorbidities. Both, 25-OH-D_3 and 25-OH-D_2 forms tended to respond differently in patients with bacteriological or fungal infection and in patients presenting sepsis. On the other hand, it was observed that 25-OH-D_2 levels decreased a mean of 41.6% ± 89.6% versus 7.0% ± 23.4% for the 25-OH-D_3 form during the ICU stay, which would suggest that the lack of vitamin D support during ICU stay could have allowed this more pronounced decrease in case of the 25-OH-D_2 form, since it would depend on the intake through diet (before the admission) or its supplementation (during ICU stay). A greater decrease in 25-OH-D_2 relative to 25-OH-D_3 could be also related to the lower affinity of 25-OH-D_2 for vitamin D–binding protein, leading to a shorter half-life and a higher rate of clearance from the circulation [51], and in some cases, it even caused a decline, thereby, precipitating in vitamin D deficiency [52]. This, together with the fact that there is literature that already reports a possible different role of 25-OH-D_3 and 25-OH-D_2 forms [51,53], although not in critical patients, could evidence the different correlations obtained with bacterial/fungal infection or sepsis and invasive mechanical ventilation previously described. Therefore, it would suggest that a lower vitamin D status at admission and worsening during three days of ICU stay may be a modifiable risk factor and an early predictive marker of adverse outcomes in hospitalized patients with COVID-19.

On associating the concentrations of both 25-OH-D and 25-OH-D_3 with other biochemical severity parameters, significantly lower vitamin D levels were correlated to higher D-dimer and PCT levels and a lower percentage of lymphocytes (Table 3). A recent meta-analysis has demonstrated that patients with severe COVID-19 tend to present increased leukocyte and neutrophil counts, neutrophil–lymphocyte ratio, PCT and CRP levels, and a decreased number of total lymphocytes, among parameters, compared to nonsevere individuals [54]. Furthermore, blood hypercoagulability is common among hospitalized patients with COVID-19. Elevated D-dimer levels are consistently reported in this scenario, and a gradual increase of this parameter in the course of the disease is particularly associated with patient worsening. Similarly, lower fibrinogen levels were found in non-survivor patients with COVID-19 [55]. In this line, the relationship between fibrinogen and 25-OH-D levels is often reported in the literature in noncritical patients [56,57]. In our study, 25-OH-D and 25-OH-D_3 levels were inversely correlated with D-dimer levels at baseline. Furthermore, 25-OH-D_3 levels have been correlated with fibrinogen levels at baseline. Our results may reflect a better vitamin D status (mainly due to vitamin D_3) in patients with a more appropriate hematological profile. We observed a positive correlation at baseline between albumin (which was below the reference values) and the levels of both 25-OH-D and 25-OH-D_2. Recently, low albumin levels have been regarded as more of a disease severity marker than as a marker of malnutrition, when such low levels are detected upon admission to hospital [58].

The present study has limitations and strengths. As limitations, the present study enrolled fewer patients than desired due to the difficulty in obtaining the sample and the patient's own clinical situation and severity both at admission and during the ICU stay. Therefore, the data should be treated with caution in order to generalize the findings of the study. Thus, on a comparative level, the effect size was shown for a better understanding. We had no reliable data on exposure to sunlight, dietary factors, or vitamin D supplementation—all of which affect vitamin D status. The overall negative results may be related to the heterogeneity of the subjects and their underlying disease conditions or severity, which may all influence the plasma 25-OH-D levels. Our findings cannot be generalized to other populations or ethnic groups, especially considering the wide range of COVID-19 prevalence. Replicating this study in a larger, prospective, and heterogeneous population and taking into account a control group, would allow for other stratified analyses based on demographic and biochemical characteristics, taking seasonality into account, and could further corroborate our findings. Additional research is therefore needed to validate our findings. As strengths, the present study used LC-MS/MS, which is the gold standard for assessing the levels of 25-OH-D [59], affording greater sensitivity, flexibility, and specificity than the enzymoimmunoassay techniques commonly used in clinical practice, which tend to overestimate the 25-OH-D values in cases of deficiency [60,61].

Recent studies have reported encouraging results after vitamin D intervention [62,63]. However, further evidence is needed to confirm that improving vitamin D status is of benefit in reducing disease severity and mortality and the probability of developing a critical clinical condition. It is essential to ensure close patient monitoring before establishing intervention guidelines [64]. This study is one of the few that have been conducted in this context, assessing the short-term evolution of the 25-OH-D levels (through 25-OH-D_2 and 25-OH-D_3 levels) and its impact in critical patients with COVID-19.

5. Conclusions

Our data reflect a high prevalence of hypovitaminosis D in all the critical patients at ICU admission, which increased after only three days of ICU stay. On the other hand, the associations observed between 25-OH-D levels, through 25-OH-D_3 and 25-OH-D_2 values and key clinical outcomes and biochemical altered parameters, suggests that it might be helpful to assess vitamin D status in patients with SARS-CoV-2 infection. Given the different response of the 25-OH-D_3 and 25-OH-D_2 forms, it would be useful to analyze them to elucidate the role of each form on the evolution of the critically ill patient. Further investigations are needed to define underlying mechanisms in vitamin D deficiency and useful strategies based on vitamin D interventions aimed at preserving vitamin D status and enhancing the clinical and biochemical profile of critical patients with COVID-19.

Author Contributions: Conceptualization, E.P., J.C.-P. and L.H.-Q.; methodology, J.M.-L. and J.M.P.-V.; software, R.C.-Z., J.M.-L. and E.P.; validation, Y.G.-M. and J.F.M.-C.; formal analysis, L.H.-Q. and H.V.-L.; investigation, H.V.-L. and L.H.-Q.; resources, E.P. and H.V.-L.; data curation, J.M.-L. and E.P.; writing—original draft preparation, L.H.-Q., Y.G.-M. and E.P.; writing—review and editing, H.V.-L. and J.M.-L.; visualization, L.H.-Q., Y.G.-M. and H.V.-L.; supervision, J.M.-L. and E.P.; project administration, E.P. and J.M.-L.; funding acquisition, E.P. All authors have read and agreed to the published version of the manuscript.

Funding: This research received external funding by FIS Projects from Carlos III Health Institute [REF. PI10/1993]. L.H.-Q. and H.V.-L. are under a FPU fellowship from the Spanish Ministry of Education.

Institutional Review Board Statement: The study was approved by the Ethical Committee of the hospital, and informed consent was obtained from the patients or their family, who agreed to participate in the study.

Informed Consent Statement: Informed consent was obtained from all subjects involved in the study.

Data Availability Statement: The datasets generated and analyzed during the current study are not publicly available because the database is very extensive and includes data from other studies complementary to this but are available from the corresponding author on reasonable request.

Acknowledgments: Thanks are due to all the patients who participated in our study and the personnel from the Hospital Virgen de las Nieves, and FIBAO foundation (Fundación Pública Andaluza para la Investigación Biosanitaria de Andalucía Oriental Alejandro Otero) from Granada. We also acknowledge the expertise of the translator who provided English editing.

Conflicts of Interest: The authors declare no conflict of interest. The funders had no role in the design of the study; in the collection, analyses, or interpretation of data; in the writing of the manuscript; or in the decision to publish the results.

References

1. Ali, N. Role of Vitamin D in Preventing of COVID-19 Infection, Progression and Severity. *J. Infect. Public Health* **2020**, *13*, 1373–1380. [CrossRef] [PubMed]
2. De las Heras, N.; Martín Giménez, V.M.; Ferder, L.; Manucha, W.; Lahera, V. Implications of Oxidative Stress and Potential Role of Mitochondrial Dysfunction in COVID-19: Therapeutic Effects of Vitamin D. *Antioxidants* **2020**, *9*, 897. [CrossRef] [PubMed]
3. Han, H.; Ma, Q.; Li, C.; Liu, R.; Zhao, L.; Wang, W.; Zhang, P.; Liu, X.; Gao, G.; Liu, F.; et al. Profiling Serum Cytokines in COVID-19 Patients Reveals IL-6 and IL-10 Are Disease Severity Predictors. *Emerg. Microbes Infect.* **2020**, *9*, 1123–1130. [CrossRef] [PubMed]
4. Aygun, H. Vitamin D Can Prevent COVID-19 Infection-Induced Multiple Organ Damage. *Naunyn. Schmiedebergs Arch. Pharmacol.* **2020**, *393*, 1157–1160. [CrossRef] [PubMed]
5. Abilés, J.; Aguayo, E.; Moreno-Torres, R.; Llopis, J.; Aranda, P.; Argüelles, S.; Ayala, A. Oxidative Stress Is Increased in Critically Ill Patients According to Antioxidant Vitamins Intake, Independent of Severity: A Cohort Study. *Crit. Care* **2006**, *10*, R146. [CrossRef] [PubMed]
6. Gamarra, Y.; Santiago, F.C.; Molina-López, J.; Castaño, J.; Herrera-Quintana, L.; Domínguez, Á.; Planells, E. Pyroglutamic Acidosis by Glutathione Regeneration Blockage in Critical Patients with Septic Shock. *Crit. Care* **2019**, *23*, 162. [CrossRef] [PubMed]
7. Zhao, X.; Li, Y.; Ge, Y.; Shi, Y.; Lv, P.; Zhang, J.; Fu, G.; Zhou, Y.; Jiang, K.; Lin, N.; et al. Evaluation of Nutrition Risk and Its Association with Mortality Risk in Severely and Critically Ill COVID-19 Patients. *J. Parenter. Enter. Nutr.* **2020**, *45*, 32–42. [CrossRef] [PubMed]
8. Laviano, A.; Koverech, A.; Zanetti, M. Nutrition Support in the Time of SARS-CoV-2 (COVID-19). *Nutrition* **2020**, *74*, 110834. [CrossRef] [PubMed]
9. Barazzoni, R.; Bischoff, S.C.; Breda, J.; Wickramasinghe, K.; Krznaric, Z.; Nitzan, D.; Pirlich, M.; Singer, P. ESPEN Expert Statements and Practical Guidance for Nutritional Management of Individuals with SARS-CoV-2 Infection. *Clin. Nutr.* **2020**, *39*, 1631–1638. [CrossRef] [PubMed]
10. Zabetakis, I.; Lordan, R.; Norton, C.; Tsoupras, A. COVID-19: The Inflammation Link and the Role of Nutrition in Potential Mitigation. *Nutrients* **2020**, *12*, 1466. [CrossRef]
11. Caccialanza, R.; Laviano, A.; Lobascio, F.; Montagna, E.; Bruno, R.; Ludovisi, S.; Corsico, A.G.; Di Sabatino, A.; Belliato, M.; Calvi, M.; et al. Early Nutritional Supplementation in Non-Critically Ill Patients Hospitalized for the 2019 Novel Coronavirus Disease (COVID-19): Rationale and Feasibility of a Shared Pragmatic Protocol. *Nutrition* **2020**, *74*, 110835. [CrossRef] [PubMed]
12. Patel, J.J.; Martindale, R.G.; McClave, S.A. Relevant Nutrition Therapy in COVID-19 and the Constraints on Its Delivery by a Unique Disease Process. *Nutr. Clin. Pract.* **2020**, *35*, 792–799. [CrossRef] [PubMed]
13. Alexander, J.; Tinkov, A.; Strand, T.A.; Alehagen, U.; Skalny, A.; Aaseth, J. Early Nutritional Interventions with Zinc, Selenium and Vitamin D for Raising Anti-Viral Resistance Against Progressive COVID-19. *Nutrients* **2020**, *12*, 2358. [CrossRef] [PubMed]
14. Van den Ouweland, J.M.W. Analysis of Vitamin D Metabolites by Liquid Chromatography-Tandem Mass Spectrometry. *TrAC Trends Anal. Chem.* **2016**, *84*, 117–130. [CrossRef]
15. Higashi, T.; Shimada, K.; Toyo'oka, T. Advances in Determination of Vitamin D Related Compounds in Biological Samples Using Liquid Chromatography–Mass Spectrometry: A Review. *J. Chromatogr. B* **2010**, *878*, 1654–1661. [CrossRef]
16. Gottschlich, M.M.; Mayes, T.; Khoury, J.; Kagan, R.J. Clinical Trial of Vitamin D_2 vs. D_3 Supplementation in Critically Ill Pediatric Burn Patients. *J. Parenter. Enter. Nutr.* **2017**, *41*, 412–421. [CrossRef] [PubMed]
17. Grant, W.B.; Lahore, H.; McDonnell, S.L.; Baggerly, C.A.; French, C.B.; Aliano, J.L.; Bhattoa, H.P. Evidence That Vitamin D Supplementation Could Reduce Risk of Influenza and COVID-19 Infections and Deaths. *Nutrients* **2020**, *12*, 988. [CrossRef] [PubMed]

18. Martín Giménez, V.M.; Inserra, F.; Tajer, C.D.; Mariani, J.; Ferder, L.; Reiter, R.J.; Manucha, W. Lungs as Target of COVID-19 Infection: Protective Common Molecular Mechanisms of Vitamin D and Melatonin as a New Potential Synergistic Treatment. *Life Sci.* **2020**, *254*, 117808. [CrossRef] [PubMed]
19. Mansur, J.L.; Tajer, C.; Mariani, J.; Inserra, F.; Ferder, L.; Manucha, W. Vitamin D high doses supplementation could represent a promising alternative to prevent or treat COVID-19 infection. *Clín. Investig. Arterioscler.* **2020**, *32*, 267–277. [CrossRef] [PubMed]
20. Weir, E.K.; Thenappan, T.; Bhargava, M.; Chen, Y. Does Vitamin D Deficiency Increase the Severity of COVID-19? *Clin. Med.* **2020**, *20*, e107–e108. [CrossRef] [PubMed]
21. Waldron, J.L.; Ashby, H.L.; Cornes, M.P.; Bechervaise, J.; Razavi, C.; Thomas, O.L.; Chugh, S.; Deshpande, S.; Ford, C.; Gama, R. Vitamin D: A Negative Acute Phase Reactant. *J. Clin. Pathol.* **2013**, *66*, 620–622. [CrossRef] [PubMed]
22. Heijboer, A.C.; Blankenstein, M.A.; Kema, I.P.; Buijs, M.M. Accuracy of 6 Routine 25-Hydroxyvitamin D Assays: Influence of Vitamin D Binding Protein Concentration. *Clin. Chem.* **2012**, *58*, 543–548. [CrossRef] [PubMed]
23. Teymoori-Rad, M.; Marashi, S.M. Vitamin D and Covid-19: From Potential Therapeutic Effects to Unanswered Questions. *Rev. Med. Virol.* **2020**, *31*, e2159. [CrossRef] [PubMed]
24. Bilezikian, J.P.; Bikle, D.; Hewison, M.; Lazaretti-Castro, M.; Formenti, A.M.; Gupta, A.; Madhavan, M.V.; Nair, N.; Babalyan, V.; Hutchings, N.; et al. Mechanisms in endocrinology: Vitamin D and COVID-19. *Eur. J. Endocrinol.* **2020**, *183*, R133–R147. [CrossRef] [PubMed]
25. Xu, Y.; Baylink, D.J.; Chen, C.-S.; Reeves, M.E.; Xiao, J.; Lacy, C.; Lau, E.; Cao, H. The Importance of Vitamin d Metabolism as a Potential Prophylactic, Immunoregulatory and Neuroprotective Treatment for COVID-19. *J. Transl. Med.* **2020**, *18*, 322. [CrossRef] [PubMed]
26. Carpagnano, G.E.; Di Lecce, V.; Quaranta, V.N.; Zito, A.; Buonamico, E.; Capozza, E.; Palumbo, A.; Di Gioia, G.; Valerio, V.N.; Resta, O. Vitamin D Deficiency as a Predictor of Poor Prognosis in Patients with Acute Respiratory Failure Due to COVID-19. *J. Endocrinol. Investig.* **2020**, *44*, 765–771. [CrossRef] [PubMed]
27. Meltzer, D.O.; Best, T.J.; Zhang, H.; Vokes, T.; Arora, V.; Solway, J. Association of Vitamin D Status and Other Clinical Characteristics With COVID-19 Test Results. *JAMA Netw. Open* **2020**, *3*, e2019722. [CrossRef] [PubMed]
28. Holick, M.F.; Binkley, N.C.; Bischoff-Ferrari, H.A.; Gordon, C.M.; Hanley, D.A.; Heaney, R.P.; Murad, M.H.; Weaver, C.M. Evaluation, Treatment, and Prevention of Vitamin D Deficiency: An Endocrine Society Clinical Practice Guideline. *J. Clin. Endocrinol. Metab.* **2011**, *96*, 1911–1930. [CrossRef] [PubMed]
29. Zhao, J.Y.; Yan, J.Y.; Qu, J.M. Interpretations of "Diagnosis and Treatment Protocol for Novel Coronavirus Pneumonia (Trial Version 7)". *Chin. Med. J.* **2020**, *133*, 1347–1349. [CrossRef]
30. Cohen, J. A Power Primer. *Psychol. Bull.* **1992**, *112*, 155–159. [CrossRef] [PubMed]
31. Rapp, J.; Lieberman-Cribbin, W.; Tuminello, S.; Taioli, E. Male Sex, Severe Obesity, Older Age, and Chronic Kidney Disease Are Associated With COVID-19 Severity and Mortality in New York City. *Chest* **2020**, *159*, 112–115. [CrossRef] [PubMed]
32. Chiappetta, S.; Sharma, A.M.; Bottino, V.; Stier, C. COVID-19 and the Role of Chronic Inflammation in Patients with Obesity. *Int. J. Obes.* **2020**, *44*, 1790–1792. [CrossRef] [PubMed]
33. Ponti, G.; Maccaferri, M.; Ruini, C.; Tomasi, A.; Ozben, T. Biomarkers associated with COVID-19 disease progression. *Crit. Rev. Clin. Lab. Sci.* **2020**, *57*, 389–399. [CrossRef] [PubMed]
34. Christopher, K.B. Vitamin D and Critical Illness Outcomes. *Curr. Opin. Crit. Care* **2016**, *22*, 332–338. [CrossRef] [PubMed]
35. Amrein, K.; Zajic, P.; Schnedl, C.; Waltensdorfer, A.; Fruhwald, S.; Holl, A.; Purkart, T.; Wünsch, G.; Valentin, T.; Grisold, A.; et al. Vitamin D Status and Its Association with Season, Hospital and Sepsis Mortality in Critical Illness. *Crit. Care* **2014**, *18*, R47. [CrossRef] [PubMed]
36. Holick, M.F. The Vitamin D Deficiency Pandemic: Approaches for Diagnosis, Treatment and Prevention. *Rev. Endocr. Metab. Disord.* **2017**, *18*, 153–165. [CrossRef]
37. Kaufman, H.W.; Niles, J.K.; Kroll, M.H.; Bi, C.; Holick, M.F. SARS-CoV-2 Positivity Rates Associated with Circulating 25-Hydroxyvitamin D Levels. *PLoS ONE* **2020**, *15*, e0239252. [CrossRef] [PubMed]
38. Benskin, L.L. A Basic Review of the Preliminary Evidence That COVID-19 Risk and Severity Is Increased in Vitamin D Deficiency. *Front. Public Health* **2020**, *8*, 513. [CrossRef] [PubMed]
39. Ilie, P.C.; Stefanescu, S.; Smith, L. The Role of Vitamin D in the Prevention of Coronavirus Disease 2019 Infection and Mortality. *Aging Clin. Exp. Res.* **2020**, *32*, 1195–1198. [CrossRef] [PubMed]
40. Daneshkhah, A.; Agrawal, V.; Eshein, A.; Subramanian, H.; Roy, H.K.; Backman, V. Evidence for possible association of vitamin D status with cytokine storm and unregulated inflammation in COVID-19 patients. *Aging Clin. Exp. Res.* **2020**, *32*, 2141–2158. [CrossRef] [PubMed]
41. Lips, P.; Cashman, K.D.; Lamberg-Allardt, C.; Bischoff-Ferrari, H.A.; Obermayer-Pietsch, B.; Bianchi, M.L.; Stepan, J.; Fuleihan, G.E.; Bouillon, R. Current vitamin D status in European and Middle East coun-tries and strategies to prevent vitamin D deficiency: A position statement of the European Calcified Tissue Society. *Eur. J. Endocrinol.* **2019**, *180*, P23–P54. [CrossRef] [PubMed]
42. Maghbooli, Z.; Sahraian, M.A.; Ebrahimi, M.; Pazoki, M.; Kafan, S.; Tabriz, H.M.; Hadadi, A.; Montazeri, M.; Nasiri, M.; Shirvani, A.; et al. Vitamin D Sufficiency, a Serum 25-Hydroxyvitamin D at Least 30 Ng/ML Reduced Risk for Adverse Clinical Outcomes in Patients with COVID-19 Infection. *PLoS ONE* **2020**, *15*, e0239799. [CrossRef] [PubMed]

53. Cereda, E.; Bogliolo, L.; Klersy, C.; Lobascio, F.; Masi, S.; Crotti, S.; De Stefano, L.; Bruno, R.; Corsico, A.G.; Di Sabatino, A.; et al. Vitamin D 25OH Deficiency in COVID-19 Patients Admitted to a Tertiary Referral Hospital. *Clin. Nutr.* **2020**, *40*, 2469–2472. [CrossRef] [PubMed]
54. Vassiliou, A.G.; Jahaj, E.; Pratikaki, M.; Orfanos, S.E.; Dimopoulou, I.; Kotanidou, A. Low 25-Hydroxyvitamin D Levels on Admission to the Intensive Care Unit May Predispose COVID-19 Pneumonia Patients to a Higher 28-Day Mortality Risk: A Pilot Study on a Greek ICU Cohort. *Nutrients* **2020**, *12*, 3773. [CrossRef]
55. Vázquez-Lorente, H.; Herrera-Quintana, L.; Molina-López, J.; Gamarra-Morales, Y.; López-González, B.; Miralles-Adell, C.; Planells, E. Response of Vitamin D after Magnesium Intervention in a Postmenopausal Population from the Province of Granada, Spain. *Nutrients* **2020**, *12*, 2283. [CrossRef] [PubMed]
56. Swanson, C.M.; Nielson, C.M.; Shrestha, S.; Lee, C.G.; Barrett-Connor, E.; Jans, I.; Cauley, J.A.; Boonen, S.; Bouillon, R.; Vanderschueren, D.; et al. Higher 25(OH)D2 Is Associated with Lower 25(OH)D3 and 1,25(OH)2D3. *J. Clin. Endocrinol. Metab.* **2014**, *99*, 2736–2744. [CrossRef] [PubMed]
57. Wang, L.; Liu, X.; Hou, J.; Wei, D.; Liu, P.; Fan, K.; Zhang, L.; Nie, L.; Li, X.; Huo, W.; et al. Serum Vitamin D Affected Type 2 Diabetes Though Altering Lipid Profile and Modified the Effects of Testosterone on Diabetes Status. *Nutrients* **2020**, *13*, 90. [CrossRef]
58. Cannell, J.J.; Vieth, R.; Umhau, J.C.; Holick, M.F.; Grant, W.B.; Madronich, S.; Garland, C.F.; Giovannucci, E. Epidemic Influenza and Vitamin D. *Epidemiol. Infect.* **2006**, *134*, 1129–1140. [CrossRef] [PubMed]
59. Buetti, N.; Ruckly, S.; de Montmollin, E.; Reignier, J.; Terzi, N.; Cohen, Y.; Shiami, S.; Dupuis, C.; Timsit, J.-F. COVID-19 Increased the Risk of ICU-Acquired Bloodstream Infections: A Case–Cohort Study from the Multicentric OUTCOMEREA Network. *Intensive Care Med.* **2021**, *47*, 180–187. [CrossRef]
60. Infante, M.; Buoso, A.; Pieri, M.; Lupisella, S.; Nuccetelli, M.; Bernardini, S.; Fabbri, A.; Iannetta, M.; Andreoni, M.; Colizzi, V.; et al. Low Vitamin D Status at Admission as a Risk Factor for Poor Survival in Hospitalized Patients with COVID-19: An Italian Retrospective Study. *J. Am. Coll. Nutr.* **2021**, 1–16. [CrossRef] [PubMed]
61. Houghton, L.A.; Vieth, R. The Case against Ergocalciferol (Vitamin D2) as a Vitamin Supplement. *Am. J. Clin. Nutr.* **2006**, *84*, 694–697. [CrossRef] [PubMed]
62. Holick, M.F. The D-Sparging of Vitamin D2: How Physiologically and Pharmacologically Relevant Is It for the Clinician? *J. Clin. Endocrinol. Metab.* **2020**, *105*, e1913–e1915. [CrossRef] [PubMed]
63. Bigman, G. Vitamin D Metabolites, D3 and D2, and Their Independent Associations with Depression Symptoms among Adults in the United States. *Nutr. Neurosci.* **2020**, 1–9. [CrossRef]
64. Feng, X.; Li, S.; Sun, Q.; Zhu, J.; Chen, B.; Xiong, M.; Cao, G. Immune-Inflammatory Parameters in COVID-19 Cases: A Systematic Review and Meta-Analysis. *Front. Med.* **2020**, *7*, 301. [CrossRef] [PubMed]
65. Terpos, E.; Ntanasis-Stathopoulos, I.; Elalamy, I.; Kastritis, E.; Sergentanis, T.N.; Politou, M.; Psaltopoulou, T.; Gerotziafas, G.; Dimopoulos, M.A. Hematological Findings and Complications of COVID-19. *Am. J. Hematol.* **2020**, *95*, 834–847. [CrossRef] [PubMed]
66. Parikh, S.; Guo, D.; Pollock, N.K.; Petty, K.; Bhagatwala, J.; Gutin, B.; Houk, C.; Zhu, H.; Dong, Y. Circulating 25-Hydroxyvitamin D Concentrations Are Correlated with Cardiometabolic Risk Among American Black and White Adolescents Living in a Year-Round Sunny Climate. *Diabetes Care* **2012**, *35*, 1133–1138. [CrossRef] [PubMed]
67. Saghir Afifeh, A.M.; Verdoia, M.; Nardin, M.; Negro, F.; Viglione, F.; Rolla, R.; De Luca, G. Determinants of Vitamin D Activation in Patients with Acute Coronary Syndromes and Its Correlation with Inflammatory Markers. *Nutr. Metab. Cardiovasc. Dis.* **2020**, *31*, 36–43. [CrossRef] [PubMed]
68. Berger, M.M.; Reintam-Blaser, A.; Calder, P.C.; Casaer, M.; Hiesmayr, M.J.; Mayer, K.; Montejo, J.C.; Pichard, C.; Preiser, J.-C.; van Zanten, A.R.H.; et al. Monitoring Nutrition in the ICU. *Clin. Nutr.* **2019**, *38*, 584–593. [CrossRef] [PubMed]
69. Vázquez-Lorente, H.; Herrera-Quintana, L.; Quintero-Osso, B.; Molina-López, J.; Planells, E. Current Trends in the Analytical Determination of Vitamin D. *Nutr. Hosp.* **2019**, *36*, 1418–1423. [PubMed]
70. Tahsin-Swafiri, S.; Blanco-Navarro, I.; Pérez-Sacristán, B.; Millán, I.; Granado-Lorencio, F. The Prevalence of Vitamin Deficiency in Clinical Practice Is Assay-Dependent. *Clin. Nutr.* **2012**, *31*, 1011–1014. [CrossRef]
71. Rousseau, A.-F.; Damas, P.; Janssens, M.; Kalin, S.; Ledoux, D.; Le Goff, C.; Gadisseur, R.; Delanaye, P.; Cavalier, E. Critical Care and Vitamin D Status Assessment: What about Immunoassays and Calculated Free 25OH-D? *Clin. Chim. Acta* **2014**, *437*, 43–47. [CrossRef] [PubMed]
72. Annweiler, C.; Hanotte, B.; Grandin de l'Eprevier, C.; Sabatier, J.-M.; Lafaie, L.; Célarier, T. Vitamin D and Survival in COVID-19 Patients: A Quasi-Experimental Study. *J. Steroid Biochem. Mol. Biol.* **2020**, *204*, 105771. [CrossRef] [PubMed]
73. Entrenas Castillo, M.; Entrenas Costa, L.M.; Vaquero Barrios, J.M.; Alcalá Díaz, J.F.; Miranda, J.L.; Bouillon, R.; Quesada Gómez, J.M. Effect of calcifediol treatment and best available therapy versus best available therapy on intensive care unit admission and mortality among patients hospitalized for COVID-19: A pilot randomized clinical study. *J. Steroid Biochem. Mol. Biol.* **2020**, *203*, 105751. [CrossRef] [PubMed]
74. Ebadi, M.; Montano-Loza, A.J. Perspective: Improving Vitamin D Status in the Management of COVID-19. *Eur. J. Clin. Nutr.* **2020**, *74*, 856–859. [CrossRef] [PubMed]

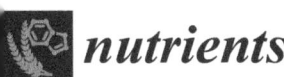

Article

Long-Term Evolution of Malnutrition and Loss of Muscle Strength after COVID-19: A Major and Neglected Component of Long COVID-19

Marine Gérard [1], Meliha Mahmutovic [1], Aurélie Malgras [1], Niasha Michot [1], Nicolas Scheyer [1], Roland Jaussaud [2], Phi-Linh Nguyen-Thi [3] and Didier Quilliot [1,*]

[1] Transversal Nutrition Unit, University of Lorraine, Nancy University Hospital, 54500 Vandoeuvre-les-Nancy, France; gerard_marine@hotmail.fr (M.G.); m.mahmutovic@chru-nancy.fr (M.M.); a.malgras@chru-nancy.fr (A.M.); n.michot@chru-nancy.fr (N.M.); n.scheyer@chru-nancy.fr (N.S.)

[2] Internal Medicine and Clinical Immunology Department, University of Lorraine, Nancy University Hospital, 54500 Vandoeuvre-les-Nancy, France; R.Jaussaud@chru-nancy.fr

[3] Medical Evaluation Department, Department of Clinical Research Support PARC, University of Lorraine, Nancy University Hospital, 54500 Vandoeuvre-les-Nancy, France; pl.nguyen-thi@chru-nancy.fr

* Correspondence: d.quilliot@chru-nancy.fr

Abstract: Post-acute consequences of COVID-19, also termed long COVID, include signs and symptoms persisting for more than 12 weeks with prolonged multisystem involvement; most often, however, malnutrition is ignored. Method: The objective was to analyze persistent symptoms, nutritional status, the evolution of muscle strength and performance status (PS) at 6 months post-discharge in a cohort of COVID-19 survivors. Results: Of 549 consecutive patients hospitalized for COVID-19 between 1 March and 29 April 2020, 23.7% died and 288 patients were at home at D30 post-discharge. At this date, 136 of them (47.2%) presented persistent malnutrition, a significant decrease in muscle strength or a PS $\geq$ 2. These patients received dietary counseling, nutritional supplementation, adapted physical activity guidance or physiotherapy assistance, or were admitted to post-care facilities. At 6 months post-discharge, 91.0% of the 136 patients (n = 119) were evaluated and 36.0% had persistent malnutrition, 14.3% complained of a significant decrease in muscle strength and 14.9% had a performance status > 2. Obesity was more frequent in patients with impairment than in those without (52.8% vs. 31.0%; $p = 0.0071$), with these patients being admitted more frequently to ICUs (50.9% vs. 31.3%; $p = 0.010$). Among those with persistent symptoms, 10% had psychiatric co-morbidities (mood disorders, anxiety, or post-traumatic stress syndrome), 7.6% had prolonged pneumological symptoms and 4.2% had neurological symptoms. Conclusions: Obese subjects as well as patients who have stayed in intensive care have a higher risk of functional loss or undernutrition 6 months after a severe COVID infection. Malnutrition and loss of muscle strength should be considered in the clinical assessment of these patients.

Keywords: long COVID-19; muscle strength; malnutrition; self-evaluation; obesity; cohort study; performance status; intensive care unit

1. Introduction

Post-acute consequences of COVID-19, also termed long COVID, include signs and symptoms that develop during or after an infection consistent with COVID-19, and persist for more than 12 weeks with prolonged multisystem involvement and significant disability. The most commonly described symptoms are sensory (loss of taste and anosmia), neurological (loss of concentration and "brain fog") and cardiorespiratory problems (fatigue, dyspnea, reduced exercise capacity). In most instances, malnutrition is left ignored as these patients are often overweight at the time of diagnosis [1].

Recent studies have reported a high prevalence of malnutrition among hospitalized patients with COVID-19 depending on the screening and diagnostic tool used [2], and levels are estimated at about 50% (31.7–66.5%) [2]. This prevalence furthermore appears particularly high in patients requiring a stay in intensive care [1,3]. Several factors could explain malnutrition during this acute phase, including marked systemic inflammation driving hypermetabolism and muscle catabolism, and prolonged periods of bedrest driving disuse atrophy. Up to 40% of patients with COVID-19 experience gastrointestinal symptoms ranging from nausea, vomiting, anorexia, diarrhea and abdominal distention, especially in ICU COVID patients [4], which can further deter eating and impact the tolerance of nutritional support [5]. Olfactory and gustatory dysfunction [6] may also contribute to weight loss [7,8].

Muscle loss and/or loss of muscle function appear to be the major nutritional challenges during this acute period. Both myalgia and muscle loss have been strongly correlated with disease severity among COVID-19 patients [9]. Protein turnover is also increased in critical illness in the early stages of COVID-19, in response to massive proteolytic stimuli [10]. Suggested mechanisms include direct muscle invasion by ECoV particles and immune-mediated muscle injury, presenting as myositis, although satisfactory proof of the direct invasion of SARS-CoV-2 into muscle cells is still lacking [11]. Lastly, muscle deconditioning due to immobility and corticosteroid treatment has been associated with diffuse atrophy at muscle biopsy [12]. A retrospective case study from China revealed that 10.7% of patients showed skeletal muscle injury during this acute phase as well as various neurological manifestations (36.4%) [13].

As a result, studies have mainly focused on the importance of nutritional intervention during the acute phase of COVID-19 in order to prevent clinical deterioration (review in [14]). However, the consequences of unintentional weight loss and resulting sarcopenia can also have major long-term functional impacts [15]. A large number of patients are being discharged from hospital following COVID-19 without a systematic assessment of their recovery and need for rehabilitation or further investigation to detect complications, in particular functional complaints related to loss of muscle strength, persistence of malnutrition and fatigue [16]. Medical teams have become increasingly aware of the importance of multidisciplinary care, taking into account fatigue and functional disability, but nevertheless overlooking the nutritional aspect and the importance of the decrease in muscle strength [1]. Nowadays, muscle weakness and fatigue appear as a frequent complaint among these patients [4,5].

In clinical practice, impairment of muscle strength is difficult to assess since, unlike weight, there is no objective assessment of muscle strength prior to disease. Such objective evaluation can be quite straightforward, i.e., using the grip test or chair lifting test. However, these tests are not easily implemented in the context of severe infection or in the patient's home, and do not establish whether the alteration is linked to the disease or whether it existed beforehand. In view of the latter, we found it useful to use a self-evaluation muscle strength scale, asking the patient how he/she rated his/her muscle strength compared to before the disease. In a preliminary study, we found a concordance between the outcome of this subjective functional evaluation (Self Evaluation of Strength (SES)) and that of the grip test [17].

During the first wave of the pandemic, we rapidly established a post-COVID follow-up service collecting data to identify unmet health needs and to identify those requiring additional rehabilitation and/or investigation for complications. All of these patients received dietary counseling and adapted physical activity guidance, some of whom with severe disability and being re-admitted to post-care facilities. The others received physiotherapy assistance and nutritional supplementation.

The aim of this study was to evaluate, at 6 months post-discharge, the evolution of health status in the group of patients who had a persistent impairment at day 30: namely, patients with persistent weight loss (>5%) or impaired muscle strength (SES < 7/10), or with a Performance Status (PS) > 2. The objective was to analyze the frequency and nature of their symptoms persisting since the initial infection, their nutritional status as well as the evolution of their muscle strength and performance status.

2. Methods

2.1. Study Design and Participants

This study, conducted as part of a prospective cohort study, included all adult inpatients ($\geq$18 years old) who were diagnosed with COVID-19 and admitted to an ICU or non-ICU unit for COVID-19 patients at the Nancy Brabois University Hospital between 1 March 2020 and 29 April 2020 and subsequently discharged alive from hospital. The diagnosis of COVID-19 was based on a positive SARS-CoV-2 RT-PCR test on a nasopharyngeal sample and/or on a typical chest CT scan [18]. The study was approved by the Research Commission of the University Hospital of Nancy and the requirement for informed consent was waived by the ethics commission. The ClinicalTrials.gov (accessed on 16 August 2021) identifier is NCT04451694.

To manage the flow of incoming patients, a certain number were transferred to other hospitals after a few days. At discharge from the intensive or acute care unit, some patients were admitted to post-acute care facilities for ongoing skilled nursing care and rehabilitation.

All hospital-discharged patients were offered a teleconsultation 30 days after discharge (D30) to assess their nutritional status and muscle function, the degree of disability linked to the degree of malnutrition and subjective functional loss, as well as limitation of daily activity estimated by the WHO performance status score. Consequently, patients with persistent weight loss (>5%) at D30 or with impaired muscle strength (Self Evaluation of Strength < 7/10) or a performance status (PS) $\geq$ 2 (group of impairment patients) were invited to be evaluated 6 months after discharge (by teleconsultation or in person).

2.2. Demographics, Comorbidities and Hospitalization Data Collection

Patient characteristics and hospitalization data were collected by manual review of electronic medical records. Epidemiological, demographic, laboratory and outcome data were extracted from electronic medical records during hospitalization. Sociodemographic data included age, sex, living alone or with others, occupational activity (active vs. unemployed and retired), smoking status (active or not) and daily alcohol consumption. Health characteristics included comorbidities (hypertension, diabetes mellitus, cerebrovascular disease, cardiovascular disease, chronic lung disease) as well as COVID-19 symptoms (anosmia and dysgeusia, diarrhea, dyspnea, asthenia, food aversion).

Hospitalization characteristics included: ICU admission (yes/no), time between symptom onset and hospitalization (days) and length of stay (days).

2.3. Recorded Symptoms

Asthenia at discharge, at day 30 and at 6 months post-discharge was evaluated using a fatigue visual analogue scale (VAS) (0–10) [19].

Dyspnea at discharge, at day 30 and at 6 months post-discharge was evaluated by the French adaptation of the American Thoracic Society Scale, according to 5 levels (from 1 to 5) [20].

Health status at day 30 and at 6 months was assessed using the WHO/Zubrod Performance Status Scale which rates patients from 0 to 4 [21].

Neurological symptoms were also explored (neuropathy, headache, impaired memory and concentration or cognitive impairment).

Depression, anxiety and PTSD diagnoses were based on DSM-V criteria [22,23].

2.4. Nutritional Assessment

Nutritional status prior to hospitalization, on admission, at discharge, at day 30 and at 6 months post-discharge was assessed using anthropometric measurements (BMI: body mass index = body weight/height^2) and weight loss (%) compared to weight prior to illness. In hospital, patients were weighed and their height was measured. On day 30 and at 6 months post-discharge, patients were instructed to use their own weighing scales.

2.5. SEFI and Self-Assessment of Muscle Function (SES) at Discharge, at Day 30 and at 6 Months Post-Discharge

Food intake was assessed using the 10-point verbal (AVeS) or visual (AViS) analogue scales (self-evaluation of food intake (SEFI)) [24], graded from 0 to 10. As suggested by Bouette et al. [24], an SEFI < 7 was considered as the cut-off value.

Self-assessment of strength (SES) was assessed at discharge, at day 30 and at 6 months post-discharge using the 10-point verbal (AVeS) or visual (AViS) analogue scales via teleconsultation for evaluating arm and leg strength in comparison to patient strength prior to hospitalization. In practice, patients were asked to evaluate their arm and leg strength in comparison with their strength prior to COVID-19. As suggested by Krznaric et al. [14], patients were asked about their degree of difficulty in lifting or carrying a weight, walking across the room, rising from a chair or bed, and to evaluate these difficulties using a 10-point verbal or visual analogue scale (10 = same strength as before illness and 0 = total loss of strength).

Assessment of physical activity was carried out by completing the International Physical Activity Questionnaire-Short Form (IPAQ-SF) [25] in order to estimate activity prior to COVID-19, with activity classified as low, moderate and high physical activity [25].

2.6. Malnutrition Diagnosis

Malnutrition diagnosis was made according to the GLIM criteria and French recommendations (at least 1 phenotypic criterion and 1 etiological criterion) [26,27]. Severe malnutrition was defined following the French recommendations as weight loss > 10% of weight before COVID-19 infection or a BMI < 17 (<18.5 for patients > 70 years old). Moderate malnutrition was defined as weight loss > 5% of weight before COVID-19 or BMI < 18.5 (<21 for patients > 70 years old) [27,28].

2.7. Statistical Analysis

Continuous variables are expressed as mean ± SD and categorical variables as absolute values and percentages. A paired Student's t-test, chi-square (χ^2), ANOVA, Fisher's exact test, and Wilcoxon tests were used to compare the values of variables between groups as appropriate. Pearson's chi-square test or Fisher's exact test was used to assess the association between each of the discrete variables and the impairment status. $p < 0.05$ was considered statistically significant. Data were recorded on Excel files. Statistical analysis was performed using Statistical Analysis Software 9.4, SAS Institute Inc, Cary, NC, USA.

3. Results

Population description (Table 1 and Figure 1).

Table 1. Characteristics of the whole population (n = 288).

Variables	n and %
Age (years)	59.8 ± 16.6
Sex (F/M)	132/156 (45.8%/54.2%)
Living alone	54 (18.8%)
Couple	132 (45.8%)
Family	96 (33.3%)
Retirement home	6 (2.1%)
BMI Class	
18.5–24.9	69 (24.3%)
25–29.9	112 (39.4%)
>30	103 (36.3%)

Table 1. *Cont.*

IPAQ (prior to COVID-19)	
Low	162 (56.3%)
Moderate	82 (28.5%)
High	44 (15.3%)
ICU	102 (35.4%)
Active smoking	12 (4.2%)
Daily alcohol	14 (4.9%)
Comorbidities	
HBP	113 (39.2%)
Coronary heart disease	41 (14.2%)
Dyslipidemia	64 (22.2%)
Diabetes mellitus	48 (16.7%)
Renal failure	23 (8.0%)
Stroke	9 (3.1%)
Asthma	14 (4.9%)
Apnea	19 (6.6%)
Chronic obstructive bronchitis	13 (4.5%)
Respiratory failure	10 (3.5%)
Active cancer	30 (10.4%)
Neurological disease	13 (4.5%)

BMI, body mass index; IPAQ, International Physical Activity Questionnaire; ICU, intensive care unit; HBP, high blood pressure.

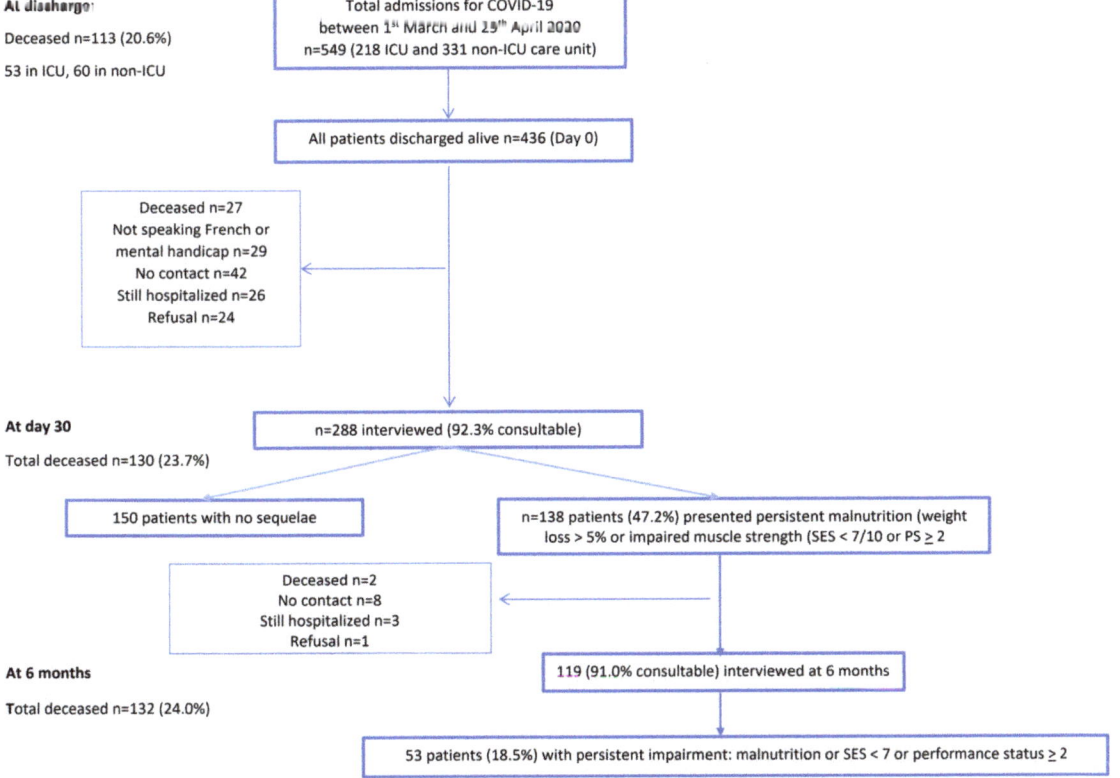

Figure 1. Flowchart of patients included in the study.

Of the 549 consecutive patients hospitalized for COVID-19 between 1 March and 29 April 2020, 23.7% died and 288 patients were at home at D30 post-discharge (Figure 1).

The mean age of the 288 interviewed patients was 59.8 ± 16.6 years, 54.2% of whom were male. The majority had a low physical activity assessed by IPAQ-SF prior to contracting COVID-19 (56.3%). Seventy-six percent of these patients were overweight or obese. According to the GLIM criteria, 20.7% were already undernourished on admission. The mean delay between the first symptom and admission was 9.7 ± 8.6 days. The most frequent comorbidities were cardiovascular diseases (hypertension, dyslipidemia, diabetes mellitus and coronary artery disease). At admission, anosmia was present in 42.7% of patients, dyspnea in 22.6%, cough in 25.0% and diarrhea in 9.3% of patients.

As reported previously [17], 13.2% of the patients hospitalized for a severe form of COVID-19 were still severely malnourished 30 days after hospital discharge (weight loss > 10% and/or BMI < 17). The highest predictive factors of persistent malnutrition were ICU stay and male sex. Moreover, 26.3% of these patients complained of impaired muscle strength and had a subjective functional loss evaluated at <7/10 using a 10-point verbal (AVeS) or visual (AViS) analogue scale. Lastly, 8.3% (n = 24) concomitantly exhibited a performance status (PS) $\geq$ 2, severe malnutrition and subjective functional loss.

At D30, 136 patients (47.2%) presented an impairment with persistent malnutrition or impaired muscle strength (SES < 7/10) or severe disability with a PS $\geq$ 2. Of the latter, 119 (91.0%) accepted phone or teleconsultations or in-person interviews at 6 months. Two patients died during this period, three were still hospitalized, eight were unreachable and there was one refusal (Figure 1).

The evolution of the characteristics of the 119 patients with impairment at D30 is shown in Table 2.

Table 2. Characteristics and evolution of nutritional status at 6 months in the sub-group of patients with impairment at day 30 after severe COVID-19 (n and %).

	Admission (n = 119)	At Discharge (n = 119)	D30 Home (n = 119)	At 6 Months (n = 119)	p
Weight (kg)	82.6 ± 19.06	76.5 ± 16.1	77.6 ± 15.9	81.2 ± 17.9	<10^{-3}
BMI	28.7 ± 5.9	26.7 ± 5.0	27.4 ± 5.0	28.3 ± 5.5	<10^{-3}
Weight variation (%)	−3.7 ± 4.9	−5.1 ± 5.9	−7.4 ± 5.0	−3.6 ± 5.9	<10^{-3}
Malnutrition					<10^{-3}
No	68/119 (57.1%)	23/119 (19.3%)	22/119 (18.5%)	76/119 (63.9%)	
Moderate	21/119 (17.6%)	42/119 (35.3%)	43/119 (36.1%)	25/119 (21.0%)	
Severe	12/119 (10.1%)	54/119 (45.4%)	54/119 (45.4%)	18/119 (15.1%)	
SEFI		7.2 ± 3.0	9.6 ± 1.2	9.8 ± 0.9	<10^{-3}
SES hands		4.2 ± 2.4	6.9 ± 2.1	9.1 ± 1.7	<10^{-3}
SES legs		4.0 ± 2.3	6.8 ± 2.1	9.1 ± 1.6	<10^{-3}
Subjective functional loss (SES < 7)%		79.8%	55.5%	14.3%	<10^{-3}
Asthenia (VAE)> 5/10 (%)			3.2 ± 3.0	1.7 ± 2.5	<10^{-3}
			35/119 (29.4%)	19/119 (16.0%)	0.020
Performance Status					<10^{-3}
0		22 (18.5%)	30 (25.2%)	70/119 (58.8%)	
1		44 (37.0%)	44 (37.0%)	27/119 (22.7%)	
2		29 (24.4%)	29 (24.4%)	9/119 (7.6%)	
3–4		24 (20.2%)	16 (13.4%)	8/119 (6.7%)	

D30, day 30; BMI, body mass index; SEFI, self-evaluation of food intake; SES, self-evaluation of strength.

As shown in Table 2, patients with impairment at D30 regained an average of 3.6 kg body weight between D30 and 6 months, with mean weight and BMI returning to near baseline values (admission); on average, patients remained 1.4 kg lighter than on admission. Forty-three patients (36.0% of the 119 patients with impairment at D30) displayed persistent malnutrition at 6 months, with 18 patients exhibiting severe malnutrition (15.1%). On average, seventeen patients (14.3% of the 119 patients with impairment at D30) complained of a significant decrease in muscle strength (SES < 7/10 with a mean ± SD = 5.0 ± 2.6 for arm and 4.9 ± 2.6 for legs). Seventeen patients also had a performance status ≥ 2 (14.9% of the 119 patients with impairment at D30). SES increased between D30 and 6 months post-discharge, nearing the index value prior to COVID infection.

3.1. Long COVID Symptoms at 6 Months Post-Discharge

The most frequent symptoms were asthenia (16.0% had fatigue score > 5/10 at 6 months) and psychiatric disorders; 12 patients (10.0%) experienced mood disorders, anxiety, or post-traumatic stress syndrome. Nine patients (7.6%) presented prolonged pneumological symptoms (dyspnea), and five patients (4.2%) had neurological symptoms (neuropathy, headache, impaired memory and concentration or cognitive impairment).

3.2. Characteristics of Patients with Impairment at 6 Months Post-Discharge, Comparison with Recovered Patients

Overall, at 6 months, 53 patients presented a persistent impairment, as assessed by malnutrition and/or SES < 7 or performance status ≥ 2. The mean characteristics of this population with persistent impairment are described in Table 3 and were compared with the recovered patients (at discharge or at D30).

Table 3. Comparison of the characteristics of recovered patients and of the group of patients with impairment at 6 months.

Variables	Recovered Patients N = 217 (80.4%)	Patients with Impairments at 6 Months N = 53 (19.6%)	p
Symptoms at discharge			
Dyspnea ≥ 2	21 (9.6%)	3 (5.7%)	NS
Anosmia at discharge	95 (43.8%)	18 (34%)	NS
Diarrhea	10 (4.6%)	2 (3.8%)	NS
cough	16 (7.4%)	4 (7.5%)	NS
Obesity (BMI ≥ 30) (%) at admission	31.0%	52.8%	0.007
ICU admission	31.3%	50.9%	0.010
SEFI at discharge	7.4 ± 2.9	6.1 ± 3.0	0.003
Dietary aversion at discharge	19 (8.8%)	8 (15.1%)	NS
Weight loss (%)			
Before admission	−2.8% ± 4.1%	−5.5 ± 7.0	0.001
Total at discharge	−5.2% ± 4.7%	−10.5 ± 6%	<0.001
Malnutrition at discharge (%)	102 (49.3%)	43 (82.6%)	0.001
Moderate	62 (30.0%)	15 (28.8%)	
Severe	40 (19.3%)	28 (53.8%)	
SES at discharge			
Arms	5.3 ± 2.6	4.3 ± 2.4	0.013
Legs	5.2 ± 2.7	4.0 ± 2.0	0.004
SES < 7	138 (71.9%)	46 (92%)	0.003

Fisher's exact test for qualitative variables, Student's t test for quantitative variables. SEFI, self-evaluation of food intake; SES, self-evaluation of strength.

Comorbidity prevalence did not significantly differ between these two groups, except for obesity which was more frequent in the group with impairment at 6 months post-discharge (52.8% vs. 31.0%; p = 0.007), with these patients being admitted more frequently to ICUs (50.9% vs. 31.3%; p = 0.010). These patients had more difficulties eating after discharge (SEFI: 6.1 ± 3.0 vs. 7.4 ± 2.9 p = 0.0032) and exhibited greater weight loss, with an increased prevalence of malnutrition. SES scores were lower at discharge in this group (4.3 ± 2.4 vs. 5.3 ± 2.6 for arms; p = 0.013, and 4.0 ± 2.0 vs. 5.2 ± 2.7 for legs; p = 0.0045) with no other significant difference being observed.

4. Discussion

This is the first report on a prospective observational cohort study of COVID-19 specifically exploring nutritional status, subjective functional loss and disability at 6 months after discharge. We showed that, at D30, 138/288 of these patients (48%) presented persistent malnutrition (33%), subjective functional loss (26.3%) and/or performance status ≥ 2 (24.3%). At 6 months, 15% of the initial cohort remained malnourished despite nutritional counseling during hospitalization and ensuing dietary guidance, oral nutritional supplements, or relocation to rehabilitation centers, 6% complained of a significant decrease in muscle strength and 6% had a performance status > 2, or 18.5% of this cohort.

Contrary to our results, a study conducted in a cohort of severe COVID-19 patients assessing nutritional status 3 months after discharge from hospital [29] reported that only 8.4% of patients were malnourished at discharge and none at 3 months. Malnutrition was correlated with severity of the disease, indirectly inferable from an assessment of length of hospital stay and need for admission to ICU. However, in this latter study, malnutrition diagnosis was based on the 2015 ESPEN consensus [30], including different criteria for malnutrition than those of the international consensus (GLIM criteria [26]), in particular the postulation that patients with a BMI above 22 are not malnourished. There are several arguments against this latter assertion. The first is that patients suffering from obesity have, because of metabolic modifications (insulin resistance, fatty acid metabolism, hyperglycemia, etc.), higher protein catabolism than subjects of normal weight in the event of traumatism [31], which was also reported in acute COVID patients with obesity [32]. Secondly, accelerated muscle loss is a major factor of morbidity and mortality in obese COVID-19 patients [33]. On the contrary, in our study, obese subjects had a higher risk of functional loss or undernutrition 6 months after a severe COVID infection, as well as patients with a stay in intensive care.

In our cohort, 20.7% of patients were already undernourished at admission. Malnutrition tended to have begun during the initial phases of the disease occurring at home since, upon admission, patients declared significant involuntary weight loss when compared to their habitual weight [29]. However, it is not excluded that malnutrition may precede the infection. A recent study showed that patients with a recent history of malnutrition could be at higher risk of severe COVID-19 [34]. The majority of our patients had comorbidities that could lead to malnutrition. However, we did not observe any influence of these comorbidities on the evolution of their nutritional status. Weight loss and undernutrition were seemingly associated very early with a major decrease in food intake, which remained strongly impaired in half of the patients at hospital discharge, despite nutritional support. Caccialanza et al. [35] also showed that this reduced self-reported food intake prior to hospitalization and/or expected by physicians in the days after admission was associated with negative clinical outcomes in non-critically ill, hospitalized COVID-19 patients. The other component is the increased energy expenditure secondary to a major inflammatory syndrome that leads to hypercatabolism which, associated with reduced food intake and immobilization, significantly contributes to muscle atrophy and sarcopenia.

Acute sarcopenia may mostly affect patient prognosis and incur post-COVID-19 functional and physical deterioration. The degree of muscle mass and functional loss can be influenced by a multiplicity of factors, including the patient's general pre-infection medical and functional condition, especially in older adults [10]. However, this functional condition prior to infection is typically not analyzed and/or is unknown. The subjective assessment of muscle strength by an analogue or numeric scale could therefore be useful to follow the evolution of muscle strength in these patients. Some patients still appeared very weak 6 months after the infection, despite advice to increase physical activity with protein support, or referral to physiotherapists or adapted physical activity therapists. Most of our patients had low physical activity assessed by IPAQ-SF prior to contracting COVID-19 (56.3%), which may represent a risk factor for severe COVID-infection [36,37].

Fifteen percent of patients presented neuro-psychiatric symptoms requiring treatment. These disorders are well-described in the literature and could be linked to a direct action of the virus on the nervous system [38,39].

Among the strengths and weaknesses of this analysis, the subjective evaluation of muscle strength is subject to debate. The strong point of such evaluation is to assess muscle function in the long term and to judge the evolution of muscle strength, without knowledge of the level of strength prior to the disease. We evaluated this tool in a small cohort of hospitalized patients [17] and while we were unable to identify the actual threshold of functional impairment, our assessment was nevertheless based on the threshold determined according to the questionnaire of Krznaric et al. [14] and on other subjective visual or numeric scales [40]. This threshold must, however, be validated in a large cohort study, notably in comparison with the evolution of muscle strength objectively measured by dynamometry.

Weighing patients at home is also a weak point due to the lack of weight scale control. Nevertheless, this measurement error was, *a priori*, the same for the patient's usual weight prior to infection.

Lastly, we hypothesized that patients who were not impaired at discharge or who improved their nutritional status and muscle strength between discharge and D30 had little risk of having a worse outcome thereafter and were thus not contacted after 6 months. However, three additional deaths were observed during this latter period, albeit all linked to an underlying disease.

In conclusion, undernutrition and loss of muscle strength are symptoms of long COVID and should be considered in the clinical assessment of these patients. Although there are no current specific treatments for use in patients who have been hospitalized for COVID-19, treatments should focus on nutritional support and rehabilitation exercises whenever possible to prevent long-term disability as a result of acute illness due to COVID-19, as well as on the management of sarcopenia. The data described herein may assist in the identification of patients outside of expected recovery trajectories who could benefit from additional rehabilitation and/or further investigation to detect post-COVID nutritional complications. Of these outlying patients, obese subjects appear particularly at risk, as well as patients who have stayed in intensive care.

Author Contributions: M.G. Conceptualization—Investigation—Software; M.M., A.M., N.M. and N.S. Investigation; R.J. Supervision; P.-L.N.-T. Conceptualization—Formal Analysis—Methodology; D.Q. Conceptualization—Project administration—Formal analysis—Methodology—Supervision—Writing—original draft—Writing—review & editing. All authors have read and agreed to the published version of the manuscript.

Funding: This research received no external funding.

Institutional Review Board Statement: The study was approved by the Research Commission of the University Hospital of Nancy and the requirement for informed consent was waived by the ethics commission.

Data Availability Statement: The data that support the findings of this study are available from the corresponding author upon reasonable request.

Acknowledgments: This study was conducted with the help of the French Society for Clinical Nutrition and Metabolism. Trial participants were thanked for their contribution to this study and for consenting that the data will be published anonymously.

Conflicts of Interest: All authors declare no conflict of interest in relation with this study.

References

1. Venturelli, S.; Benatti, S.V.; Casati, M.; Binda, F.; Zuglian, G.; Imeri, G.; Conti, C.; Biffi, A.M.; Spada, M.S.; Bondi; et al. Surviving COVID-19 in Bergamo province: A post-acute outpatient re-evaluation. *Epidemiol. Infect.* **2021**, *149*, e32. [CrossRef] [PubMed]
2. Abate, S.M.; Chekole, Y.A.; Estifanos, M.B.; Abate, K.H.; Kabthymer, R.H. Prevalence and outcomes of malnutrition among hospitalized COVID-19 patients: A systematic review and meta-analysis. *Clin. Nutr. ESPEN* **2021**, *43*, 174–183. [CrossRef] [PubMed]
3. Anker, M.S.; Landmesser, U.; von Haehling, S.; Butler, J.; Coats, A.J.S.; Anker, S.D. Weight loss, malnutrition, and cachexia in COVID-19: Facts and numbers. *J. Cachexia Sarcopenia Muscle* **2021**, *12*, 9–13. [CrossRef] [PubMed]
4. Ye, L.; Yang, Z.; Liu, J.; Liao, L.; Wang, F. Digestive system manifestations and clinical significance of coronavirus disease 2019: A systematic literature review. *J. Gastroenterol. Hepatol.* **2021**, *36*, 1414–1422. [CrossRef]
5. Liu, R.; Paz, M.; Siraj, L.; Boyd, T.; Salamone, S.; Lite, T.V.; Leung, K.M.; Chirinos, J.D.; Shang, H.H.; Townsend, M.J.; et al. Feeding intolerance in critically ill patients with COVID-19. *Clin. Nutr.* **2021**, *29*, S261–S5614.
6. Tong, J.Y.; Wong, A.; Zhu, D.; Fastenberg, J.H.; Tham, T. The Prevalence of Olfactory and Gustatory Dysfunction in COVID-19 Patients: A Systematic Review and Meta-analysis. *Otolaryngol. Head Neck Surg.* **2020**, *163*, 3–11. [CrossRef]
7. Roos, D.S.; Oranje, O.J.M.; Freriksen, A.F.D.; Berendse, H.W.; Boesveldt, S. Flavor perception and the risk of malnutrition in patients with Parkinson's disease. *J. Neural Transm.* **2018**, *125*, 925–930. [CrossRef]
8. Li, T.; Zhang, Y.; Gong, C.; Wang, J.; Liu, B.; Shi, L.; Duan, J. Prevalence of malnutrition and analysis of related factors in elderly patients with COVID-19 in Wuhan, China. *Eur. J. Clin. Nutr.* **2020**, *74*, 871–875. [CrossRef]
9. Liu, H.; Chen, S.; Liu, M.; Nie, H.; Lu, H. Comorbid Chronic Diseases are Strongly Correlated with Disease Severity among COVID-19 Patients: A Systematic Review and Meta-Analysis. *Aging Dis.* **2020**, *11*, 668–678. [CrossRef]
10. Piotrowicz, K.; Gasowski, J.; Michel, J.P.; Veronese, N. Post-COVID-19 acute sarcopenia: Physiopathology and management. *Aging Clin. Exp. Res.* **2021**, *33*, 2887–2898. [CrossRef]
11. Wong, D.W.L.; Klinkhammer, B.M.; Djudjaj, S.; Villwock, S.; Timm, M.C.; Buhl, E.M.; Wucherpfennig, S.; Cacchi, C.; Braunschweig, T.; Knuchel-Clarke, R.; et al. Multisystemic Cellular Tropism of SARS-CoV-2 in Autopsies of COVID-19 Patients. *Cells* **2021**, *10*, 1900. [CrossRef]
12. Msigwa, S.S.; Wang, Y.; Li, Y.; Cheng, X. The neurological insights of the emerging coronaviruses. *J. Clin. Neurosci.* **2020**, *78*, 1–7. [CrossRef]
13. Mao, L.; Jin, H.; Wang, M.; Hu, Y.; Chen, S.; He, Q.; Chang, J.; Hong, C.; Zhou, Y.; Wang, D.; et al. Neurologic Manifestations of Hospitalized Patients With Coronavirus Disease 2019 in Wuhan, China. *JAMA Neurol.* **2020**, *77*, 683–690. [CrossRef]
14. Cereda, E.; Clave, P.; Collins, P.F.; Holdoway, A.; Wischmeyer, P.E. Recovery Focused Nutritional Therapy across the Continuum of Care: Learning from COVID-19. *Nutrients* **2021**, *13*, 3293. [CrossRef]
15. Seessle, J.; Waterboer, T.; Hippchen, T.; Simon, J.; Kirchner, M.; Lim, A.; Muller, B.; Merle, U. Persistent symptoms in adult patients one year after COVID-19: A prospective cohort study. *Clin. Infect. Dis.* **2021**, *5*, ciab611.
16. Adeloye, D.; Elneima, O.; Daines, L.; Poinasamy, K.; Quint, J.K.; Walker, S.; Brightling, C.E.; Siddiqui, S.; Hurst, J.R.; Chalmers, J.D.; et al. The long-term sequelae of COVID-19: An international consensus on research priorities for patients with pre-existing and new-onset airways disease. *Lancet Respir. Med.* **2021**, *17*, S2213-2600.
17. Quilliot, D.; Gerard, M.; Bonsack, O.; Malgras, A.; Vaillant, M.F.; Di Patrizio, P.; Jaussaud, R.; Ziegler, O.; Nguyen-Thi, P.L. Impact of severe SARS-CoV-2 infection on nutritional status and subjective functional loss in a prospective cohort of COVID-19 survivors. *BMJ Open* **2021**, *11*, e048948. [CrossRef]
18. Cheng, M.P.; Papenburg, J.; Desjardins, M.; Kanjilal, S.; Quach, C.; Libman, M.; Dittrich, S.; Yansouni, C.P. Diagnostic Testing for Severe Acute Respiratory Syndrome-Related Coronavirus 2: A Narrative Review. *Ann. Intern. Med.* **2020**, *172*, 726–734. [CrossRef]
19. Hewlett, S.; Hehir, M.; Kirwan, J.R. Measuring fatigue in rheumatoid arthritis: A systematic review of scales in use. *Arthritis Rheum.* **2007**, *57*, 429–439. [CrossRef]
20. Society, A.T. Recommended respiratory disease questionnaires for use with adults and children in epidemiological research. *Am. Rev. Respir. Dis.* **1978**, *118*, 7–35.
21. Oken, M.M.; Creech, R.H.; Tormey, D.C.; Horton, J.; Davis, T.E.; McFadden, E.T.; Carbone, P.P. Toxicity and response criteria of the Eastern Cooperative Oncology Group. *Am. J. Clin. Oncol.* **1982**, *5*, 649–655. [CrossRef]
22. American Psychiatric Association: DSM-V Development. Available online: https://www.psychiatry.org/psychiatrists/practice/dsm/updates-to-dsm-5//updates-to-dsm-5-criteria-text (accessed on 20 July 2021).
23. American Psychiatric Association. *Diagnostic and Statistical Manual of Mental Disorders*, 5th ed.; Arlington, V.A.P.A., Ed.; American Psychiatric Association: Washington, DC, USA, 2013; pp. 271–272.
24. Thibault, R.; Goujon, N.; Le Gallic, E.; Clairand, R.; Sebille, V.; Vibert, J.; Schneider, S.M.; Darmaun, D. Use of 10-point analogue scales to estimate dietary intake: A prospective study in patients nutritionally at-risk. *Clin. Nutr.* **2009**, *28*, 134–140. [CrossRef]
25. Craig, C.L.; Marshall, A.L.; Sjostrom, M.; Bauman, A.E.; Booth, M.L.; Ainsworth, B.E.; Pratt, M.; Ekelund, U.; Yngve, A.; Sallis, J.F.; et al. International physical activity questionnaire: 12-country reliability and validity. *Med. Sci. Sports Exerc.* **2003**, *35*, 1381–1395. [CrossRef]
26. Cederholm, T.; Jensen, G.L.; Correia, M.; Gonzalez, M.C.; Fukushima, R.; Higashiguchi, T.; Baptista, G.; Barazzoni, R.; Blaauw, R.; Coats, A.; et al. GLIM criteria for the diagnosis of malnutrition—A consensus report from the global clinical nutrition community. *Clin. Nutr.* **2019**, *38*, 1–9. [CrossRef]

27. HAS. Diagnostic de la Dénutrition de l'Enfant et de l'Adulte. Saint-Denis La Plaine. 2019. Available online: https://www.has-sante.fr/upload/docs/application/pdf/2019-11/reco277_recommandations_rbp_denutrition_cd_2019_11_13_v0.pdf (accessed on 20 July 2021).
28. Thibault, R.; Quilliot, D.; Seguin, P.; Tamion, F.; Schneider, S.; Déchelotte, P. Nutritional care at hospital during the Covid-19 viral epidemic: Expert opinion from the French-speaking Society for Clinical Nutrition and Metabolism (SFNCM). *Nut. Clin. Métab.* **2020**, *34*, 97–104. [CrossRef]
29. Fiorindi, C.; Campani, F.; Rasero, L.; Campani, C.; Livi, L.; Giovannoni, L.; Amato, C.; Giudici, F.; Bartoloni, A.; Fattirolli, F.; et al. Prevalence of nutritional risk and malnutrition during and after hospitalization for COVID-19 infection: Preliminary results of a single-centre experience. *Clin. Nutr. ESPEN* **2021**, *45*, 351–355. [CrossRef]
30. Cederholm, T.; Bosaeus, I.; Barazzoni, R.; Bauer, J.; Van Gossum, A.; Klek, S.; Muscaritoli, M.; Nyulasi, I.; Ockenga, J.; Schneider, S.M.; et al. Diagnostic criteria for malnutrition—An ESPEN Consensus Statement. *Clin. Nutr.* **2015**, *34*, 335–340. [CrossRef]
31. Jeevanandam, M.; Young, D.H.; Schiller, W.R. Obesity and the metabolic response to severe multiple trauma in man. *J. Clin. Invest.* **1991**, *87*, 262–269. [CrossRef]
32. Gualtieri, P.; Falcone, C.; Romano, L.; Macheda, S.; Correale, P.; Arciello, P.; Polimeni, N.; Lorenzo, A. Body Composition Findings by Computed Tomography in SARS-CoV-2 Patients: Increased Risk of Muscle Wasting in Obesity. *Int. J. Mol. Sci.* **2020**, *21*, 4670. [CrossRef]
33. Zhang, X.; Xie, X.; Dou, Q.; Liu, C.; Zhang, W.; Yang, Y.; Deng, R.; Cheng, A.S.K. Association of sarcopenic obesity with the risk of all-cause mortality among adults over a broad range of different settings: A updated meta-analysis. *BMC Geriatr.* **2019**, *19*, 183. [CrossRef]
34. Kurtz, A.; Grant, K.; Marano, R.; Arrieta, A.; Grant, K., Jr.; Feaster, W.; Steele, C.; Ehwerhemuepha, L. Long-term effects of malnutrition on severity of COVID-19. *Sci. Rep.* **2021**, *11*, 14974. [CrossRef] [PubMed]
35. Caccialanza, R.; Formisano, E.; Klersy, C.; Ferretti, V.; Ferrari, A.; Demontis, S.; Mascheroni, A.; Masi, S.; Crotti, S.; Lobascio, F.; et al. Nutritional parameters associated with prognosis in non-critically ill hospitalized COVID-19 patients: The NUTRI-COVID19 study. *Clin. Nutr.* **2021**, *25*, S261–S5614.
36. Wu, C.; Chen, X.; Cai, Y.; Xia, J.; Zhou, X.; Xu, S.; Huang, H.; Zhang, L.; Zhou, X.; Du, C.; et al. Risk Factors Associated With Acute Respiratory Distress Syndrome and Death in Patients With Coronavirus Disease 2019 Pneumonia in Wuhan, China. *JAMA Intern. Med.* **2020**, *180*, 934–943. [CrossRef] [PubMed]
37. Williamson, E.J.; Walker, A.J.; Bhaskaran, K.; Bacon, S.; Bates, C.; Morton, C.E.; Curtis, H.J.; Mehrkar, A.; Evans, D.; Inglesby, P.; et al. Factors associated with COVID-19-related death using OpenSAFELY. *Nature* **2020**, *584*, 430–436. [CrossRef]
38. Ousseiran, Z.H.; Fares, Y.; Chamoun, W.T. Neurological manifestations of COVID-19: A systematic review and detailed comprehension. *Int. J. Neurosci.* **2021**, *27*, 1–16. [CrossRef]
39. Majolo, F.; Silva, G.L.D.; Vieira, L.; Anli, C.; Timmers, L.; Laufer, S.; Goettert, M.I. Neuropsychiatric Disorders and COVID-19: What We Know So Far. *Pharmaceuticals* **2021**, *14*, 933. [CrossRef]
40. Bouette, G.; Esvan, M.; Apel, K.; Thibault, R. A visual analogue scale for food intake as a screening test for malnutrition in the primary care setting: Prospective non-interventional study. *Clin. Nutr.* **2020**, *40*, 174–180. [CrossRef]

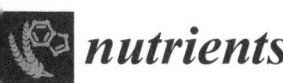

Article

Oropharyngeal Dysphagia and Impaired Motility of the Upper Gastrointestinal Tract—Is There a Clinical Link in Neurocritical Care?

Paul Muhle [1,2,*], Karen Konert [1], Sonja Suntrup-Krueger [1,2], Inga Claus [1], Bendix Labeit [1,2], Mao Ogawa [3], Tobias Warnecke [1], Rainer Wirth [4] and Rainer Dziewas [5]

[1] Department of Neurology with Institute for Translational Neurology, Albert-Schweitzer-Campus, 1 A, University Hospital Muenster, 48149 Muenster, Germany; karen.konert@uni-muenster.de (K.K.); sonja.suntrup-krueger@ukmuenster.de (S.S.-K.); inga.claus@ukmuenster.de (I.C.); bendixruven.labeit@ukmuenster.de (B.L.); tobias.warnecke@ukmuenster.de (T.W.)
[2] Institute for Biomagnetism and Biosignalanalysis, University Hospital Muenster, Malmedyweg 15, 48149 Muenster, Germany
[3] Department of Rehabilitation Medicine I, School of Medicine, Fujita Health University, Toyoake 470-1192, Japan; positiclub111@yahoo.co.jp
[4] Department of Geriatric Medicine, Marien Hospital Herne, University Hospital Ruhr-Universität Bochum, 44625 Herne, Germany; r.wirth@web.de
[5] Department of Neurology, Klinikum Osnabrück, Am Finkenhügel 1, 49076 Osnabrück, Germany; rainer.dziewas@klinikum-os.de
* Correspondence: muhlep@uni-muenster.de

Abstract: Patients in the neurological ICU are at risk of suffering from disorders of the upper gastrointestinal tract. Oropharyngeal dysphagia (OD) can be caused by the underlying neurological disease and/or ICU treatment itself. The latter was also identified as a risk factor for gastrointestinal dysmotility. However, its association with OD and the impact of the neurological condition is unclear. Here, we investigated a possible link between OD and gastric residual volume (GRV) in patients in the neurological ICU. In this retrospective single-center study, patients with an episode of mechanical ventilation (MV) admitted to the neurological ICU due to an acute neurological disease or acute deterioration of a chronic neurological condition from 2011–2017 were included. The patients were submitted to an endoscopic swallowing evaluation within 72 h of the completion of MV. Their GRV was assessed daily. Patients with $\geq$1 d of GRV $\geq$500 mL were compared to all the other patients. Regression analysis was performed to identify the predictors of GRV $\geq$500 mL/d. With respect to GRV, the groups were compared depending on their FEES scores (0–3). A total of 976 patients were included in this study. A total of 35% demonstrated a GRV of $\geq$500 mL/d at least once. The significant predictors of relevant GRV were age, male gender, infratentorial or hemorrhagic stroke, prolonged MV and poor swallowing function. The patients with the poorest swallowing function presented a GRV of $\geq$500 mL/d significantly more often than the patients who scored the best. Conclusions: Our findings indicate an association between dysphagia severity and delayed gastric emptying in critically ill neurologic patients. This may partly be due to lesions in the swallowing and gastric network.

Keywords: gastric residual volume; dysphagia; flexible endoscopic evaluation of swallowing; gastric emptying; intensive care; neurology; swallowing

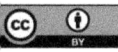

1. Introduction

The upper gastrointestinal (GI) tract consists of the mouth, pharynx, esophagus, stomach and duodenum. To provide sufficient nutrition and fluid intake, a finely tuned interaction between the structures of the GI tract is crucial [1–4], starting with the oropharyngeal phase of swallowing. Oropharyngeal dysphagia (OD) is a key feature of different neurological diseases, such as stroke, neuromuscular and neurodegenerative disorders [5].

Particularly in the context of neurocritical care, OD is associated with an increased risk of complications, such as malnutrition and aspiration pneumonia, and is also intimately linked to an overall poor prognosis [2,6,7]. The pathophysiology of OD is complex and may, according to the specific disease in question, involve damage to the central and/or peripheral levels of the swallowing network [2]. Furthermore, in the critically ill, direct trauma to the pharyngeal and laryngeal mucosa caused, for example, by endotracheal or nasogastric tubes, may worsen peripheral sensory feedback and thereby aggravate swallowing impairment [8].

GI motility is also frequently disordered in the critically ill, with up to 60% of patients having been reported to experience GI dysmotility of some form and necessitating therapeutic intervention [3,4]. GI dysmotility of the upper GI tract has significant clinical consequences, being associated with diminished provision of enteral nutrition and subsequent malnutrition, gastroesophageal reflux, and aspiration, as well as longer length of stay (LOS) in the intensive care unit (ICU) and increased mortality [9]. The pathophysiology of GI dysmotility in the critically ill is complex and, to a large extent, still unclear [4]. Interestingly, apart from the consequences of ICU treatment itself and, in particular, the GI side-effects of opioids and sedatives, alterations of hormonal pathways and impaired intrinsic modulation via enteric nerves [10], there is some evidence that dysfunction of the different parts of the nervous system may also contribute to GI dysmotility. Thus, probably because they also cause lesions to the cortical representation of the esophagus [11,12], acute strokes were shown to be related to esophageal dysmotility [13,14] and gastroesophageal reflux [15], ultimately increasing the risk of aspiration and subsequent pneumonia in affected patients [16]. In addition, patients with brain injuries have frequently been reported to present with delayed gastric emptying, resulting in gastric feeding intolerance and its sequelae [17–22].

In the present study, therefore, we investigate whether there is a correlation between OD and GI dysmotility, in particular delayed gastric emptying, in a comparatively large cohort of critically ill neurological patients requiring treatment in the ICU and mechanical ventilation (MV).

2. Materials and Methods
2.1. Study Design and Setting

This retrospective single-center investigation was conducted using the data of patients admitted to the neurological ICU of Münster University Hospital between January 2011 and December 2017. The inclusion criteria were: admittance to the neurological ICU due to an acute neurological disease, or the acute deterioration of a chronic neurological condition, an episode of MV and flexible fiberoptic endoscopic evaluation of swallowing (FEES) within 72 h of the completion of MV (either extubation or, in tracheotomized patients, the completion of weaning). The exclusion criteria were FEES $\geq$ 72 h after end of MV, palliative care and reduced vigilance ($\leq$8 points on the Glasgow Coma scale), due to its impact on swallowing function. The data were derived from the clinical documentation system.

2.2. Patient Characteristics and Clinical Parameters

The epidemiological data, including sex and age, the Body Mass Index, the modified Rankin Scale (mRS) [23] on admission and discharge, the Functional Oral Intake Scale on discharge (FOIS) [24], the RASS (Richmond-Agitation-Sedation-Scale) [25] at the time of initial FEES after the completion of weaning from MV, the Acute Physiology And Chronic Health Evaluation (APACHE) II [26] on admission and discharge, the occurrence of pneumonia [27], sepsis [28] or ileus, the duration of treatment with anti-infectives and, in the case of ischemic or hemorrhagic stroke, the supra- and/or infratentorial lesion location were extracted from the patients' files. Furthermore, if the volume of enteral nutrition (EN) was reduced and/or prokinetics were administered due to high gastric residual volume (GRV), this was recorded as well.

2.3. Dysphagia Assessment

According to our in-house guidelines, all the patients were examined at their bedside in an upright position by an experienced neurologist, together with a speech-language pathologist. The FEES were assessed according to the items 'secretion management', 'spontaneous swallowing' and 'laryngeal sensibility/cough'. These items were scored, as previously described, according to the "Standardized Endoscopic Swallowing Evaluation for Tracheostomy Decannulation in Critically Ill Neurologic Patients" (SESETD) [29,30]. For this purpose and for better comparability across the patient collective, the items were similarly rated in non-tracheotomized patients as well. The item 'saliva management' was considered failed if massive pooling (not only coating) causing an impaired view of the vocal folds and/or silent penetration and/or aspiration of pooled saliva (permanently without any reaction) occurred. 'Spontaneous swallows' were considered failed if ≤ 2 swallows occurred during 2 min of observation. If no reaction to touch of the arytenoids with the tip of the endoscope on both sides could be elicited, the item 'laryngeal sensibility' was rated as "not passed". Deriving from these three single items with passing = 1 point and failing = 0 points, a sum score was built, reaching from 0 to 3, as previously described [30]. All the examinations were part of local routine clinical care. The FEES were carried out using a 3.1-mm-diameter flexible fiberoptic rhinolaryngoscope (11101 RP2, Karl Storz, Tuttlingen, Germany), a combined light source and camera system (rp CAM-X, rpSzene®, Rehder/Partner, Hamburg, Germany) and a Medical Panel PC (WMP-226, Wincomm Corporation, Hsinchu, Taiwan) for display and recording. The videos were produced in standard definition quality. The data acquisition and analysis were approved by the local ethics committee.

2.4. Evaluation of Gastric Residual Volume

The amount of GRV was recorded daily (6 a.m. to 6 a.m.). For this purpose, the GRV drained into a reservoir connected to the gastric tube following gravity, according to our clinical routine and as previously described [31,32]. The reservoir was connected to the nasogastric tube (NGT) every 12 h for 1 h 30 min after the conclusion of EN. If vomiting or a significant amount of GRV were detected by our nursing staff, the EN was paused for 12 h. The patients were managed in a semi-recumbent position (30–45°) during the drainage of the GRV to prevent aspiration. Patients who had received in vivo thrombolysis and/or thrombectomy or surgery (e.g., external ventricular drainage) were kept nil-by-mouth for the first 24 h and EN was started thereafter. A GRV $\geq$500 mL/d on at least one day during the stay on the neurological ICU was defined as significant. This cut-off was chosen according to current recommendations and previous studies assuming this amount of GRV to be clinically relevant [31,32].

2.5. Statistical Analysis

The characteristics and clinical parameters of patients with vs. without increased GRV were compared. To test for a normal distribution of continuous variables, the Kolmogorov–Smirnov test was applied. For normally distributed data, the t-test was performed for group comparison, otherwise the Mann–Whitney U-test was used. The categorical variables were tested using the Fisher exact test in case the contingency tables included fewer than five cases and the chi^2-test was used in case of a larger sample size. The significance level was set at 0.05. The significant variables in these univariate analyses were later included in a multivariate binary logistic regression analysis to identify the independent predictors of relevant GRV. The variables that were only gathered at discharge were not included. Pearson correlation was applied to test for an association between initial FEES sum score and days with significant GRV. All the analyses were performed using SPSS 26.0 (IBM, Armonk, NY, USA).

3. Results

Of the 1461 patients admitted to the neurological ICU with an episode of MV during the observational period, for further analysis, 295 had to be excluded (see patient recruitment diagram, Figure 1). Hence, 976 patients (423 females) were included in this study (Figure 1) of whom 627 (64.2%) were tracheotomized.

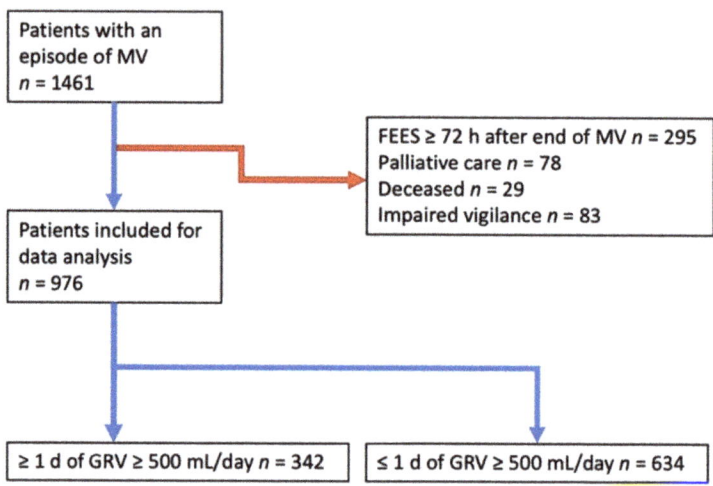

Figure 1. Recruitment flowchart; MV = mechanical ventilation; FEES = flexible endoscopic evaluation of swallowing; GRV = gastric residual volume; mL = milliliters.

The epidemiological and clinical parameters are summarized in Table 1. On the initial FEES following the conclusion of MV, 360 patients received a score of 0, indicating severe dysphagia (36.9%); 145 passed one of the three items used to evaluate swallowing function (14.9%); and 173 received a score of 2 (17.7%). A total of 297 patients passed all three items (30.4%).

Table 1. Epidemiological and clinical parameters and group test according to GRV.

	All n = 976	Max. GRV < 500 mL/d n = 634 (65.0%)	Max. GRV ≥ 500 mL/d n = 342 (35.0%)	p-Value
Age, mean (SD)	64.79 (±16.06)	66.78 (±16.06)	61.08 (±15.41)	<0.001 †
Female/Male, n (%)	423 (43.3)/553 (56.7)	301 (47.5)/333 (52.5)	122 (35.7)/220 (64.3)	<0.001 ‡
Body mass index, mean (SD)	26.61 (±5.15)	26.41 (±4.88)	26.92 (±5.59)	0.116 †
Ischemic stroke, n (%)	546 (55.9)	355 (60.0)	191 (55.8)	0.932 ‡
Hemorrhagic stroke, n (%)	155 (15.9)	85 (13.4)	70 (20.5)	0.004 ‡
Lesion location strokes				
Supratentorial, n (%)	569 (58.3)	367 (57.9)	202 (59.1)	0.722 ‡
Infratentorial, n (%)	132 (13.5)	73 (11.5)	59 (17.3)	0.014 ‡
Meningitis/Encephalitis, n (%)	76 (7.8)	55 (8.7)	21 (6.1)	0.159 ‡
GBS/AMAN, n (%)	24 (2.5)	15 (2.4)	9 (2.6)	0.798 ‡

Table 1. Cont.

	All n = 976	Max. GRV < 500 mL/d n = 634 (65.0%)	Max. GRV ≥ 500 mL/d n = 342 (35.0%)	p-Value
Myopathy/Myasthenia/Myositis, n (%)	13 (1.3)	9 (1.4)	4 (1.2)	1.000 §
Epilepsy, n (%)	82 (8.4)	58 (9.1)	24 (7.0)	0.252 ‡
Amyotrophic lateral sclerosis, n (%)	11 (1.1)	9 (1.4)	2 (0.6)	0.346 §
Others, n (%)	69 (7.1)	46 (7.3)	23 (6.7)	0.758 ‡
mRS on admission, mean [median]	4.57 [5 (4–5)]	4.59 [5 (4–5)]	4.54 [5 (4–5)]	0.135 †
APACHE II on admission, mean [median]	13.67 [13 (10–17)]	14.02 [14 (10–18)]	13.04 [13 (9–17)]	0.008 †
Mechanical ventilation (h), mean (SD)	334.05 (±355.18)	264.88 (±314.32)	462.28 (±389.77)	<0.001 †
LOS ICU (d), mean (SD)	27.94 (±20.62)	23.71 (±19.33)	35.76 (±20.67)	<0.001 †
FEES sum score after end of MV, mean [median]	1.42 [1 (0–3)]	1.55 [2 (0–3)]	1.17 [1 (0–2)]	<0.001 †
Aspiration/pooling, n (%)	463 (47.4)	269 (42.4)	194 (56.7)	<0.001 ‡
Swallowing frequency <2x/2 min, n (%)	457 (46.8)	268 (42.3)	189 (55.3)	<0.001 ‡
Failing sensory testing, n (%)	625 (64.0)	381 (60.1)	244 (71.3)	<0.001 ‡
Antiinfective treatment (d), mean (SD)	19.71 (±13.73)	17.40 (±13.34)	23.99 (±14.26)	<0.001 †
Pneumonia, n (%)	691 (70.8)	434 (68.5)	257 (75.1)	0.028 †
Sepsis, n (%)	78 (8.0)	39 (6.2)	39 (11.41)	0.004 ‡
Diabetes mellitus, n (%)	226 (23.2)	154 (24.3)	72 (21.1)	0.253 ‡
Medication due to high GRV, n (%)	465 (47.8)	203 (32.0)	334 (97.7)	<0.001 ‡
NGT/PEG on discharge, n (%)	533 (58.7)	318 (54.1)	215 (67.2)	<0.001 ‡
FOIS at discharge, mean [median]	3.25 [3 (1–5)]	3.49 [3 (1–6)]	2.83 [2 (1–5)]	<0.001 †
Deceased on ICU, n (%)	59 (6.0)	38 (6.0)	21 (6.1)	0.927 ‡
mRS at discharge, mean [median]	4.33 [5 (4–5)]	4.29 [5 (4–5)]	4.41 [5 (4–5)]	0.168 †

SD = standard deviation; h = hours; d = days; LOS = length of stay; ICU = intensive care unit; GRV = gastric residual volume; GBS = Guillain-Barré syndrome; AMAN = acute motor axonal neuropathy; mRS = modified Rankin Scale; FEES = flexible endoscopic evaluation of swallowing; EN = enteral nutrition; NGT = nasogastric tube, FOIS = Functional Oral Intake Scale; † = Mann–Whitney U-test; ‡ = chi²-test; § = Fisher-exact test.

We observed a significant negative correlation between FEES score and the number of days with relevant GRV (Pearson correlation coefficient −0.125, $p < 0.01$). The number of days of GRV ≥500 mL/d according to the initial FEES score after the conclusion of MV can be seen in Figure 2.

Comparing groups without vs. with significant GRV, the latter demonstrated a longer LOS in the ICU ($p < 0.001$) and duration of MV ($p < 0.001$), suffered from hemorrhagic stroke ($p = 0.004$) and infratentorial lesions more often ($p = 0.014$), were younger ($p < 0.001$), included more males ($p < 0.001$), received a lower APACHE II on admission ($p = 0.008$), scored worse on the initial FEES after the conclusion of weaning ($p < 0.001$), including every single item of the sum score, suffered more often from pneumonia ($p = 0.028$) or sepsis ($p = 0.004$) and were discharged from the hospital with PEG or NGT significantly more often ($p < 0.001$). Multivariate logistic regression analysis (Table 2) indicated the following factors as significant independent predictors of GRV ≥500 mL/d on at least one day: dysphagia severity as evaluated by the FEES sum score ($p = 0.010$), duration of MV

(p = 0.004), hemorrhagic stroke (p = 0.042), infratentorial lesion location of stroke (p = 0.019), age (p < 0.001) and male gender (p = 0.018).

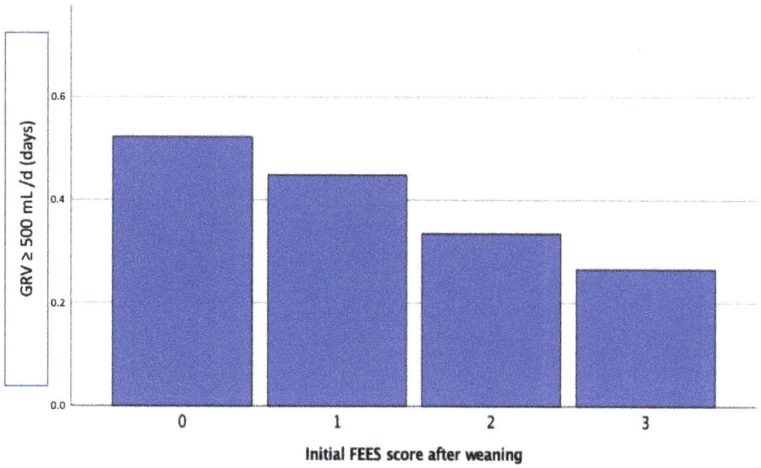

Figure 2. Days of gastric residual volume ≥500 mL/d, according to sum score on the first flexible endoscopic evaluation of swallowing (FEES) within 72 h of the conclusion of mechanical ventilation. Score 0: n = 360; Score 1: n = 146; Score 2: n = 173; Score 3: n = 297; GRV = gastric residual volume; mL = milliliters.

Table 2. Multivariate binary logistic regression analysis; outcome variable: GRV ≥ 500 mL/d on at least one day.

	Regression Coefficient	Adjusted Odds Ratio [95% CI]	p-Value
Age	−0.019	0.981 [0.971–0.991]	**<0.001**
Male gender (cat.)	0.351	1.421 [1.061–1.903]	**0.018**
Hemorrhagic stroke (cat.)	0.394	1.483 [1.015–2.166]	**0.042**
Infratentorial lesion location (stroke) (cat.)	0.491	1.634 [1.083–2.465]	**0.019**
Mechanical ventilation (hours)	0.001	1.001 [1.001–1.002]	**0.004**
LOS on the ICU (days)	0.012	1.102 [0.996–1.028]	0.146
FEES sum score initial FEES after end of weaning (cat.)	−0.155	0.857 [0.762–0.963]	**0.010**
APACHE II	−0.025	0.975 [0.948–1.002]	0.073
Days of antiinfective treatment	0.004	0.996 [0.978–1.015]	0.688
Sepsis (cat.)	0.322	1.380 [0.820–2.324]	0.226

cat = categorical; LOS = length of stay; ICU = Intensive Care Unit.

4. Discussion

In this study, we assessed the relationship between the occurrence and degree of GI dysmotility and OD in ventilated patients in the neurological ICU and tried to identify predictors of GI dysmotility in this cohort. In support of our hypothesis, our first main finding was that the impairment of swallowing function diagnosed at the conclusion of MV was associated with relevant GRV as a surrogate marker of GI dysmotility. While the GI tract possesses intrinsic neural plexus that allow a certain degree of autonomy over digestion and nutrient absorption, the central nervous system provides extrinsic input that regulates, modulates and controls these functions [33]. The small and large intestines exert comparatively independent neural control; the stomach, however, is considerably dependent on extrinsic neural inputs, particularly from the parasympathetic and sympathetic pathways connected to nuclei located in the caudal brainstem [33,34]. In line with this, relevant GRV was observed in patients with an infratentorial lesion significantly more often in our data. Recently, Rebollo et al. identified delayed connectivity between the brain and the slow electrical rhythm generated in the stomach using gastric-BOLD coupling, indicating a functional brain–gut link [35]. Within the brain, different nodes of this 'gastric network' were coupled to the gastric rhythm with different phase delays, indicating a temporal sequence of activations within this network—which, in principle, is similar to the central control of the swallowing network [36]. Interestingly, the gastric network partly comprises regions ('nodes') that are similarly found to be activated during swallowing, e.g., the primary and secondary somatosensory cortex and the supplementary motor area, as well as the insula [37–39]. Thus, the close clinical relation of both functions, in the present study may have been due to lesions that affected swallowing as well as the gastric network.

Our second main finding was that prolonged MV was a significant predictor of impaired gastric emptying, which was in line with previous findings [40]. There are indications that positive pressure mechanical ventilation leads to splanchnic vasoconstriction and gut-hypoperfusion, which is linked with increased plasma catecholamines and proinflammatory cytokine levels, both of which are related to delayed gastric emptying [41]. Furthermore, alterations in hormone levels in the critically ill have an impact on GI motility. Lowered ghrelin levels, as well as increased levels of cholecystokinin and peptide YY, were found in the critically ill and are linked with slower gastric emptying [42,43]. Sedatives such as Propofol and the use of opioids to provide sufficient analgesia during mechanical ventilation were shown to be associated with delayed gastric emptying, as well as the use of catecholamines/vasopressors [3,40,43]. Interestingly, swallowing function has also been shown to be worse in patients with prolonged mechanical ventilation and longer ICU treatment, as well as following the use of sedatives [44], supporting the hypothesis that—at least partly—the underlying mechanisms that cause impaired swallowing function and slowed gastric motility may be similar.

The third main finding was that patients suffering from intracranial hemorrhage seem to be at a particularly high risk of slowed gastric emptying. It was previously shown that intracranial hemorrhage is a risk factor for inferior swallowing function compared to ischemic stroke in patients with and without tracheostomy [45,46]. It was proposed that besides the specific localization [47] and volume of the intracranial hemorrhage [48], this may at least partly be attributed to secondary consequences of the hemorrhage, e.g., vasospasms [49], cisternal and interventricular blood or hydrocephalus [48]. There is more evidence that increased intracranial pressure is related to delayed gastric emptying. Thus, in a study of 21 brain-injured patients requiring sedation, MV and intracranial pressure monitoring for ≥24 h, increased intracranial pressure (>20 mmHg) was associated with reduced gastric emptying, as measured by the paracetamol absorption technique, possibly due to a decreased parasympathetic tonus [18]. In a study by Kao et al., 80% of head-injury patients exhibited abnormal gastric emptying halfway through liquid meals compared to healthy age-matched control subjects [20]. Using electrogastrography, it was further shown that brain trauma or coma cause gastric dysrhythmias and intolerance to feeding, supporting the hypothesis of an altered functional brain–gut link that causes delayed gastric emptying in patients with acquired brain injury [21].

As our fourth and fifth main findings, younger age and male gender were demonstrated to be related to delayed gastric emptying. Findings on the effects of ageing in the context of gastric motor function are inconsistent. Studies in healthy as well as critically ill patients found indications of declining gastric motor function with increasing age [43,50], whereas others identified a trend towards increased gastric emptying depending on increasing age in healthy adults [51]. In the neuro-ICU setting, as mentioned above, the influence of the intensive care treatment as well as the underlying condition causing the need for treatment may have caused the differing findings in the recent study. This can similarly be assumed for the gender differences. In general, gastric motility seems to be slower in healthy women than in healthy men [52] but there are indications that gastric motility may be less gender-specific depending on the consistency of administered boluses [53]. For a better understanding, the role of age as well as gender in the intensive care setting needs be investigated more closely.

The clinical relevance of GRV is still a matter of discussion. Generally, the intermittent measurement of GRV is a widely used practice to evaluate impaired gastric motility and feeding intolerance [4]. Several studies, including a meta-analysis, indicated that not monitoring GRV was not inferior to routine GRV measurement with regard to ICU-related infections, LOS in the ICU, length of MV and mortality. Furthermore, not monitoring GRV even improved the delivery of enteral nutrition [54–56]. These data were mainly derived from mixed cohorts. In stroke patients, who often suffer from dysphagia and impaired protective reflexes, Chen et al. observed that aspiration occurred significantly less often if GRV was monitored and the infusion rate of the EN was adjusted accordingly [57]. In our cohort of critically ill neurologic patients, relevant amounts of GRV were associated with pneumonia and sepsis. Pneumonia in the context of delayed gastric emptying in the critically ill is thought to be caused by aspiration due to gastro-esophageal reflux, which itself is a consequence of reduced esophageal sphincter tonus and increased residual volume in the stomach [4]. Dysphagia is another risk factor for pneumonia, notably as a result of aspiration [2]. Since patients with relevant GRV presented with a worse swallowing function, both disorders may foster each other. In line with this, patients with GI dysmotility presented a worse FOIS score at discharge and were more likely to be discharged with a feeding tube. Moreover, during systemic inflammation, intestinal edema deriving from capillary leakage influences GI function and cytokine release during sepsis, impedes intestinal myocyte function and inhibits enteric neuromuscular transmission [58–62].

Certain limitations to our study should be considered. First, the retrospective design may have introduced a bias into our data, which possibly include imprecise documentation of the patients' records. Second, all the patients were recruited on a single neurological ICU; hence, the transfer of findings to other environments and, in particular, to groups of patients with a different spectrum of diseases may be only be possible only to a limited extent. Third, bedside measures were previously shown to be imprecise in the identification of motility disorders [63]. While the intermittent measurement of GRV may be the most common practice through which gastric motility disorders are evaluated, indirect tests, such as the carbohydrate absorption (3-OMG), the radio-isotope breath ($_{13}CO_2$) or the aforementioned paracetamol absorption test, as well as gastric scintigraphy, evaluate gastric dysmotility with more precision, although they are not always applicable in the ICU setting [4]. Fourth, with regards to the impact of our findings, no long-term outcome assessment was available.

5. Conclusions

The findings in this study indicate an association between delayed gastric emptying and dysphagia severity in critically ill neurologic patients in the ICU. Beside the effects of intensive care treatment, there are indications that central lesions in the swallowing and gastric network both add to the deterioration of swallowing function as well as to the impairment of upper GI motility.

Author Contributions: P.M.: writing—original draft preparation, data curation, investigation K.K.: data curation, investigation; S.S.-K.: investigation, writing—original draft preparation, formal analysis; I.C.: data curation, writing—reviewing and editing; B.L.: visualization, validation, writing—reviewing and editing; M.O.: data curation, validation, writing—reviewing; T.W.: conceptualization, methodology, supervision; R.W.: methodology, writing—reviewing; R.D.: conceptualization, supervision, project administration, writing—reviewing. All authors have read and agreed to the published version of the manuscript.

Funding: This work was supported by the Deutsche Forschungsgemeinschaft [grant number SU 922/1–1, WO1425/6–1, DZ 78/1–1].

Institutional Review Board Statement: The study was conducted according to the guidelines of the Declaration of Helsinki, and approved by the Ethics Committee of the Ärztekammer Westfalen-Lippe and the Westfalian Wilhelms-University (2016-391-f-S; date: 12 August 2016).

Informed Consent Statement: Patient consent was waived due to the retrospective design of the study.

Data Availability Statement: The data presented in this study are available on request from the corresponding author. The data are not publicly available due to hospital policy.

Conflicts of Interest: The authors declare no conflict of interest.

References

1. Dodds, W.J.; Stewart, E.T.; Logemann, J.A. Physiology and radiology of the normal oral and pharyngeal phases of swallowing. *AJR Am. J. Roentgenol.* **1990**, *154*, 953–963. [CrossRef]
2. Zuercher, P.; Moret, C.S.; Dziewas, R.; Schefold, J.C. Dysphagia in the intensive care unit: Epidemiology, mechanisms, and clinical management. *Crit. Care* **2019**, *23*, 103. [CrossRef] [PubMed]
3. Deane, A.M.; Chapman, M.J.; Reintam Blaser, A.; McClave, S.A.; Emmanuel, A. Pathophysiology and Treatment of Gastrointestinal Motility Disorders in the Acutely Ill. *Nutr. Clin. Pract.* **2019**, *34*, 23–36. [CrossRef]
4. Ladopoulos, T.; Giannaki, M.; Alexopoulou, C.; Proklou, A.; Pediaditis, E.; Kondili, E. Gastrointestinal dysmotility in critically ill patients. *Ann. Gastroenterol.* **2018**, *31*, 273–281. [CrossRef]
5. Dziewas, R.; Baijens, L.; Schindler, A.; Verin, E.; Michou, E.; Clave, P. European Society for Swallowing Disorders FEES Accreditation Program for Neurogenic and Geriatric Oropharyngeal Dysphagia. *Dysphagia* **2017**, *32*, 725–733. [CrossRef]
6. Schröder, J.B.; Glahn, J.; Dziewas, R. ICU-related dysphagia. Epidemiology, pathophysiology, diagnostics and treatment. *ICU Manag* **2015**, *15*, 108–111.
7. Schefold, J.C.; Berger, D.; Zurcher, P.; Lensch, M.; Perren, A.; Jakob, S.M.; Parviainen, I.; Takala, J. Dysphagia in Mechanically Ventilated ICU Patients (DYnAMICS): A Prospective Observational Trial. *Crit. Care Med.* **2017**, *45*, 2061–2069. [CrossRef] [PubMed]
8. Scheel, R.; Pisegna, J.M.; McNally, E.; Noordzij, J.P.; Langmore, S.E. Endoscopic Assessment of Swallowing after Prolonged Intubation in the ICU Setting. *Ann. Otol. Rhinol. Laryngol.* **2016**, *125*, 43–52. [CrossRef]
9. Blaser, A.R.; Starkopf, J.; Kirsimagi, U.; Deane, A.M. Definition, prevalence, and outcome of feeding intolerance in intensive care: A systematic review and meta-analysis. *Acta Anaesthesiol. Scand.* **2014**, *58*, 914–922. [CrossRef] [PubMed]
10. Phillips, L.K.; Deane, A.M.; Jones, K.L.; Rayner, C.K.; Horowitz, M. Gastric emptying and glycaemia in health and diabetes mellitus. *Nat. Rev. Endocrinol.* **2015**, *11*, 112–128. [CrossRef] [PubMed]
11. Aziz, Q.; Thompson, D.G.; Ng, V.W.; Hamdy, S.; Sarkar, S.; Brammer, M.J.; Bullmore, E.T.; Hobson, A.; Tracey, I.; Gregory, L.; et al. Cortical processing of human somatic and visceral sensation. *J. Neurosci.* **2000**, *20*, 2657–2663. [CrossRef]
12. Dziewas, R.; Soros, P.; Ishii, R.; Chau, W.; Henningsen, H.; Ringelstein, E.B.; Knecht, S.; Pantev, C. Cortical processing of esophageal sensation is related to the representation of swallowing. *Neuroreport* **2005**, *16*, 439–443. [CrossRef] [PubMed]
13. Micklefield, G.H.; Jorgensen, E.; Blaeser, I.; Jorg, J.; Kobberling, J. Esophageal manometric studies in patients with an apoplectic stroke with/without oropharyngeal dysphagia. *Dtsch. Med. Wochenschr.* **1999**, *124*, 239–244. [CrossRef]
14. Micklefield, G.; Jorgensen, E.; Blaeser, I.; Jorg, J.; Kobberling, J. Motility disorders of the esophagus in patients with apoplectic infarct during the acute illness phase. *Med. Klin.* **1999**, *94*, 245–250. [CrossRef]
15. Satou, Y.; Oguro, H.; Murakami, Y.; Onoda, K.; Mitaki, S.; Hamada, C.; Mizuhara, R.; Yamaguchi, S. Gastroesophageal reflux during enteral feeding in stroke patients: A 24-hour esophageal pH-monitoring study. *J. Stroke Cerebrovasc. Dis.* **2013**, *22*, 185–189. [CrossRef]
16. Langdon, P.C.; Lee, A.H.; Binns, C.W. High incidence of respiratory infections in 'nil by mouth' tube-fed acute ischemic stroke patients. *Neuroepidemiology* **2009**, *32*, 107–113. [CrossRef] [PubMed]
17. Lucena, A.F.; Tiburcio, R.V.; Vasconcelos, G.C.; Ximenes, J.D.; Cristino Filho, G.; Graca, R.V. Influence of acute brain injuries on gut motility. *Rev. Bras. Ter. Intensiva* **2011**, *23*, 96–103. [CrossRef] [PubMed]
18. McArthur, C.J.; Gin, T.; McLaren, I.M.; Critchley, J.A.; Oh, T.E. Gastric emptying following brain injury: Effects of choice of sedation and intracranial pressure. *Intensive Care Med.* **1995**, *21*, 573–576. [CrossRef]
19. Bochicchio, G.V.; Bochicchio, K.; Nehman, S.; Casey, C.; Andrews, P.; Scalea, T.M. Tolerance and efficacy of enteral nutrition in traumatic brain-injured patients induced into barbiturate coma. *JPEN J. Parenter. Enter. Nutr.* **2006**, *30*, 503–506. [CrossRef]
20. Kao, C.H.; ChangLai, S.P.; Chieng, P.U.; Yen, T.C. Gastric emptying in head-injured patients. *Am. J. Gastroenterol.* **1998**, *93*, 1108–1112. [CrossRef] [PubMed]
21. Thor, P.J.; Goscinski, I.; Kolasinska-Kloch, W.; Madroszkiewicz, D.; Madroszkiewicz, E.; Furgala, A. Gastric myoelectric activity in patients with closed head brain injury. *Med. Sci. Monit.* **2003**, *9*, CR392–CR395. [PubMed]

22. Dickerson, R.N.; Mitchell, J.N.; Morgan, L.M.; Maish, G.O., 3rd; Croce, M.A.; Minard, G.; Brown, R.O. Disparate response to metoclopramide therapy for gastric feeding intolerance in trauma patients with and without traumatic brain injury. *JPEN J. Parenter. Enter. Nutr.* **2009**, *33*, 646–655. [CrossRef] [PubMed]
23. Van Swieten, J.C.; Koudstaal, P.J.; Visser, M.C.; Schouten, H.J.; van Gijn, J. Interobserver agreement for the assessment of handicap in stroke patients. *Stroke* **1988**, *19*, 604–607. [CrossRef]
24. Crary, M.A.; Mann, G.D.; Groher, M.E. Initial psychometric assessment of a functional oral intake scale for dysphagia in stroke patients. *Arch. Phys. Med. Rehabil.* **2005**, *86*, 1516–1520. [CrossRef]
25. Sessler, C.N.; Gosnell, M.S.; Grap, M.J.; Brophy, G.M.; O'Neal, P.V.; Keane, K.A.; Tesoro, E.P.; Elswick, R.K. The Richmond Agitation-Sedation Scale: Validity and reliability in adult intensive care unit patients. *Am. J. Respir. Crit. Care Med.* **2002**, *166*, 1338–1344. [CrossRef] [PubMed]
26. Knaus, W.A.; Draper, E.A.; Wagner, D.P.; Zimmerman, J.E. Apache II: A severity of disease classification system. *Crit. Care Med.* **1985**, *13*, 818–829. [CrossRef]
27. Mann, G.; Hankey, G.J.; Cameron, D. Swallowing disorders following acute stroke: Prevalence and diagnostic accuracy. *Cerebrovasc. Dis.* **2000**, *10*, 380–386. [CrossRef]
28. Bone, R.C.; Balk, R.A.; Cerra, F.B.; Dellinger, R.P.; Fein, A.M.; Knaus, W.A.; Schein, R.M.; Sibbald, W.J. Definitions for sepsis and organ failure and guidelines for the use of innovative therapies in sepsis. The ACCP/SCCM Consensus Conference Committee. American College of Chest Physicians/Society of Critical Care Medicine. *Chest* **1992**, *101*, 1644–1655. [CrossRef] [PubMed]
29. Warnecke, T.; Suntrup, S.; Teismann, I.K.; Hamacher, C.; Oelenberg, S.; Dziewas, R. Standardized endoscopic swallowing evaluation for tracheostomy decannulation in critically ill neurologic patients. *Crit. Care Med.* **2013**, *41*, 1728–1732. [CrossRef]
30. Warnecke, T.; Muhle, P.; Claus, I.; Schröder, J.B.; Labeit, B.; Lapa, S.; Suntrup-Krueger, S.; Dziewas, R. Inter-rater and test-retest Reliability of the "Standardized Endoscopic Swallowing Evaluation for Tracheostomy Decannulation in Critically Ill Neurologic Patients". *Neurol. Res. Pract.* **2020**, *2*, 9. [CrossRef]
31. Montejo, J.C.; Minambres, E.; Bordeje, L.; Mesejo, A.; Acosta, J.; Heras, A.; Ferre, M.; Fernandez-Ortega, F.; Vaquerizo, C.I.; Manzanedo, R. Gastric residual volume during enteral nutrition in ICU patients: The REGANE study. *Intensive Care Med.* **2010**, *36*, 1386–1393. [CrossRef] [PubMed]
32. Reintam Blaser, A.; Starkopf, J.; Alhazzani, W.; Berger, M.M.; Casaer, M.P.; Deane, A.M.; Fruhwald, S.; Hiesmayr, M.; Ichai, C.; Jakob, S.M.; et al. Early enteral nutrition in critically ill patients: ESICM clinical practice guidelines. *Intensive Care Med.* **2017**, *43*, 380–390. [CrossRef] [PubMed]
33. Browning, K.N.; Travagli, R.A. Central nervous system control of gastrointestinal motility and secretion and modulation of gastrointestinal functions. *Compr. Physiol.* **2014**, *4*, 1339–1368. [CrossRef] [PubMed]
34. Deane, A.; Chapman, M.J.; Fraser, R.J.; Bryant, L.K.; Burgstad, C.; Nguyen, N.Q. Mechanisms underlying feed intolerance in the critically ill: Implications for treatment. *World J. Gastroenterol.* **2007**, *13*, 3909–3917. [CrossRef]
35. Rebollo, I.; Devauchelle, A.D.; Beranger, B.; Tallon-Baudry, C. Stomach-brain synchrony reveals a novel, delayed-connectivity resting-state network in humans. *Elife* **2018**, *7*, e33321. [CrossRef] [PubMed]
36. Teismann, I.K.; Dziewas, R.; Steinstraeter, O.; Pantev, C. Time-dependent hemispheric shift of the cortical control of volitional swallowing. *Hum. Brain Mapp.* **2009**, *30*, 92–100. [CrossRef] [PubMed]
37. Nachev, P.; Kennard, C.; Husain, M. Functional role of the supplementary and pre-supplementary motor areas. *Nat. Rev. Neurosci.* **2008**, *9*, 856–869. [CrossRef]
38. Hamdy, S.; Mikulis, D.J.; Crawley, A.; Xue, S.; Lau, H.; Henry, S.; Diamant, N.E. Cortical activation during human volitional swallowing: An event-related fMRI study. *Am. J. Physiol.* **1999**, *277*, G219–G225. [CrossRef]
39. Dziewas, R.; Soros, P.; Ishii, R.; Chau, W.; Henningsen, H.; Ringelstein, E.B.; Knecht, S.; Pantev, C. Neuroimaging evidence for cortical involvement in the preparation and in the act of swallowing. *Neuroimage* **2003**, *20*, 135–144. [CrossRef]
40. Rhoney, D.H.; Parker, D., Jr.; Formea, C.M.; Yap, C.; Coplin, W.M. Tolerability of bolus versus continuous gastric feeding in brain-injured patients. *Neurol. Res.* **2002**, *24*, 613–620. [CrossRef]
41. Mutlu, G.M.; Mutlu, E.A.; Factor, P. GI complications in patients receiving mechanical ventilation. *Chest* **2001**, *119*, 1222–1241. [CrossRef] [PubMed]
42. Luttikhold, J.; de Ruijter, F.M.; van Norren, K.; Diamant, M.; Witkamp, R.F.; van Leeuwen, P.A.; Vermeulen, M.A. Review article: The role of gastrointestinal hormones in the treatment of delayed gastric emptying in critically ill patients. *Aliment. Pharmacol. Ther.* **2013**, *38*, 573–583. [CrossRef]
43. Heyland, D.K.; Tougas, G.; King, D.; Cook, D.J. Impaired gastric emptying in mechanically ventilated, critically ill patients. *Intensive Care Med.* **1996**, *22*, 1339–1344. [CrossRef] [PubMed]
44. Macht, M.; Wimbish, T.; Bodine, C.; Moss, M. ICU-acquired swallowing disorders. *Crit. Care Med.* **2013**, *41*, 2396–2405. [CrossRef]
45. Catalino, M.P.; Lin, F.C.; Davis, N.; Anderson, K.; Olm-Shipman, C.; Dedrick Jordan, J. Early versus late tracheostomy after decompressive craniectomy for stroke. *J. Intensive Care* **2018**, *6*, 6. [CrossRef]
46. Suntrup, S.; Warnecke, T.; Kemmling, A.; Teismann, I.K.; Hamacher, C.; Oelenberg, S.; Dziewas, R. Dysphagia in patients with acute striatocapsular hemorrhage. *J. Neurol.* **2012**, *259*, 93–99. [CrossRef]
47. Keser, T.; Kofler, M.; Katzmayr, M.; Schiefecker, A.J.; Rass, V.; Ianosi, B.A.; Lindner, A.; Gaasch, M.; Beer, R.; Rhomberg, P.; et al. Risk Factors for Dysphagia and the Impact on Outcome after Spontaneous Subarachnoid Hemorrhage. *Neurocrit. Care* **2019**, *33*, 132–139. [CrossRef]

48. Rhie, S.H.; Choi, J.W.; Jeon, S.J.; Kang, S.D.; Joo, M.C.; Kim, M.S. Characteristics of Patients with Aneurysmal Subarachnoid Hemorrhage and Risk Factors Related to Dysphagia. *Ann. Rehabil. Med.* **2016**, *40*, 1024–1032. [CrossRef]
49. Dunn, K.; Rumbach, A. Incidence and Risk Factors for Dysphagia following Non-traumatic Subarachnoid Hemorrhage: A Retrospective Cohort Study. *Dysphagia* **2019**, *34*, 229–239. [CrossRef] [PubMed]
50. Horowitz, M.; Maddern, G.J.; Chatterton, B.E.; Collins, P.J.; Harding, P.E.; Shearman, D.J. Changes in gastric emptying rates with age. *Clin. Sci. (Lond)* **1984**, *67*, 213–218. [CrossRef] [PubMed]
51. Saad, R.J.; Semler, J.R.; Wilding, G.E.; Chey, W.D. The Effect of Age on Regional and Whole Gut Transit Times in Healthy Adults. *Gastroenterology* **2010**, *138*, 127. [CrossRef]
52. Mori, H.; Suzuki, H.; Matsuzaki, J.; Taniguchi, K.; Shimizu, T.; Yamane, T.; Masaoka, T.; Kanai, T. Gender Difference of Gastric Emptying in Healthy Volunteers and Patients with Functional Dyspepsia. *Digestion* **2017**, *95*, 72–78. [CrossRef] [PubMed]
53. Bennink, R.; Peeters, M.; Van den Maegdenbergh, V.; Geypens, B.; Rutgeerts, P.; De Roo, M.; Mortelmans, L. Comparison of total and compartmental gastric emptying and antral motility between healthy men and women. *Eur. J. Nucl. Med.* **1998**, *25*, 1293–1299. [CrossRef]
54. Reignier, J.; Mercier, E.; Le Gouge, A.; Boulain, T.; Desachy, A.; Bellec, F.; Clavel, M.; Frat, J.P.; Plantefeve, G.; Quenot, J.P.; et al. Effect of not monitoring residual gastric volume on risk of ventilator-associated pneumonia in adults receiving mechanical ventilation and early enteral feeding: A randomized controlled trial. *JAMA* **2013**, *309*, 249–256. [CrossRef]
55. Wang, Z.; Ding, W.; Fang, Q.; Zhang, L.; Liu, X.; Tang, Z. Effects of not monitoring gastric residual volume in intensive care patients: A meta-analysis. *Int. J. Nurs. Stud.* **2019**, *91*, 86–93. [CrossRef] [PubMed]
56. Poulard, F.; Dimet, J.; Martin-Lefevre, L.; Bontemps, F.; Fiancette, M.; Clementi, E.; Lebert, C.; Renard, B.; Reignier, J. Impact of not measuring residual gastric volume in mechanically ventilated patients receiving early enteral feeding: A prospective before-after study. *JPEN J. Parenter. Enteral. Nutr.* **2010**, *34*, 125–130. [CrossRef] [PubMed]
57. Chen, S.; Xian, W.; Cheng, S.; Zhou, C.; Zhou, H.; Feng, J.; Liu, L.; Chen, L. Risk of regurgitation and aspiration in patients infused with different volumes of enteral nutrition. *Asia Pac. J. Clin. Nutr.* **2015**, *24*, 212–218. [CrossRef]
58. Ohno, T.; Mochiki, E.; Kuwano, H. The roles of motilin and ghrelin in gastrointestinal motility. *Int. J. Pept.* **2010**, *2010*. [CrossRef]
59. Nguyen, N.Q.; Fraser, R.J.; Bryant, L.K.; Chapman, M.J.; Wishart, J.; Holloway, R.H.; Butler, R.; Horowitz, M. The relationship between gastric emptying, plasma cholecystokinin, and peptide YY in critically ill patients. *Crit. Care* **2007**, *11*, R132. [CrossRef] [PubMed]
60. Crona, D.; MacLaren, R. Gastrointestinal hormone concentrations associated with gastric feeding in critically ill patients. *JPEN J. Parenter. Enteral. Nutr.* **2012**, *36*, 189–196. [CrossRef] [PubMed]
61. Camilleri, M.; Papathanasopoulos, A.; Odunsi, S.T. Actions and therapeutic pathways of ghrelin for gastrointestinal disorders. *Nat. Rev. Gastroenterol. Hepatol.* **2009**, *6*, 343–352. [CrossRef] [PubMed]
62. Overhaus, M.; Togel, S.; Pezzone, M.A.; Bauer, A.J. Mechanisms of polymicrobial sepsis-induced ileus. *Am. J. Physiol. Gastrointest. Liver Physiol.* **2004**, *287*, G685–G694. [CrossRef] [PubMed]
63. Ukleja, A. Altered GI motility in critically Ill patients: Current understanding of pathophysiology, clinical impact, and diagnostic approach. *Nutr. Clin. Pract.* **2010**, *25*, 16–25. [CrossRef] [PubMed]

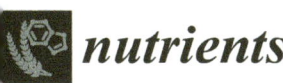

Article

Impact of COVID-19 Lockdown on Anthropometric Variables, Blood Pressure, and Glucose and Lipid Profile in Healthy Adults: A before and after Pandemic Lockdown Longitudinal Study

José Ignacio Ramírez Manent [1,2], Bárbara Altisench Jané [1,*], Pilar Sanchís Cortés [2,3], Carla Busquets-Cortés [4,5], Sebastiana Arroyo Bote [4,5], Luis Masmiquel Comas [1,2] and Ángel Arturo López González [2,4,5]

[1] General Practitioner Department, Balearic Islands Health Service, 07003 Palma, Illes Balears, Spain; jignacioramirez@telefonica.net (J.I.R.M.); lmasmiquel@hsll.es (L.M.C.)
[2] Health Institute of the Balearic Islands (IDISBA), Balearic Islands Health Research Institute Foundation, 07003 Palma, Illes Balears, Spain; pilar.sanchis@uib.es (P.S.C.); angarturo@gmail.com (Á.A.L.G.)
[3] Chemistry Department, University Balearic Islands, 07003 Palma, Illes Balears, Spain
[4] Faculty of Odontology, University School ADEMA Palma, 07003 Palma, Illes Balears, Spain; cbusquets@eua.edu.es (C.B.-C.); sarroyobote@hotmail.com (S.A.B.)
[5] Investigation Group IUNICS, Health Research Institute of the Balearic Islands (IDISBA), 07003 Palma, Illes Balears, Spain
* Correspondence: baltisench@gmail.com

Abstract: In December 2019, 27 cases of pneumonia were reported in Wuhan. In 2020, the causative agent was identified as a virus called SARS-CoV-2. The disease was called "coronavirus disease 2019" (COVID-19) and was determined as a Public Health Emergency. The main measures taken to cope with this included a state of lockdown. The aim of this study was to assess how the unhealthy lifestyles that ensued influenced different parameters. A prospective study was carried out on 6236 workers in a Spanish population between March 2019 and March 2021. Anthropometric, clinical, and analytical measurements were performed, revealing differences in the mean values of anthropometric and clinical parameters before and after lockdown due to the pandemic, namely increased body weight (41.1 ± 9.9–43.1 ± 9.9), BMI (25.1 ± 4.7–25.9 ± 4.7), and percentage of body fat (24.5 ± 9.1–26.9 ± 8.8); higher total cholesterol levels, with a statistically significant increase in LDL levels and a reduction in HDL; and worse glucose levels (90.5 ± 16.4–95.4 ± 15.8). Lockdown can be concluded to have had a negative effect on health parameters in both sexes in all age ranges, causing a worsening of cardiovascular risk factors.

Keywords: COVID-19; cardiovascular risk factors; lockdown; disease

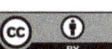

1. Introduction

In December 2019, 27 cases of severe pneumonia of unknown cause were reported in the city of Wuhan (Hubei, China), which had in common their appearance in a wholesale market for fish and live animals [1]. On 7 January 2020, the causative agent was identified as a new virus (Coronaviridae), called SARS-CoV-2 [2]. The disease caused by this virus became internationally known as "coronavirus disease 2019" (COVID-19). The most common clinical manifestations were fever, cough, fatigue, and gastrointestinal symptoms. Respiratory or gastrointestinal symptoms could coexist or be found in isolation [3–5]. Depending on individual genetics, ethnic origin, age and geographical location, it has been seen that the clinical manifestations and morbidity and mortality from COVID-19 are different [6–8]. On 30 January 2020, COVID-19 was determined as a Public Health Emergency of International Importance (ESPII) and later, on 11 March 2020, declared a global pandemic by the WHO [5].

The rapid spread and severity of the COVID-19 pandemic became a threat to public health, with the lack of effective drugs or vaccines at that time leading governments of more than 100 countries to apply strict measures in their efforts to limit and control the spread of the disease [9,10]. Measures such as a lockdown, quarantine, or isolation of their populations were put in place, in such a way that in April 2020 more than a third of the world's population was under some type of lockdown [11]. In Spain this was established by Royal Decree 463/2020 of March 14, declaring a state of emergency [12].

This state of lockdown had a negative impact on the physical and mental health of the population, with a decrease in physical activity and a significant change in eating patterns at all ages [13–18]. Lifestyle modifications and withdrawal from work, university, or school are all related to boredom and were discovered to cause bingeing or loss of appetite [13,19,20]. A decrease in the consumption of fish, seafood, fruit, and vegetables was found, along with [21] a rise in the consumption of salty and sugary snacks (including desserts, sweets, chips, nuts, crackers, popcorn, peanuts, pistachios, sunflower seeds, etc.) [22,23]. There was also a high prevalence of sleep [24–26] and physical activity disorders [6], which are related to unbalanced nutritional patterns in adults and adolescents [27,28].

Consequently, there was an increase in weight in the world population range from 11.1% to 72.4% during the lockdown period. In Spain, the weight gain reported by patients themselves ranged between 12.8% and 44% [29]. People who put on weight during the lockdown also had a more sedentary lifestyle most of the time - watching television and doing on-screen leisure activities, using smartphones, the internet, or socializing online. This weight gain related to COVID-19 will cause an increased risk of developing metabolic disorders in the population with a previous diagnosis of disease [30], but also in the population who had not suffered from these disorders beforehand [31]. Moreover, it has been observed that the population with previous pathology has a higher risk of becoming severely ill if infected by the virus [31,32].

Our objective was to evaluate how these unhealthy lifestyles influenced different anthropometric parameters, blood glucose levels, lipid profile, and blood pressure in a sample of 6236 workers in Spain, with the aim that if at some future time a similar situation occurs, we would be able to take adequate preventive measures to reduce its side effects on people's health and the development of disease.

2. Materials and Methods

A prospective study was carried out on 6283 workers in the Balearic Islands and the Valencian Community in companies from different productive sectors, the most represented were working at hotels, construction, commerce, health and public administration, transport, education and the cleaning industry between March 2019 and March 2021. Employees were selected from among those who attended the periodic occupational medical check-ups during those years. Of these, 47 were excluded (19 since they did not agree to participate and 28 since they did not undergo the second medical examination), leaving 6236 finally included in the study (Figure 1).

Inclusion criteria

- Aged between 18 and 69 years;
- Being an active worker;
- Healthy population, without underlying diseases that do not allow passing the annual medical check-up;
- Belonging to one of the companies collaborating in the study;
- Agreeing to participate in the study.

Anthropometric, clinical, and analytical measurements were performed by the health personnel of the different occupational health units participating in the study, after homogenizing the measurement techniques. To measure weight, expressed in kilograms, and height, expressed in cm, a scale with a measuring rod was used, namely model SECA 700 with a capacity of 200 kg and 50-g divisions, with a SECA 220 telescopic measuring rod with millimetric division and a 60–200 cm interval.

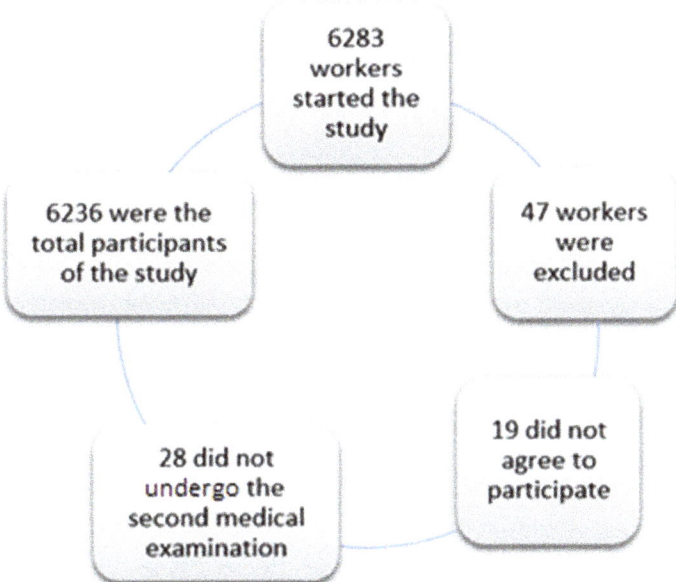

Figure 1. Flowchart of participants.

Abdominal waist circumference was measured in cm with a measuring tape (SECA model 20, with an interval of 1–200 cm and millimeter division). The person stood feet together and trunk erect, abdomen relaxed, and upper limbs hanging on both sides of the body. The tape measure was placed parallel to the floor at the level of the last floating rib. Hip circumference was measured with a SECA model 200 tape with a measuring interval of 12–200 cm and millimeter division. The same position was adopted as for waist circumference and the measuring tape was passed horizontally at hip level. Waist/height and waist/hip indices were obtained by dividing waist circumference by height and hip circumference, respectively. The cut-off point for the former was 0.50 while for the latter it was 0.85 for females and 0.95 for males [33].

Blood pressure was measured in the supine position with a calibrated OMRON M3 automatic sphygmomanometer after 10 min of rest. Three measurements were taken at one-minute intervals and the mean of the three was calculated. Blood tests were obtained by peripheral venepuncture after a 12-h fast, sent to reference laboratories, and processed within 48–72 h. Automated enzymatic methods were used for blood glucose, total cholesterol, and triglycerides. Values are expressed in mg/dL. HDL was determined by precipitation with dextran sulphate Cl2Mg, and values are expressed in mg/dL. LDL was calculated using the Friedewald formula (provided triglycerides were less than 400 mg/dL). Values are expressed in mg/dL.

Friedewald's formula:

$$LDL = \text{total cholesterol} - HDL - \text{triglycerides}/5$$

BMI was calculated by dividing weight by height in meters squared. Obesity was considered to be over 30 [33]. Body fat percentage was determined by bioimpedance using a Tanita model MC-780MA S.

A smoker was considered to be a person who had regularly consumed at least one cigarette/day (or the equivalent in other types of consumption) in the previous month or had stopped smoking less than a year before.

Physical activity was determined by means of the International Physical Activity Questionnaire (IPAQ) [34], a seven-question self-administered questionnaire that assesses the type of physical activity performed in daily life during the previous seven days which was performed at each medical check-up.

2.1. Statistical Analysis

A descriptive analysis of the categorical variables was carried out by calculating the frequency and distribution of responses for each one. For quantitative variables, the mean and standard deviation were calculated, whereas for qualitative variables, the percentage was calculated. Bivariate association analysis was performed using the X^2 test (with correction of Fisher's exact statistic when conditions so required) and Student's t test for independent samples. For multivariate analysis, binary logistic regression was used with the Wald method, with calculation of the odds ratio and the Hosmer-Lemeshow goodness-of-fit test. The statistical analysis was performed with the SPSS 27.0 (IBM, New York, USA) program, with an accepted statistical significance level of 0.05.

2.2. Ethical Considerations and Aspects

The study was approved by the Clinical Research Ethics Committee of the Balearic Islands Health Area no. IB 4383/20. All procedures were performed in accordance with the ethical standards of the institutional research committee and with the 2013 Declaration of Helsinki. All patients signed written informed consent documents before participating in the study.

3. Results

Lockdown began for all participants on 15 March 2020, and post-lockdown anthropometric measurements were carried out by the same health personnel from the different occupational health units. Of the 6283 workers, 51.9% were female and 48.1% were male, constituting a proportional representation of both sexes. Participant characteristics, including anthropometric characteristics, physical activity, and smoking before and after lockdown, are all summarized in Table 1. The number of participants was the same each year, being a total of 6236 Spanish workers.

Table 1 shows the statistically significant differences in the mean values of anthropometric and clinical parameters before and after lockdown due to the COVID-19 pandemic.

An increase in body weight and therefore also in BMI can be seen in the population studied; as well as an increase in the percentage of body fat, and hip and waist circumference; being this the one with the highest increase. Regarding clinical parameters, the elevation of total cholesterol levels stands out, with a statistically significant increase in LDL levels (going from mean values of 117.4 mg/dL to 131 mg/dL) and a reduction in HDL levels. Triglyceride values also rose.

Comparing blood pressure levels, during lockdown there was a tendency to higher diastolic blood pressure levels. Systolic blood pressure was also affected. Glucose levels increased during lockdown such as the previously analyzed parameters.

The percentage of people who increased their smoking habit during lockdown was 2%, while an 11% decrease their physical activity, causing an elevation of 4.1% in overweight and 2.5% in obesity.

Comparing the mean values of the anthropometric, clinical, and laboratory parameters in different ranges of years according to whether this change occurred before or during the COVID-19 pandemic lockdown, it is possible to observe a tendency to a worsening of the values of the different parameters analyzed, as shown in Table 2.

Table 1. Characteristics of the population.

	Year 2018	Year 2019	Year 2020	
N = 6236	Mean ± SD	Mean ± SD	Mean ± SD	p-Value
Age (years)	41.1 ± 9.9	42.1 ± 9.9	43.1 ± 9.9	<0.001
Weight (kg)	71.7 ± 16.3	72.2 ± 16.4	73.8 ± 16.5	<0.001
BMI (kg/m^2)	25.1 ± 4.7	25.3 ± 4,7	25.9 ± 4.7	<0.001
Waist circumference (cm)	82.8 ± 14.0	84.6 ± 14.1	87.6 ± 14.1	<0.001
Hip circumference (cm)	98.7 ± 9.4	99.8 ± 9.4	101.5 ± 9.5	<0.001
Waist to Height ratio	0.49 ± 0.08	0.50 ± 0.08	0.52 ± 0.08	<0.001
Waist to hip ratio	0.84 ± 0.10	0.85 ± 0.09	0.86 ± 0.09	<0.001
Body fat (%)	24.5 ± 9.1	25.3 ± 8.7	26.9 ± 8.8	<0.001
SBP (mmHg)	120.0 ± 16.8	121.3 ± 16.3	124.6 ± 16.3	<0.001
DBP (mmHg)	76.9 ± 10.7	78.2 ± 10.5	82.8 ± 10.6	<0.001
Glycaemia (mg/dL)	90.5 ± 16.4	91.9 ± 15.7	95.4 ± 15.8	<0.001
Total cholesterol (mg/dL)	190.7 ± 37.3	194.3 ± 35.3	202.8 ± 35.7	<0.001
HDL-c (mg/dL)	53.9 ± 13.7	53.1 ± 13.4	50.7 ± 13.7	<0.001
LDL-c (mg/dL)	117.4 ± 40.3	121.4 ± 38.5	131.0 ± 39.0	<0.001
Triglycerides (mg/dL)	96.8 ± 79.2	98.7 ± 78.5	105.8 ± 78.9	<0.001
	N (%)	N (%)	N (%)	p-value
Smokers	1176 (18.9)	1202 (19.3)	1302 (20.9)	<0.001
Physical exercise	2732 (43.8)	2600 (41.7)	2044 (32.8)	<0.001
Normal weight	3500 (56.1)	3398 (54.5)	3085 (49.5)	<0.001
Overweight	1890 (30.3)	1978 (31.7)	2144 (34.4)	
Obesity	846 (13.6)	860 (13.8)	1007 (16.1)	
Waist to height ratio high	2526 (40.5)	2826 (45.3)	3368 (54.0)	<0.001
Waist to hip ratio high	1460 (23.4)	1612 (25.8)	1944 (31.2)	<0.001
Body fat normal	4115 (66.0)	3996 (64.1)	3722 (59.7)	<0.001
Body fat high	1394 (22.4)	1428 (22.9)	1466 (23.5)	

SBP: systolic blood pressure; DBP: diastolic blood pressure; HDL: high density lipoproteins; LDL: low density lipoproteins.

Figure 2 shows the graphs of the parameters related to cardiovascular risk factors. It can be observed that over the years, the trend in all of them was towards an increase in mean values, with an exponential, statistically significant increase during the year of the pandemic due to COVID-19. It can be seen an increase in BMI levels, percentage of fat mass, laboratory values of glucose and total cholesterol, as well as higher blood pressure levels. The alteration encountered in mean blood pressure values was less pronounced compared to the rest of the parameters analyzed, which underwent greater changes, causing an increase in cardiovascular risk in the population studied.

Table 2. Changes in anthropometric, clinical, laboratory, and healthy habit variables in different pre-COVID and COVID years.

	2018–2019 Change	2019–2020 Change
Weight (kg)	0.47 ± 1.04	1.61 ± 1.28
BMI (kg/m^2)	0.16 ± 0.37	0.57 ± 0.46
Waist circumference (cm)	1.82 ± 4.87	2.92 ± 1.17
Hip circumference (cm)	1.14 ± 0.85	1.69 ± 1.15
Waist to Height ratio	0.01 ± 0.03	0.02 ± 0.01
Waist to hip ratio	0.01 ± 0.05	0.01 ± 0.02
Body fat (%)	0.88 ± 2.14	1.58 ± 1.68
SBP (mmHg)	1.28 ± 4.08	3.26 ± 3.68
DBP (mmHg)	1.35 ± 1.48	4.62 ± 1.82
Glycaemia (mg/dL)	1.47 ± 5.16	3.49 ± 2.30
Total cholesterol (mg/dL)	3.59 ± 17.30	8.52 ± 13.40
HDL-c (mg/dL)	−0.82 ± 3.97	−2.44 ± 1.78
LDL-c (mg/dL)	4.04 ± 17.64	9.54 ± 13.41
Triglycerides (mg/dL)	1.83 ± 8.74	7.09 ± 4.63

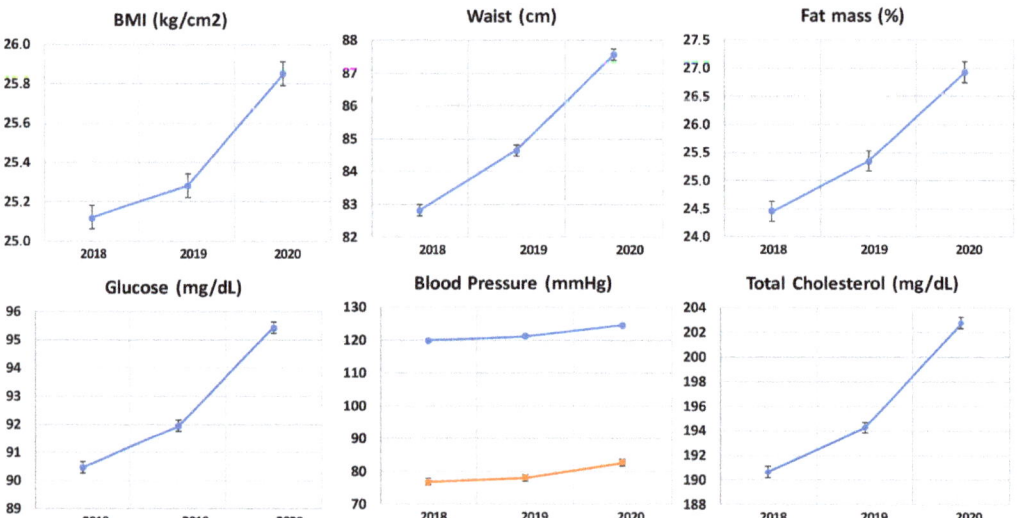

Figure 2. Changes in cardiovascular risk factors in 2018, 2019, and 2020: BMI, waist, lean mass, glucose, blood pressure, and total cholesterol.

Comparing the different cardiovascular risk parameters that had worse mean values after COVID (and considering an increased risk when the category changed to a worse one according to the corresponding risk factor), it can be observed in Figure 3 that by analyzing the parameters according to relative risk, with a 95% confidence interval, and odds ratio, the changes in the mean values of triglyceride levels were not related to the other parameters analyzed. In the other variables analyzed, blood pressure levels were those with the highest RR (1.261–1.306) along with OR (1.283). The rest of the parameters can be seen in the figure.

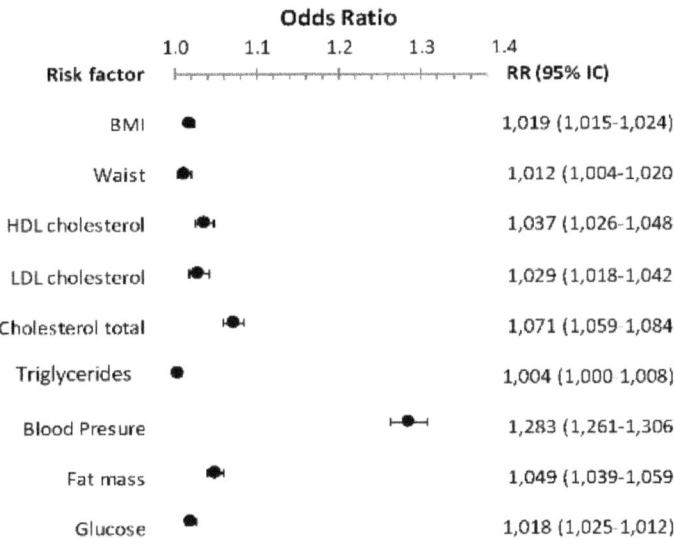

Figure 3. Relative Risk (RR) of patients who had worsened cardiovascular risk factors in the 2019–2020 season when compared with the 2018–2019 season. Patients were considered to have worsened when they changed to a worse category in the corresponding risk factor: BMI (normal, overweight, obesity); glycemic status (normal, prediabetes, diabetes); blood pressure status (normal, pre-AHT, AHT1, AHT2); waist (normal, high); fat mass (normal, high); total cholesterol (normal, high); LDL (normal, high, very high); HDL (normal, low); and TG (normal, high).

The parameters of BMI, glycemic status, blood pressure, waist circumference, and percentage of fat mass were analyzed in relation to age, sex, BMI, glycemic status, and blood pressure levels. It can be observed in Table 3 that upon analyzing by age variable, there is a statistically significant worsening of the values of BMI, glycemic status, blood pressure, and waist circumference, which does not occur in the percentage of fat mass, although this relationship is not statistically significant with age. In the group over 50 years of age, the RR is higher.

When analyzing by sex, the BMI values obtained are not considered statistically significant, although there is statistical significance for the rest of the variables studied. It should be noted that, in males, there is no causal relationship with an increase in percentage of fat mass, while in females there is.

There is no clear association between overweight or obesity and glucose levels, with a RR < 1 and a p-value of 0.241. In terms of BMI, despite having a causal relationship with the percentage of fat mass with a RR > 1, the values obtained have a p-value of 0.704, therefore this relationship and the levels obtained could be caused by other factors as they are not statistically significant. Changes in BMI are not always related to a higher percentage of fat mass; patients with high muscle mass and a low percentage of fat mass, for instance, could also have altered BMI values since this parameter does not differentiate between muscle or fat.

By analyzing glycemic status, workers with prediabetes did reveal a direct relationship with alterations in percentage of fat mass, but not with blood pressure levels or waist circumference. When relating baseline blood glucose levels to BMI, despite observing a causal relationship with a RR > 1, the values obtained were not statistically significant (p-value 0.065) and would therefore not be interpretable for this reason.

Blood pressure levels do not have a statistically significant relationship with glycemic status. Although the relationship between blood pressure and waist circumference and percentage of fat mass have been statistically related to a p-value < 0.001, in the group of workers with type 1 hypertension, there was no increase in blood glucose levels as there was no direct association with the anthropometric parameters analyzed.

When analyzing according to age of participants, a statistically significant increase in total cholesterol levels was observed, with a greater association in workers aged 40–50 years) with a p-value of < 0.001. There are also statistically significant differences with p-value < 0.001 in LDL cholesterol levels with a lower association in workers over 50 years old), as can be seen in Table 4.

When the relationship between age, HDL cholesterol, and triglyceride levels is analyzed, the differences are not statistically significant with a p-value of > 0.05, so the changes in the parameters could be due to other factors and not by age.

According to the sex of the patient studied, a statistically significant worsening stands out with a direct association for the clinical parameters of total cholesterol, HDL cholesterol, and LDL cholesterol in both males and females, but not for triglyceride levels where the differences between males) and females are not statistically significant.

In the population studied that was overweight or obese, the increased analytical values of total cholesterol and the decrease in HDL cholesterol were statistically significant (p-value < 0.05) even though in the group of overweight patients, there was no direct association with HDL cholesterol values. No statistically significant relationship was found with LDL cholesterol or triglyceride levels in the overweight and obese population.

The glycemic level of the workers studied was found to have a direct, statistically significant association with a p-value of < 0.05 for HDL cholesterol and LDL cholesterol, but not with total cholesterol or triglyceride levels. In the group of patients with prediabetes, no direct relationship with changes in LDL cholesterol was observed.

If we analyze according to blood pressure levels, patients with normal blood pressure or type II hypertension are associated with a higher risk (RR: 1.106; 95% CI 1.081–1.132) and (RR: 1.053; 95% CI 0.620–1.787) for total cholesterol and a RR: 1.005; 95% CI 0.987–1.024 and RR: 1.003; 95% CI 0.955–1.053 for HDL cholesterol, respectively; but with a non-statistically significant association for LDL cholesterol levels with a p-value of 0.072.

Regarding triglyceride levels, according to blood pressure levels, no direct relationship was found in patients with hypertension, but was found in normotensive patients with a p-value of 0.036.

In relation to physical activity, the changes caused by lockdown, measured through the IPAQ questionnaire, can be seen in Table 5. A decrease in physical activity is observed in both sexes for the group that exercised before lockdown, as well as an increase in sedentary lifestyle in groups that did not perform physical activity before lockdown on a regular basis.

The decrease in physical activity is statistically significant for both sexes, with a p-value < 0.0001 compared to the time before the pandemic.

Table 3. Relative risk of patients with increased BMI, waist, fat mass, glycemic status, and hypertension status divided into categories of age, sex, BMI, glycemic status, and hypertension status. Patients were considered to have worsened when they changed to an upper category in the corresponding risk factor: BMI (normal, overweight, obesity); glycemic status (normal, prediabetes, diabetes); blood pressure status (normal, pre-AHT, AHT1, AHT2); waist (normal, high); fat mass (normal, high, very high); total cholesterol (normal, high); LDL (normal, high); HDL (normal, low); TG (normal, high).

	BMI RR	BMI (95% CI)	p-Value of Interaction	Glycemic Status RR	Glycemic Status (95% CI)	p-Value of Interaction	Blood Pressure RR	Blood Pressure (95% CI)	p-Value of Interaction	Waist RR	Waist (95% CI)	p-Value of Interaction	Fat Mass RR	Fat Mass (95% CI)	p-Value of Interaction
Age			<0.001			<0.001			<0.001			<0.001			0.907
<35	1.008	(1.001–1.014)		1.010	(1.001–1.019)		1.223	(1.186–1.261)		1.009	(0.997–1.020)		1.084	(1.062–1.106)	
35–40	1.021	(1.012 1.030)		1.021	(1.008–1.035)		1.287	(1.234–1.343)		1.013	(1.000–1.027)		1.037	(1.015–1.060)	
40–50	1.020	(1.013–1.028)		1.022	(1.011–1.034)		1.323	(1.283–1.365)		1.017	(1.004–1.029)		1.022	(1.007–1.037)	
>50	1.029	(1.018–1.041)		1.021	(1.004–1.038)		1.284	(1.235–1.336)		0.999	(0.975–1.023)		1.064	(1.042–1.087)	
Gender			0.453			<0.001			<0.001			<0.001			<0.001
man	1.024	(1.017–1.031)		1.022	(1.011–1.033)		1.372	(1.335–1.411)		1.002	(0.991–1.013)		0.971	(0.957–0.985)	
women	1.015	(1.010–1.021)		1.014	(1.007–1.021)		1.212	(1.186–1.238)		1.022	(1.011–1.032)		1.125	(1.112–1.139)	
BMI						0.241			<0.001			<0.001			0.704
Normal	-	-		0.986	(1.007–1.021)		1.230	(1.204–1.257)		1.008	(1.004–1.011)		1.075	(1.061–1.089)	
Overweight	-	-		0.998	(0.980–1.024)		1.293	(1.252–1.335)		1.044	(1.022–1.066)		1.009	(0.993–1.025)	
Obesity	-	-		0.968	(1.019–1.045)		1.516	(1.431–1.606)		0.954	(0.927–0.982)		1.038	(1.014–1.063)	
Glucemic status			0.065			0.004			0.001			0.235			0.013
NORMAL	1.015	(1.011–1.020)			(-)		1.061	(1.050–1.073)		1.017	(1.009–1.025)		1.029	(1.016–1.043)	
prediabetes	1.041	(1.027–1.055)			(-)		0.989	(0.967–1.011)		0.977	(0.954–1.002)		1.028	(1.001–1.056)	
diabetes	1.031	(0.996–1.067)			(-)		0.993	(0.934–1.056)		1.050	(0.978–1.129)		1.070	(0.979–1.170)	
Blood Pressure			<0.001			0.280						<0.001			<0.001
normal	1.011	(1.006 1.017)		1.015	(1.004 1.025)			(-)		1.018	(1.005 1.031)		1.102	(1.019–1.048)	
preHTA	1.023	(1.016–1.030)		1.016	(1.007–1.025)			(-)		1.016	(1.005–1.028)		1.033	(1.019–1.048)	
HTA 1	1.019	(1.007–1.030)		1.021	(1.004–1.038)			(-)		0.990	(0.972–1.009)		0.994	(0.970–1.019)	
HTA 2	1.033	(1.008–1.059)		1.042	(1.010–1.073)			(-)		1.002	(0.964–1.042)		1.026	(0.983–1.072)	

Table 4. Relative Risk of patients with increased total cholesterol, LDL, TG and a decrease in HDL levels, divided by categories of age, sex, BMI, glycemic status and hypertension status. Patients were deemed to have worsened when they changed to an upper category in the corresponding risk factor: BMI (normal, overweight, obesity); glycemic status (normal, prediabetes, diabetes); blood pressure status (normal, pre-AHT, AHT1, AHT2); waist (normal, high); fat mass (normal, high, very high); total cholesterol (normal, high); LDL (normal, high); HDL (normal, low); and TG (normal, high).

	Total Cholesterol RR	Total Cholesterol (95% CI)	p-Value of Interaction	HDL RR	HDL (95% CI)	p-Value of Interaction	LDL RR	LDL (95% CI)	p-Value of Interaction	TG RR	TG (95% CI)	p-Value of Interaction
Age			0.001			0.958			<0.001			0.902
<35	1.049	(1.020–1.139)		1.047	(1.027–1.068)		1.047	(1.025–1.069)		1.012	(1.004–1.021)	
35–40	1.049	(1.021–1.078)		1.028	(0.998–1.059)		1.017	(0.991–1.044)		1.004	(0.994–1.015)	
40–50	1.089	(1.066–1.113)		1.028	(1.011–1.046)		1.048	(1.026–1.069)		0.999	(0.994–1.004)	
>50	1.008	(0.982–1.035)		1.044	(1.022–1.068)		0.982	(0.955–1.011)		1.000	(0.990–1.010)	

Table 4. Cont.

		Total Cholesterol			HDL			LDL			TG	
		RR	(95% CI)	p-Value of Interaction	RR	(95% CI)	p-Value of Interaction	RR	(95% CI)	p-Value of Interaction	RR	(95% CI)	p-Value of Interaction
Gender	Men	1.061	(1.044–1.080)	<0.001	1.078	(1.059–1.097)	0.000	1.018	(1.001–1.035)	0.040	0.999	(0.993–1.006)	0.643
	Women	1.081	(1.062–1.099)		1.002	(0.990–1.014)		1.041	(1.024–1.058)		1.008	(1.003–1.012)	
BMI category	Normal	1.092	(1.074–1.110)	0.027	1.046	(1.033–1.060)	0.000	1.040	(1.024–1.057)	0.327	1.004	(0.999–1.010)	0.220
	Overweight	1.049	(1.027–1.071)		0.989	(0.958–1.021)		1.011	(0.979–1.045)		1.006	(0.999–1.013)	
	Obesity	1.041	(1.007–1.075)		1.038	(1.017–1.060)		1.011	(0.979–1.045)		0.995	(0.984–1.006)	
Glucemic status	Normal	1.066	(1.052–1.080)	0.113	1.004	(1.000–1.009)	0.015	1.277	(1.253–1.301)	0.003	1.034	(1.023–1.046)	0.596
	prediabetes	1.111	(1.079–1.143)		0.996	(0.987–1.006)		1.299	(1.237–1.365)		1.066	(1.033–1.099)	
	diabetes	1.002	(0.932–1.077)		1.042	(1.001–1.084)		1.506	(1.272–1.783)		0.866	(0.774–0.969)	
Blood Pressure	normal	1.106	(1.081–1.132)	<0.001	1.005	0.987 1.024 (1.039–1.071)	0.006	1.040	(1.018 1.062) (1.009–1.044)	0.072	1.004	0.996 1.013 (1.001–1.012)	0.036
	preHTA	0.545	(0.464–0.641)		1.055			1.026			1.007		
	HTA 1	0.639	(0.478–0.853)		1.059	(1.030–1.089)		1.022	(0.992–1.053)		0.997	(0.990–1.004)	
	HTA 2	1.053	(0.620–1.787)		1.003	(0.955–1.053)		1.023	(0.979–1.069)		0.999	(0.981–1.017)	

Table 5. Percentage of physical activity, before and during lockdown in men and women separated into groups according to whether or not they previously performed physical activity.

	Year 2018	Year 2019	Year 2020	p-Value
Women non physical exercise	57.0	57.4	69.2	<0.0001
Women yes physical exercise	43.0	42.6	30.8	
Men non physical exercise	55.3	59.3	65.1	<0.0001
Men yes physical exercise	44.7	40.7	34.9	

4. Discussion

The global pandemic caused by COVID-19 has had a great impact on health population [35]. Not only due to the infection caused by the virus, which has left complications and consequences of the disease from which some people are yet to fully recover, but also due to the pathology derived from lockdown, social distancing, and isolation, in which chronic diseases have worsened [36–39]. These measures taken by governments to protect public health have produced a psychological impact on the population that has caused overeating, a more sedentary lifestyle, and modification of several anthropometric, clinical, and laboratory health parameters affecting all body systems [40,41].

In this study, we objectify the changes produced in the population due to lockdown, in a population of Spanish workers. Although it is true that, in recent decades, the population has had a tendency to obesity and overweight due to a sedentary lifestyle [13,16], what can be seen in this study is that, during lockdown, many of the parameters that influence cardiovascular risk were affected, such as obesity, alcoholism, and a sedentary lifestyle, changing their values, leading to a greater risk of suffering from cardiovascular diseases. Our results are similar to those published by other authors from different countries such as Lithuania, China, Korea, Israel, UK, amongst others [40–45].

In the study carried out by Paltrinieri et al., the changes produced during lockdown in relation to physical activity, diet, alcohol consumption, and tobacco were studied through a self-administered survey. The results showed there had been a reduction in physical activity without a change in diet [46]. In our study, these modifications were studied through anthropometric, clinical, and laboratory parameters, and their changes could be observed with a statistically significant increase in both obesity and overweight, as seen in our results.

A simultaneous to the increase in cardiovascular risk, as detailed in Table 1, the 4.1% increase in the rate of overweight and obesity, as well as the 11% decrease in physical activity and 2% increase in smoking brought about the development of other diseases, both acute and chronic, which have modified the health status of the population and increased morbidity and mortality from other causes, not only due to infection with COVID-19. These consequences were also pointed out by Palmer et al. [47,48].

The results of our study reveal statistically significant differences when comparing clinical, laboratory, and anthropometric parameters in a population of workers due to a lockdown. The increase in body weight and therefore BMI is a consequence of the dietary habits and sedentary lifestyle of the population during this period [49,50]. An increase in percentage of fat mass and waist and abdominal perimeter was also observed [42,44,45]. There are studies in the literature that compare body weight during and after lockdown, such as the study by Blautani S, et al. which shows that it was not the entire population that suffered an increase in body weight, with 18.2% of the population in their study losing weight during lockdown. At the end of lockdown, those who had gained weight continued to gain, so it is likely that their health effects associated to body changes will persist over time [51] if lifestyle modifications are not made [52].

Not only were anthropometric parameters affected, but alterations were also found in biochemical parameters. In the lipid profile, for instance, an increase in total cholesterol levels was detected, which corresponded to an additional increase in LDL cholesterol levels and decrease in HDL cholesterol levels, with statistically significant differences. These results are similar to those published in other studies, although their sample sizes were much smaller than ours [40,53].

Plasma glucose levels deteriorated, probably in connection with the increased rate of obesity, overweight, and decrease in physical exercise [54]. In patients with blood glucose levels in the range of diabetes mellitus, a statistically significant decrease of LDL cholesterol levels was detected, although this was not statistically significant in patients with prediabetes values, in whom there was no clear relationship with changes in LDL cholesterol values. At a general level, there was an increase of triglyceride levels with statistically significant results. The combined increase in serum triglycerides points to the role of a variation in eating habits and reinforces the need not to attenuate attention to an adequate lifestyle program, with regular physical activity and a correct dietary approach, even when successful pharmacological treatment is ongoing [54]. A high-carbohydrate diet is known to raise fasting triglyceride levels more than a high-fat diet, which is also related to greater mortality [55]. Our results are similar to those obtained in previous studies [40,53].

Regarding blood pressure levels, lockdown also caused a deterioration in people who were not previously hypertensive, probably due to their lifestyle during these months and the worsening of the population's health status owing to a change in dietary habits and physical activity. In the literature consulted, we have found very few studies that refer to changes in blood pressure during lockdown due to COVID-19. However, the studies published are similar to our results [40,56].

The lockdown adversely affected multiple risk factors for disease, especially cardiovascular disease. Plasma concentrations for LDL and HDL cholesterol, respectively increased and decreased. Concurrently, blood glucose concentrations and blood pressures increased. According to the increases in ratio of waist to hip circumferences, these effects were associated with increased central obesity [57]. Notably, low HDL cholesterol, a large waist circumference, hyperglycemia, hypertension, and hypertriglyceridemia are components of metabolic syndrome, a global measure of risk for cardiovascular disease and developing type 2 diabetes mellitus [58]. According to the latest guidelines, the metabolic syndrome is described as a set of analytical and anthropometric alterations, in which the patient must have at least three altered parameters in order to be diagnosed of metabolic syndrome. These parameters are: waist circumference in men $\geq$102 cm and $\geq$88 cm in women, triglyceride values $\geq$150 mg/dL or being on pharmacological treatment, HDL levels <40 mg/dL in men and <50 mg/dL in women. Blood pressure values $\geq$130/85 mmHg or being on pharmacological treatment with antihypertensives and fasting blood glucose levels $\geq$100 mg/dL or being on antihyperglycemic treatment [59].

According to the results obtained in our study, which have been explained previously, a global worsening of these parameters could be detected, secondary to the change in lifestyle caused by lockdown. The increased metabolic syndrome has been able to develop the appearance of different cardiovascular and metabolic complications that have caused an increase in morbidity and mortality, as well as an increased risk of COVID-19 infection with greater potential for severity as has been seen in recent studies [60–62] as shown in the study carried out by Li B et al., which shows how the population with cardiovascular risk factors has a higher risk of severe infection by COVID-19 [63].

Periodic medical check-ups, in the case of our study, of Spanish workers, has allowed the detection of these alterations and the possibility of applying preventive measures to avoid the development of diseases in the future as well as complications in the event of infection by COVID-19 [60,61].

In the different tables of results, the worsening of blood pressure levels, glycaemia, waist-abdominal perimeter as well as analytical levels of triglycerides and HDL cholesterol are observed. Early application of preventive measures in the different altered parameters could prevent the development of metabolic syndrome and its possible complications [59,62,64].

Despite being known as a syndrome, there is no single approach, since the objective is to apply preventive or therapeutic measures individually according to the altered parameters [65,66] in each individual, always starting with lifestyle modifications, a factor that has been greatly influenced by lockdown due to the increase in sedentary lifestyle, with a decrease in physical activity [67–69] and the complications driven by COVID-19.

The aim of treating or preventing these altered analytical and anthropometric parameters produced by the state of lockdown would be to prevent the development of cardiovascular diseases and therefore reduce cardiovascular risk at the population and its potential morbidity and mortality. In the study conducted by Yangjing X, et al., people with established cardiovascular disease or altered cardiovascular risk parameters are shown to have a worse prognosis when faced with COVID-19 infection [70].

In our study, many of these cardiovascular risks are seen to have modified their levels during lockdown, leading to an increase in cardiovascular risk. Also, the fact of decreasing physical activity and increasing sedentary lifestyle is associated with an increase and worsening in the different parameters studied and also with a tendency to obesity and therefore to the complications derived from it, causing an increase in cardiovascular risk factors in the population [71], as has also been seen in other studies such as the ones from Hendren et al. or Hu L et al. [72,73].

In our study, we found a significant decrease in physical activity both in men and women, being higher in women. Our results are consistent with other published studies [74,75], and differ from those obtained by Castañeda-Barbarro et al.'s. in which a greater decrease in physical exercise in men is found [76].

Regular physical activity helps reduce cardiovascular risk [68], by reducing the percentage of fat mass and improving laboratory and clinical values such as blood pressure, insulin resistance ... helping in the prevention of developing diseases derived from an unhealthy lifestyle and preventing cardiovascular diseases [69,77].

With all this, it can be stated that the COVID-19 pandemic has increased the risk of developing pathologies derived from lifestyle modifications, in addition to raising the risk of COVID-19 infection by altering parameters that increase the risk of illness [54,69,78].

5. Strengths and Limitations

Several studies compare the effects of the pandemic and COVID-19 infection with changes in obesity and overweight parameters, as well as cardiovascular risk factors and other pathologies, but we have not found any study in which so many parameters are compared in the same population as in our study.

Further, none of the studies that present the evaluation of the different parameters separately have a sample size such as ours, with 6283 patients.

The limitations found in this study are the fact that it was carried out in a specific geographic area, with a Caucasian working population, over a certain period of time, which could limit the generalization of the results to other areas where lifestyles may be different.

Selection bias is another limitation of our study, since it is limited to workers who voluntarily attended company medical examinations during those years.

Therefore, the results do not apply to other populations, and specific studies would have to be carried out.

6. Conclusions

Health behaviors have been negatively affected during lockdown, leading to an increase in sedentary behavior in all age groups, an unhealthy diet, and, therefore, associated with weight gain, as well as an increased consumption of tobacco.

With the parameters and results described above, it can be concluded that the months of lockdown caused a statistically significant deterioration of several health parameters due to increased sedentary behavior in a similar way in males and females in all age ranges, although the over 40-year-old group is the one where the worst values of the variables analyzed were observed, causing an increase in the magnitude of multiple risk factors for cardiovascular disease and the appearance of new pathologies that have resulted in an increase in morbidity and mortality due to all causes.

Author Contributions: Conceptualization: J.I.R.M., B.A.J. and Á.A.L.G. Data collection and analysis: P.S.C., C.B.-C., S.A.B. and L.M.C. Methodology: J.I.R.M., B.A.J. and Á.A.L.G. Draft: B.A.J., Á.A.L.G. Revision: J.I.R.M., B.A.J., P.S.C., C.B.-C., S.A.B. and L.M.C. All authors have read and agreed to the published version of the manuscript.

Funding: This research received no external funding. The funders had no role in the design of the study; in the collection, analyses, or interpretation of data; in the writing of the manuscript, or in the decision to publish the results.

Institutional Review Board Statement: The study was carried out after the authorization of the Ethical Committee of the Balearic Islands, with the prior informed consent of the study subjects and following the norms of the Helsinki Declaration. The confidentiality of the subjects included will be guaranteed at all times in accordance with the provisions of the Organic Law 3/2018, of December 5, on the Protection of Personal Data and guarantee of digital rights and Regulation (EU) 2016/679 of the European Parliament and the Council of 27 April 2016 on Data Protection (RGPD).

Informed Consent Statement: Informed consent was obtained from all subjects involved in the study.

Data Availability Statement: Data available on request due to restrictions (privacy or ethical).

Conflicts of Interest: The authors declare they have no conflict of interest.

References

1. Chen, N.; Zhou, M.; Dong, X.; Qu, J.; Gong, F.; Han, Y.; Qiu, Y.; Wang, J.; Liu, Y.; Wei, Y.; et al. Epidemiological and clinical characteristics of 99 cases of 2019 novel coronavirus pneumonia in Wuhan, China: A descriptive study. *Lancet* **2020**, *395*, 507–513. [CrossRef]
2. Wuhan Seafood Market Pneumonia Virus Isolate Wuhan-Hu-1, Complete Genome. 23 January 2020; [citado 7 February 2020]. Available online: http://www.ncbi.nlm.nih.gov/nuccore/MN908947.3 (accessed on 2 November 2021).
3. Huang, C.; Wang, Y.; Li, X.; Ren, L.; Zhao, J.; Hu, Y.; Zhang, L.; Fan, G.; Xu, J.; Gu, X.; et al. Clinical features of patients infected with 2019 novel coronavirus in Whuam, China. *Lancet* **2020**, *395*, 497–506. [CrossRef]
4. Galanopoulos, M.; Gkeros, F.; Doukatas, A.; Karianakis, G.; Pontas, C.; Tsoukalas, N.; Viazis, N.; Liatsos, C.; Mantzaris, G.J. COVID-19 pandemic: Pathophysiology and manifestations from the gastrointestinal tract. *World J. Gastroenterol.* **2020**, *26*, 4579–4588. [CrossRef] [PubMed]
5. Guan, W.-J.; Ni, Z.-Y.; Hu, Y.; Liang, W.-H.; Ou, C.-Q.; He, J.-X.; Liu, L.; Shan, H.; Lei, C.-l.; Hui, D.S.C.; et al. Clinical Characteristics of Coronavirus Disease 2019 in China. *N. Engl. J. Med.* **2020**, *382*, 1708–1720. [CrossRef]
6. Centers for Disease Control and Prevention. Coronavirus Disease 2019 (COVID-19)—Cases, Data, & Surveillance. Available online: https://www.cdc.gov/coronavirus/2019-ncov/cases-updates/cases-in-us.html (accessed on 16 November 2021).
7. Wu, F.; Zhao, S.; Yu, B.; Chen, Y.-M.; Wang, W.; Song, Z.-G.; Hu, Y.; Tao, Z.-W.; Tian, J.-H.; Pei, Y.-Y.; et al. A new coronavirus associated with human respiratory disease in China. *Nature* **2020**, *579*, 265–269. [CrossRef]
8. Zhang, G.; Zhang, J.; Wang, B.; Zhu, X.; Wang, Q.; Qiu, S. Analysis of clinical characteristics and laboratory findings of 95 cases of 2019 novel coronavirus pneumonia in Wuhan, China: A retrospective analysis. *Respir. Res.* **2020**, *21*, 1–10. [CrossRef]
9. Pollard, C.A.; Morran, M.P.; Nestor-Kalinoski, A.L. The COVID-19 pandemic: A global health crisis. *Physiol. Genom.* **2020**, *52*, 549–557. [CrossRef]
10. Ward, M.P.; Li, X.; Tian, K. Novel coronavirus 2019, an emerging public health emergency. *Transbound. Emerg. Dis.* **2020**, *67*, 469–470. [CrossRef]
11. Koh, D. COVID-19 lockdowns throughout the world. *Occup. Med.* **2020**, *70*, 322. [CrossRef]
12. Real Decreto 463/2020, de 14 de Marzo, por el que se Declara el Estado de Alarma para la Gestión de la Situación de crisis Sanitaria Ocasionada por el COVID-19. Available online: https://www.boe.es/buscar/doc.php?id=BOE-A-2020-3692 (accessed on 2 February 2022).
13. Owen, A.J.; Tran, T.; Hammarberg, K.; Kirkman, M.; Fisher, J.; The COVID-19 Restrictions Impact Research Group. Poor appetite and overeating reported by adults in Australia during the coronavirus-19 disease pandemic: A population-based study. *Public Health Nutr.* **2021**, *24*, 275–281. [CrossRef]
14. Constandt, B.; Thibaut, E.; De Bosscher, V.; Scheerder, J.; Ricour, M.; Willem, A. Exercising in times of lockdown: An analysis of the impact of COVID-19 on levels and patterns of exercise among adults in Belgium. *Int. J. Environ. Res. Public Health* **2020**, *17*, 4144. [CrossRef]
15. Levi, S. The Pandemic Has More Than Doubled Food-Delivery Apps' Business. Now What? 2020. Available online: https://www.marketwatch.com/story/the-pandemic-has-more-than-doubled-americans-use-of-food-delivery-apps-but-that-doesnt-mean-the-companies-are-making-money-11606340169 (accessed on 20 November 2021).

16. Skotnicka, M.; Karwowska, K.; Kłobukowski, F.; Wasilewska, E.; Małgorzewicz, S. Dietary Habits before and during the COVID-19 Epidemic in Selected European Countries. *Nutrients* **2021**, *13*, 1690. [CrossRef]
17. Di Renzo, L.; Gualtieri, P.; Pivari, F.; Soldati, L.; Attinà, A.; Cinelli, G.; Leggeri, C.; Caparello, G.; Barrea, L.; Scerbo, F.; et al. Eating habits and lifestyle changes during COVID-19 lockdown: An Italian survey. *J. Transl. Med.* **2020**, *18*, 229. [CrossRef]
18. Bennett, G.; Young, E.; Butler, I.; Coe, S. The Impact of Lockdown During the COVID-19 Outbreak on Dietary Habits in Various Population Groups: A Scoping Review. *Front. Nutr.* **2021**, *8*, 53. [CrossRef]
19. Son, C.; Hegde, S.; Smith, A.; Wang, X.; Sasangohar, F. Effects of COVID-19 on College Students' Mental Health in the United States: Interview Survey Study. *J. Med. Internet Res.* **2020**, *22*, e21279. [CrossRef]
20. Shah, M.; Sachdeva, M.; Johnston, H. Eating disorders in the age of COVID-19. *Psychiatry Res.* **2020**, *290*, 113122. [CrossRef]
21. Rodríguez-Pérez, C.; Molina-Montes, E.; Verardo, V.; Artacho, R.; García-Villanova, B.; Guerra-Hernández, E.J.; Ruíz-López, M.D. Changes in Dietary Behaviours during the COVID-19 Outbreak Confinement in the Spanish COVIDiet Study. *Nutrients* **2020**, *12*, 1730. [CrossRef]
22. Bakaloudi, D.R.; Jeyakumar, D.T.; Jayawardena, R.; Chourdakis, M. The impact of COVID-19 lockdown on snacking habits, fast-food and alcohol consumption: A systematic review of the evidence. *Clin. Nutr.* **2021**, *17*, S0261-5614(21)00212-0. [CrossRef]
23. Deschasaux-Tanguy, M.; Druesne-Pecollo, N.; Esseddik, Y.; de Edelenyi, F.S.; Allès, B.; Andreeva, V.A.; Baudry, J.; Charreire, H.; Deschamps, V.; Egnell, M.; et al. Diet and physical activity during the coronavirus disease 2019 (COVID-19) lockdown (March–May 2020): Results from the French NutriNet-Santé cohort study. *Am. J. Clin. Nutr.* **2021**, *113*, 924–938. [CrossRef]
24. Pinto, J.; van Zeller, M.; Amorim, P.; Pimentel, A.; Dantas, P.; Eusébio, E. Sleep quality in times of COVID-19 pandemic. *Sleep Med.* **2020**, *74*, 81–85. [CrossRef]
25. Kumar, N.; Gupta, R. Disrupted Sleep During a Pandemic. *Sleep Med. Clin.* **2022**, *17*, 41–52. [CrossRef]
26. Gualano, M.R.; Lo Moro, G.; Voglino, G.; Bert, F.; Siliquini, R. Effects of COVID-19 Lockdown on Mental Health and Sleep Disturbances in Italy. *Int. J. Environ. Res. Public Health* **2020**, *17*, 4779. [CrossRef]
27. Manz, K.; Mensink, G.B.M.; Finger, J.D.; Haftenberger, M.; Brettschneider, A.-K.; Lage Barbosa, C. Associations between physical activity and food intake among children and adolescents: Results of KiGGS Wave 2. *Nutrients* **2019**, *11*, 1060. [CrossRef]
28. Taeymans, J.; Luijckx, E.; Rogan, S.; Haas, K.; Baur, H. Physical Activity, Nutritional Habits, and Sleeping Behavior in Students and Employees of a Swiss University During the COVID-19 Lockdown Period: Questionnaire Survey Study. *JMIR Public Health Surveill.* **2021**, *7*, e26330. [CrossRef]
29. Fernandez-Rio, J.; Cecchini, J.A.; Mendez Gimenez, A.; Carriedo, A. Weight changes during the COVID-19 home confinement. Effects on psychosocial variables. *Obes. Res. Clin. Pract.* **2020**, *14*, 383–385. [CrossRef]
30. Singu, S.; Acharya, A.; Challagundla, K.; Byrareddy, S.N. Impact of Social Determinants of Health on the Emerging COVID-19 Pandemic in the United States. *Front. Public Health* **2020**, *8*, 406. [CrossRef]
31. Shivalkar, S.; Pingali, M.S.; Verma, A.; Singh, A.; Singh, V.; Paital, B.; Das, D.; Varadwaj, P.K.; Samanta, S.K. Outbreak of COVID-19: A Detailed Overview and Its Consequences. *Adv. Exp. Med. Biol.* **2021**, *1353*, 23–45. [CrossRef]
32. Pal, A.; Ahirwar, A.K.; Sakarde, A.; Asia, P.; Gopal, N.; Alam, S.; Kaim, K.; Ahirwar, P.; Sorte, S.R. COVID-19 and cardiovascular disease: A review of current knowledge. *Horm. Mol. Biol. Clin. Investig.* **2021**, *42*, 99–104. [CrossRef]
33. López-González, A.A.; Ramírez Manent, J.I.; Vicente-Herrero, M.T.; García Ruiz, E.; Albaladejo Blanco, M.; López Safont, N. Prevalence of diabesity in the Spanish working population: Influence of sociodemographic variables and tobacco consumption. *An. Sist. Sanit. Navar.* **2021**. *online ahead of print*. [CrossRef]
34. Lee, P.H.; Macfarlane, D.J.; Lam, T.H.; Stewart, S.M. Validity of the international physical activity questionnaire short form (IPAQ-SF): A systematic review. *Int. J. Behav. Nutr. Phys. Act.* **2011**, *8*, 115. [CrossRef]
35. White, A. Men and COVID-19: The aftermath. *Postgrad. Med.* **2020**, *132*, 18–27. [CrossRef] [PubMed]
36. Guzik, T.J.; Mohiddin, S.A.; DiMarco, A.; Patel, V.; Savvatis, K.; Marelli-Berg, F.M.; Madhur, M.S.; Tomaszewski, M.; Maffia, P.; D'Acquisto, F.; et al. COVID-19 and the cardiovascular system: Implications for risk assessment, diagnosis, and treatment options. *Cardiovasc. Res.* **2020**, *116*, 1666–1687. [CrossRef] [PubMed]
37. Lima-Martínez, M.M.; Boada, C.C.; Madera-Silva, M.D.; Marín, W.; Contreras, M. COVID-19 and diabetes: A bidirectional relationship. *Clínica e Investigación en Arteriosclerosis (Engl. Ed.)* **2021**, *33*, 151–157. [CrossRef] [PubMed]
38. Beran, D.; Perone, S.A.; Perolini, M.C.; Chappuis, F.; Chopard, P.; Haller, D.M.; Bausch, F.J.; Maisonneuve, H.; Perone, N.; Gastaldi, G. Beyond the virus: Ensuring continuity of care for people with diabetes during COVID-19. *Prim. Care Diabetes* **2021**, *15*, 16–17. [CrossRef]
39. Martínez-Quintana, E.; Vega-Acedo, L.D.C.; Santana-Herrera, D.; Pérez-Acosta, C.; Medina-Gil, J.M.; Muñoz-Díaz, E.; Rodríguez-González, F. Mental well-being among patients with congenital heart disease and heart failure during the COVID-19 pandemic. *Am. J. Cardiovasc. Dis.* **2021**, *11*, 618–623.
40. Sohn, M.; Koo, B.K.; Yoon, H.I.; Song, K.-H.; Kim, E.S.; Bin Kim, H.; Lim, S. Impact of COVID-19 and Associated Preventive Measures on Cardiometabolic Risk Factors in South Korea. *J. Obes. Metab. Syndr.* **2021**, *30*, 248–260. [CrossRef]
41. Kaufman-Shriqui, V.; Navarro, D.A.; Raz, O.; Boaz, M. Multinational dietary changes and anxiety during the coronavirus pan-demic-findings from Israel. *Isr. J. Health Policy Res.* **2021**, *10*, 28. [CrossRef]
42. Kriaucioniene, V.; Bagdonaviciene, L.; Rodríguez-Pérez, C.; Petkeviciene, J. Associations between Changes in Health Behav-iours and Body Weight during the COVID-19 Quarantine in Lithuania: The Lithuanian COVIDiet Study. *Nutrients* **2020**, *12*, 3119. [CrossRef]

43. He, M.; Xian, Y.; Lv, X.; He, J.; Ren, Y. Changes in Body Weight, Physical Activity, and Lifestyle During the Semi-lockdown Period After the Outbreak of COVID-19 in China: An Online Survey. *Disaster Med. Public Health Prep.* **2021**, *15*, e23–e28. [CrossRef]
44. Robinson, E.; Boyland, E.; Chisholm, A.; Harrold, J.; Maloney, N.G.; Marty, L.; Mead, B.R.; Noonan, R.; Hardman, C.A. Obesity, eating behavior and physical activity during COVID-19 lockdown: A study of UK adults. *Appetite* **2021**, *156*, 104853. [CrossRef]
45. Ammar, A.; Brach, M.; Trabelsi, K.; Chtourou, H.; Boukhris, O.; Masmoudi, L.; Bouaziz, B.; Bentlage, E.; How, D.; Ahmed, M.; et al. Effects of COVID-19 Home Confinement on Eating Behaviour and Physical Activity: Results of the ECLB-COVID19 International Online Survey. *Nutrients* **2020**, *12*, 1583. [CrossRef]
46. Paltrinieri, S.; Bressi, B.; Costi, S.; Mazzini, E.; Cavuto, S.; Ottone, M.; De Panfilis, L.; Fugazzaro, S.; Rondini, E.; Rossi, P.G. Beyond Lockdown: The potential side effects of the SARS-CoV-2 pandemic on public health. *Nutrients* **2021**, *13*, 1600. [CrossRef]
47. Palmer, K.; Monaco, A.; Kivipelto, M.; Onder, G.; Maggi, S.; Michel, J.-P.; Prieto, R.; Sykara, G.; Donde, S. The potential long-term impact of the COVID-19 outbreak on patients with non-communicable diseases in Europe: Consequences for healthy ageing. *Aging Clin. Exp. Res.* **2020**, *32*, 1189–1194. [CrossRef]
48. Mattioli, A.V.; Sciomer, S.; Cocchi, C.; Maffei, S.; Gallina, S. Quarantine during COVID-19 outbreak: Changes in diet and physical activity increase the risk of cardiovascular disease. *Nutr. Metab. Cardiovasc. Dis.* **2020**, *30*, 1409–1417. [CrossRef]
49. Flanagan, E.W.; Beyl, R.A.; Fearnbach, S.N.; Altazan, A.D.; Martin, C.K.; Redman, L.M. The Impact of COVID-19 Stay-At-Home Orders on Health Behaviors in Adults. *Obesity* **2021**, *29*, 438–445. [CrossRef]
50. Bakaloudi, D.R.; Barazzoni, R.; Bischoff, S.C.; Breda, J.; Wickramasinghe, K.; Chourdakis, M. Impact of the first COVID-19 lockdown on body weight: A combined systematic review and a meta-analysis. *Clin. Nutr.* **2021**, *20*, S0261-5614(21)00207-7. [CrossRef]
51. Bhutani, S.; Vandellen, M.; Cooper, J. Longitudinal Weight Gain and Related Risk Behaviors during the COVID-19 Pandemic in Adults in the US. *Nutrients* **2021**, *13*, 671. [CrossRef]
52. Alshahrani, S.M.; Alghannam, A.F.; Taha, N.; Alqahtani, S.S.; Al-Mutairi, A.; Al-Saud, N.; Alghnam, S. The Impact of COVID-19 Pandemic on Weight and Body Mass Index in Saudi Arabia: A Longitudinal Study. *Front. Public Health* **2022**, *9*, 775022. [CrossRef]
53. Jontez, N.B.; Novak, K.; Kenig, S.; Petelin, A.; Pražnikar, Z.J.; Mohorko, N. The Impact of COVID-19-Related Lockdown on Diet and Serum Markers in Healthy Adults. *Nutrients* **2021**, *13*, 1082. [CrossRef]
54. Martinez-Ferran, M.; De La Guía-Galipienso, F.; Sanchis-Gomar, F.; Pareja-Galeano, H. Metabolic Impacts of Confinement during the COVID-19 Pandemic Due to Modified Diet and Physical Activity Habits. *Nutrients* **2020**, *12*, 1549. [CrossRef]
55. Dehghan, M.; Mente, A.; Zhang, X.; Swaminathan, S.; Li, W.; Mohan, V.; Iqbal, R.; Kumar, R.; Wentzel-Viljoen, E.; Rosengren, A.; et al. Associations of fats and carbohydrate intake with cardiovascular disease and mortality in 18 countries from five continents (PURE): A prospective cohort study. *Lancet* **2017**, *390*, 2050–2062. [CrossRef]
56. Aajal, A.; El Boussaadani, B.; Hara, L.; Benajiba, C.; Boukouk, O.; Benali, M.; Ouadfel, O.; Bendoudouch, H.; Zergoune, N.; Alkattan, D.; et al. The consequences of the lockdown on cardiovascular diseases. *Ann. Cardiol. Angeiol.* **2021**, *70*, 94–101. [CrossRef]
57. Wu, Y.; Li, H.; Tao, X.; Fan, Y.; Gao, Q.; Yang, J. Optimised anthropometric indices as predictive screening tools for metabolic syndrome in adults: A cross-sectional study. *BMJ Open* **2021**, *11*, e043952. [CrossRef]
58. Saklayen, M.G. The Global Epidemic of the Metabolic Syndrome. *Curr. Hypertens. Rep.* **2018**, *20*, 1–8. [CrossRef]
59. Bovolini, A.; Garcia, J.; Andrade, M.A.; Duarte, J.A. Metabolic Syndrome Pathophysiology and Predisposing Factors. *Int. J. Sports Med.* **2021**, *42*, 199–214. [CrossRef] [PubMed]
60. Yanai, H. Metabolic Syndrome and COVID-19. *Cardiol. Res.* **2020**, *11*, 360–365. [CrossRef] [PubMed]
61. Bansal, R.; Gubbi, S.; Muniyappa, R. Metabolic Syndrome and COVID 19: Endocrine-Immune-Vascular Interactions Shapes Clinical Course. *Endocrinology* **2020**, *161*, bqaa112. [CrossRef] [PubMed]
62. Stefan, N.; Birkenfeld, A.L.; Schulze, M.B. Global pandemics interconnected—Obesity, impaired metabolic health and COVID-19. *Nat. Rev. Endocrinol.* **2021**, *17*, 135–149. [CrossRef]
63. Li, B.; Yang, J.; Zhao, F.; Zhi, L.; Wang, X.; Liu, L.; Bi, Z.; Zhao, Y. Prevalence and impact of cardiovascular metabolic diseases on COVID-19 in China. *Clin. Res. Cardiol.* **2020**, *109*, 531–538. [CrossRef]
64. Chiu, T.-H.; Huang, Y.-C.; Chiu, H.; Wu, P.-Y.; Chiou, H.-Y.C.; Huang, J.-C.; Chen, S.-C. Comparison of Various Obesity-Related Indices for Identification of Metabolic Syndrome: A Population-Based Study from Taiwan Biobank. *Diagnostics* **2020**, *10*, 1081. [CrossRef]
65. Gonzalez-Chávez, A.; Chávez-Fernández, J.A.; Elizondo-Argueta, S.; González-Tapia, A.; Leon-Pedroza, J.I.; Ochoa, C. Metabolic Syndrome and Cardiovascular Disease: A Health Challenge. *Arch. Med. Res.* **2018**, *49*, 516–521. [CrossRef]
66. Xu, Q.; Wang, L.; Ming, J.; Cao, H.; Liu, T.; Yu, X.; Bai, Y.; Liang, S.; Hu, R.; Chen, C.; et al. Using noninvasive anthropometric indices to develop and validate a predictive model for metabolic syndrome in Chinese adults: A nationwide study. *BMC Endocr. Disord.* **2022**, *22*, 53. [CrossRef]
67. Delgado-Floody, P.; Álvarez, C.; Cadore, E.L.; Flores-Opazo, M.; Caamaño-Navarrete, F.; Izquierdo, M. Preventing metabolic syndrome in morbid obesity with resistance training: Reporting interindividual variability. *Nutr. Metab. Cardiovasc. Dis.* **2019**, *29*, 1368–1381. [CrossRef]
68. Myers, J.; Kokkinos, P.; Nyelin, E. Physical Activity, Cardiorespiratory Fitness, and the Metabolic Syndrome. *Nutrients* **2019**, *11*, 1652. [CrossRef]

69. Pinto, A.J.; Dunstan, D.W.; Owen, N.; Bonfa, E.; Gualano, B. Combating physical inactivity during the COVID-19 pandemic. *Nat. Rev. Rheumatol.* **2020**, *16*, 347–348. [CrossRef]
70. Xie, Y.; You, Q.; Wu, C.; Cao, S.; Qu, G.; Yan, X.; Han, X.; Wang, C.; Zhang, H. Impact of Cardiovascular Disease on Clinical Characteristics and Outcomes of Coronavirus Disease 2019 (COVID-19). *Circ. J.* **2020**, *84*, 1277–1283. [CrossRef]
71. Lavie, C.J.; Ozemek, C.; Carbone, S.; Katzmarzyk, P.T.; Blair, S.N. Sedentary Behavior, Exercise, and Cardiovascular Health. *Circ. Res.* **2019**, *124*, 799–815. [CrossRef]
72. Hendren, N.; De Lemos, J.; Ayers, C.; Das, S.; Rao, A.; Carter, S.; Rosenblatt, A.; Walcho, J.; Omar, W.; Khera, R.; et al. Association of Body Mass Index and Age with Morbidity and Mortality in Patients Hospitalized with COVIS-19: Results From the American Heart Association COVID-19 Cardiovascular Disease Registry. *Circulation* **2021**, *143*, 135–144. [CrossRef]
73. Hu, L.; Huang, X.; You, C.; Li, J.; Hong, K.; Li, P.; Wu, Y.; Wu, Q.; Wang, Z.; Gao, R.; et al. Prevalence of overweight, obesity, abdominal obesity and obesity-related risk factors in southern China. *PLoS ONE* **2017**, *12*, e0183934. [CrossRef]
74. García-Tascón, M.; Sahelices-Pinto, C.; Mendaña-Cuervo, C.; Magaz-González, A.M. The Impact of the COVID-19 Confinement on the Habits of PA Practice According to Gender (Male/Female): Spanish Case. *Int. J. Environ. Res. Public Health* **2020**, *17*, 6961. [CrossRef]
75. Wunsch, K.; Kienberger, K.; Niessner, C. Changes in Physical Activity Patterns Due to the COVID-19 Pandemic: A Systematic Review and Meta-Analysis. *Int. J. Environ. Res. Public Health* **2022**, *19*, 2250. [CrossRef] [PubMed]
76. Castañeda-Babarro, A.; Arbillaga-Etxarri, A.; Gutiérrez-Santamaría, B.; Coca, A. Physical Activity Change during COVID-19 Confinement. *Int. J. Environ. Res. Public Health* **2020**, *17*, 6878. [CrossRef] [PubMed]
77. Violant-Holz, V.; Gallego-Jiménez, M.G.; González-González, C.S.; Muñoz-Violant, S.; Rodríguez, M.J.; Sansano-Nadal, O.; Guerra-Balic, M. Psychological Health and Physical Activity Levels during the COVID-19 Pandemic: A Systematic Review. *Int. J. Environ. Res. Public Health* **2020**, *17*, 9419. [CrossRef] [PubMed]
78. De Rubies, V.; Lee, J.; Anwer, M.S.; Yoshida-Montezuma, Y.; Andreacchi, A.; Stone, E.; Iftikhar, S.; Motgenstern, J.; Rebinsky, R.; Neil-Sztramlo, S.; et al. Impact of disasters, including pandemics, on cardiometabolic outcomes across the life-course: A systematic review. *BMJ Open* **2021**, *11*, e047152. [CrossRef]

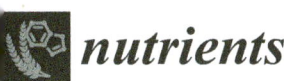

Article

Vitamin A Plasma Levels in COVID-19 Patients: A Prospective Multicenter Study and Hypothesis

Phil-Robin Tepasse [1,*,†], Richard Vollenberg [1,†], Manfred Fobker [2], Iyad Kabar [1], Hartmut Schmidt [1], Jörn Arne Meier [1], Tobias Nowacki [1] and Anna Hüsing-Kabar [1]

[1] Department of Medicine B for Gastroenterology, Hepatology, Endocrinology and Clinical Infectiology, University Hospital Muenster, 48149 Muenster, Germany; richard.vollenberg@ukmuenster.de (R.V.); iyad.kabar@ukmuenster.de (I.K.); hepar@ukmuenster.de (H.S.); joernarne.meier@ukmuenster.de (J.A.M.); tobias.nowacki@ukmuenster.de (T.N.); Anna.Huesing-Kabar@ukmuenster.de (A.H.-K.)

[2] Center for Laboratory Medicine, University Hospital Muenster, 48149 Muenster, Germany; manfred.fobker@ukmuenster.de

* Correspondence: phil-robin.tepasse@ukmuenster.de; Tel.: +49-251-834-4882

† These authors contributed equally to this work.

Abstract: COVID-19 is a pandemic disease that causes severe pulmonary damage and hyperinflammation. Vitamin A is a crucial factor in the development of immune functions and is known to be reduced in cases of acute inflammation. This prospective, multicenter observational cross-sectional study analyzed vitamin A plasma levels in SARS-CoV-2 infected individuals, and 40 hospitalized patients were included. Of these, 22 developed critical disease (Acute Respiratory Distress Syndrome [ARDS]/Extracorporeal membrane oxygenation [ECMO]), 9 developed severe disease (oxygen supplementation), and 9 developed moderate disease (no oxygen supplementation). A total of 47 age-matched convalescent persons that had been earlier infected with SARS-CoV-2 were included as the control group. Vitamin A plasma levels were determined by high-performance liquid chromatography. Reduced vitamin A plasma levels correlated significantly with increased levels of inflammatory markers (CRP, ferritin) and with markers of acute SARS-CoV-2 infection (reduced lymphocyte count, LDH). Vitamin A levels were significantly lower in hospitalized patients than in convalescent persons ($p < 0.01$). Of the hospitalized patients, those who were critically ill showed significantly lower vitamin A levels than those who were moderately ill ($p < 0.05$). Vitamin A plasma levels below 0.2 mg/L were significantly associated with the development of ARDS (OR = 5.54 [1.01–30.26]; $p = 0.048$) and mortality (OR 5.21 [1.06–25.5], $p = 0.042$). Taken together, we conclude that vitamin A plasma levels in COVID-19 patients are reduced during acute inflammation and that severely reduced plasma levels of vitamin A are significantly associated with ARDS and mortality.

Keywords: COVID-19; vitamin A; retinol; retinoic acid; ARDS; pneumonia; pandemic; SARS-CoV-2; inflammation

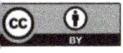

1. Introduction

Coronavirus disease 2019 (COVID-19) is a novel infectious disease that has been spreading worldwide [1]. The clinical manifestation of COVID-19 can range from asymptomatic infection to critical illness with severe pneumonia, respiratory failure, and death [2]. Worse clinical outcomes are related to dysregulated immune responses in the host, leading to the uncontrolled release of proinflammatory cytokines such as interleukin-6 (IL-6). This cytokine storm mediates the progression of lung damage and respiratory failure in a relevant number of cases [3]. The understanding of host parameters leading to the susceptibility of immune dysregulation is incomplete. A standard therapy has not yet been established. To date, the RNA-polymerase inhibitor remdesivir and the immunosuppressive corticosteroid dexamethasone are the only Food and Drug Administration (FDA) approved drugs for COVID-19 therapy with demonstrated effects on mortality and disease outcome [4,5]. Despite certain therapeutic approaches, the lethality of hospitalized, mechanically ventilated patients remains high [6].

Vitamin A is of special interest in the field of infectious diseases, especially for pulmonary infections. It is crucial for the development of normal lung tissue and tissue repair after injury due to infection [7]; therefore, it may play a role in recovery after severe COVID-19 pneumonia. Vitamin A has immune regulatory functions [8] and positively affects both the innate and adaptive immune cell response [9,10]. Malnutrition leads to relevant incidences of vitamin A deficiency worldwide. Vitamin A deficiency can disrupt vaccine-induced antibody-forming cells and negatively influences immunoglobulin development in the upper and lower respiratory tract [11]. Several studies revealed increased risks of severe illness due to respiratory tract infections in vitamin A-deficient individuals, whereas vitamin A supplementation can reduce the risks of severe illness and death, as was shown for children with measles and in influenza pneumonia in mice models [12–14]. The occurrence of severe infections and inflammation can also negatively affect vitamin A status, and several mechanisms such as urinary loss of vitamin A [15], decreased vitamin A hepatic mobilization [16], and reduced intestinal vitamin A absorption [17] during infection have been described.

Data concerning vitamin A plasma levels in COVID-19 patients are lacking. Therefore, this study aimed at characterizing vitamin A plasma levels in acute COVID-19 and analyzed the association of plasma levels with disease severity and outcome. Vitamin A plasma levels were found to be significantly reduced in COVID-19 patients during the acute phase of disease compared to plasma levels in convalescent patients, and a reduction in vitamin A levels correlated significantly with an increase in inflammatory parameters. Critically ill patients showed lower vitamin A levels compared to moderately ill patients and severely reduced vitamin A levels were associated with ARDS and mortality. Further research is necessary to investigate the role of vitamin A as a possible therapeutic agent for COVID-19.

2. Materials and Methods

2.1. Participant Selection and Patient Samples

This multicenter, prospective observational cross-sectional study included 40 hospitalized patients with laboratory-confirmed SARS-CoV-2 infection (nasopharyngeal swab and test by polymerase-chain reaction), admitted to the University Hospital Muenster and Marien-Hospital Steinfurt in Germany between March and June 2020. Details of medical history and laboratory data were collected. Blood from hospitalized patients was collected during acute phase of disease. Disease severity was defined as critical (presence of acute respiratory distress syndrome [ARDS]; $n = 22$), severe (requiring oxygen supplementation; $n = 9$) or moderate (neither ARDS was present nor oxygen supplementation required; $n = 9$). ARDS was diagnosed according to the Berlin definition (bilateral opacities on chest radiograph, exclusion of other causes of respiratory failure) [18]. COVID-19 patients were categorized according to their condition at the time of blood collection. One blood sample per patient was taken within the first 24 h after admission.

Additionally, 91 individuals with laboratory-confirmed SARS-CoV-2 infection who had recovered from infection were contacted for donation of convalescent plasma in our outpatient clinic. The blood sample was taken after recovery from disease. Of these, 47 were manually selected to match the age and gender of inpatients (Supplementary Figure S1). This group of patients had only moderate symptoms, and hospitalization was not necessary (Supplementary Figure S2).

Plasma samples were obtained from each participant after they provided informed consent. The Ethics Committee of Muenster University approved the current study (local ethics committee approval AZ 2020-220-f-S and AZ 2020-210-f-S), and the procedures were in accordance with the Helsinki Declaration of 1975 as revised in 1983. None of the patients received antiviral, experimental, or immunosuppressive therapies. Plasma samples were protected from light and frozen ($-80\ °C$) until measurement.

2.2. Vitamin A Measurement

Vitamin A (both free/unbound vitamin A and vitamin A bound to retinol binding protein [RBD]) was assayed on EDTA-plasma using a commercially available high-performance liquid chromatography kit (Chromsystems, Munich, Germany) following the manufacturer's instructions. Vitamin A levels were given in mg/L. For further analysis, participants were divided in to two groups (Group 1: vitamin A plasma levels ≥ 0.2 mg/L; Group 2: vitamin A plasma levels < 0.2 mg/L) following international guidelines on vitamin A deficiency from the World Health Organization (WHO, clinically relevant nutritional Vitamin A deficiency defined as Vitamin A plasma levels < 0.2 mg/L) [19].

2.3. Laboratory Measurements and Validation of the Clinical Status

Clinical laboratory assessment included complete blood count and levels of D-dimer, creatinine, C-reactive protein (CRP), albumin, lactate dehydrogenase (LDH), pseudo-cholinesterase (PCHe), and alanine aminotransferase (ALT). SAPS II (Simplified Acute Physiology Score [20]) was determined on the day of laboratory measurement and used to characterize the physiological conditions of hospitalized patients.

2.4. Data Analysis/Statistics

For continuous variables, we report the median with the interquartile range, and values were compared using the Mann–Whitney U (Wilcoxon) test. For categorical variables, we report absolute numbers and percentages, and values were compared with Chi-square tests of association or Fisher's exact tests. A Kruskal–Wallis test was conducted to compare more than two groups. To compare subgroups, the Bonferroni correction post hoc test was performed when variance was equal (Levene's test), and the Games-Howell test was performed when variance was different. The Pearson correlation coefficient was determined to analyze the correlation of vitamin A levels with clinical laboratory parameters. Univariable logistic regression analysis was conducted to determine the association of severely reduced vitamin A plasma levels with the risk of acute respiratory distress syndrome (ARDS) and mortality due to COVID-19 in hospitalized patients ($n = 40$). All the tests were two-tailed, and $p < 0.05$ was considered to indicate a statistically significant difference. All the statistical analyses were performed using SPSS (Version 26IBM Corp., Armonk, NY, USA).

3. Results

3.1. Cohort Characteristics

Most participants were male (77.8–100%) in all groups. The median interval between symptom onset and sample collection in hospitalized patients was 12 days (IQR 8, 3–17), in outpatients 52 days (IQR 40–75). The median age was 50–58 years and did not significantly differ between groups, nor too did the interval from the first symptom to the collection of the blood sample. Preexisting diseases were prevalent almost exclusively in the group of critically ill patients. SAPS II differed significantly between hospitalized patients, as did inflammatory and blood count parameters (for example C-reactive protein and lymphocyte count) (Table 1). The correlations of the subgroups are shown in Supplementary Figure S3.

3.2. Correlation of Vitamin A Plasma Levels with Laboratory Parameters

In the overall study group ($n = 87$), reduced vitamin A plasma levels correlated significantly with increased levels of the inflammation markers C-reactive protein ($r = -0.54$, $p < 0.001$) and ferritin ($r = -0.45$, $p < 0.001$). Reduced absolute ($r = 0.4$, $p < 0.001$) and relative lymphocyte counts ($r = 0.43$, $p < 0.001$), reduced albumin levels ($r = 0.65$, $p < 0.001$), and elevated lactate dehydrogenase levels ($r = -0.53$, $p < 0.001$) correlated significantly with reduced vitamin A plasma levels. Elevated levels of liver markers (AST: $r = -0.22$, $p < 0.05$; gamma-GT: $r = -0.29$, $p < 0.01$) also correlated significantly with reduced vitamin A levels. Reduced vitamin A levels were associated with reduced pseudocholinesterase (PCHe) levels as a parameter of the liver synthetic capacity ($r = 0.53$, $p < 0.001$) (Figure 1).

Table 1. Cohort characteristics; differences were calculated via the Kruskal–Wallis test; BMI = body mass index, SAPS II = Simplified Acute Physiology Score II; IQR = interquartile range; LDH = lactate dehydrogenase; PCHe = pseudocholinesterase, ALT = alanine aminotransferase; abs. = absolute; n.d. = not defined.

	Moderate Disease (n = 9)	Severe Disease (n = 9)	Critical Disease (n = 22)	Convalescent Patients (n = 47)	p-Value
Age, median (min–max)	54 (30–81)	50 (39–73)	58 (41–82)	54 (41–70)	0.24
Gender, male (%)	77.8	100.0	90.9	97.9	0.29
BMI, median (IQR)	24 (23–26)	24 (23–26)	27 (24–30)	26 (24–28)	0.05
Interval from first symptom to acquisition of blood sample in days, median (IQR)	8 (6–14)	13 (8.5–17)	12 (10–22)	52 (40–75)	0.15
Cardiovascular disease (abs.)	1	0	4	0	
Respiratory disease abs.)	0	0	2	0	
Kidney insufficiency (abs.)	0	0	0	0	
Metastatic neoplasm (abs.)	0	0	0	0	
Diabetes (abs.)	0	0	1	0	
Hematologic malignancy (abs.)	2	0	4	0	
Death (abs.)	0	0	9	0	
SAPS II, median (IQR)	15 (13–25)	19 (13–22)	54 (35–72)	n.d.	<0.001
Leukocytes $\times 10^9$/L, median (IQR)	4.4 (3.4–6.4)	5.4 (3.8–7.6)	9.2 (5.8–11)	5.4 (4.9–6.8)	0.21
Lymphocytes (rel., %), median (IQR)	19.5 (12.6–29.9)	21.3 (15.0–22.8)	10.3 (7.3–14.0)	29.0 (25.3–32.5)	0.003
D-Dimer (mg/L), median (IQR)	0.75 (0.32–2.31)	0.76 (0.55–2.02)	2.56 (1.42–7.42)	n.d.	0.005
Creatinine (mg/dL), median (IQR)	1.0 (0.9–1.2)	0.8 (0.8–1.0)	1 (0.6–1.7)	1 (0.9–1)	0.36
Ferritin (µg/L), median (IQR)	449 (200–665)	692 (370–938)	917 (665–1560)	188 (89–325)	0.003
Interleukin-6 (pg/mL), median (IQR)	16 (10–30)	30 (17–70)	107 (39–239)	2 (2–2)	<0.001
Procalcitonin (ng/mL), median (IQR)	0.11 (0.07–0.18)	0.08 (0.07–0.12)	0.64 (0.18–2.04)	0.05 (0.04–0.07)	<0.001
C-reactive protein (mg/dL), median (IQR)	1.6 (0.5–3.2)	6 (3.3–9.4)	14.8 (6.2–24.8)	0.5 (0.5–0.5)	<0.001
PCHe (U/L), median (IQR)	7746 (5524–9193)	6960 (6173–8321)	3668 (2749–4788)	8699 (7754–10082)	<0.001
Gamma-GT (U/L), median (IQR)	43 (30–126)	40 (30–60)	113 (54–185)	29 (21–47)	<0.001
ALT (U/L), median (IQR)	26 (22–46)	33 (29–58)	41 (29–67)	29 (24–40)	0.079
Albumin (g/dL), median (IQR)	3.9 (3.3–4.5)	3.8 (3.5–4.4)	2.3 (3.0–2.7)	4.6 (4.4–4.7)	<0.001
Vitamin A (mg/L), median (IQR)	0.48 (0.29–0.56)	0.32 (0.21–0.42)	0.25 (0.16–0.38)	0.60 (0.51–0.69)	<0.001

3.3. Vitamin A Plasma Levels in COVID-19 Patients

Vitamin A plasma levels differed significantly depending on disease severity. Hospitalized patients of all groups (mild, moderate, severe, and critical disease) revealed significantly reduced vitamin A plasma levels compared to convalescent outpatients ($p < 0.01$ to $p < 0.001$). In hospitalized patients, the vitamin A plasma levels of critically ill patients were significantly reduced compared to patients with moderate disease ($p < 0.05$). Patients with severe disease also had reduced plasma levels compared to patients with moderate disease, but this finding did not reach statistical significance (median: 0.32 vs. 0.48 mg/L) (Figure 2).

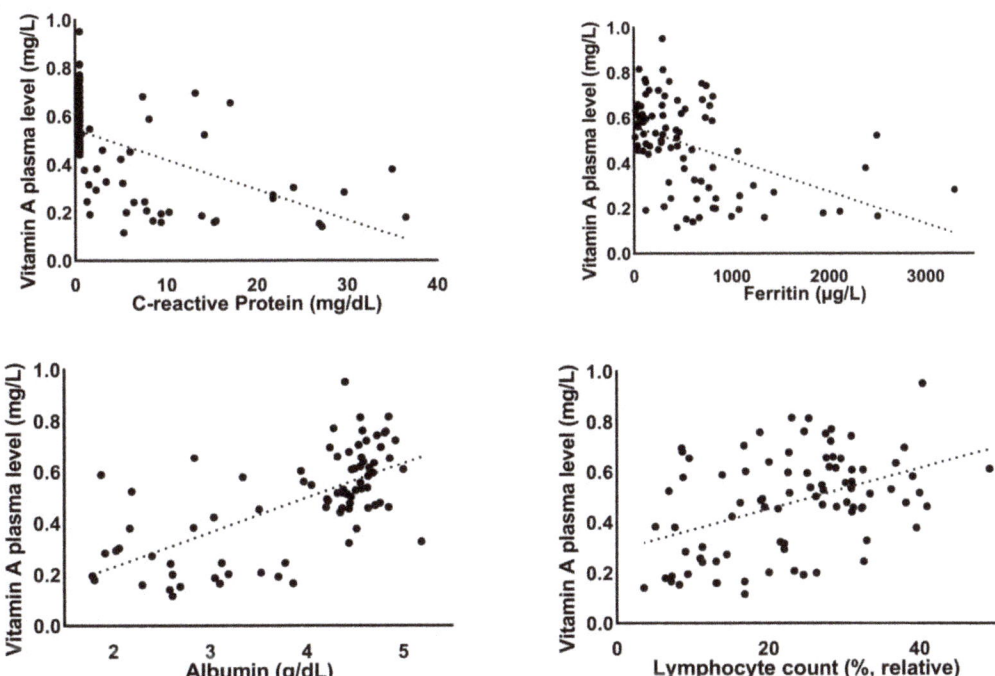

Figure 1. Correlation of vitamin A plasma levels with laboratory parameters.

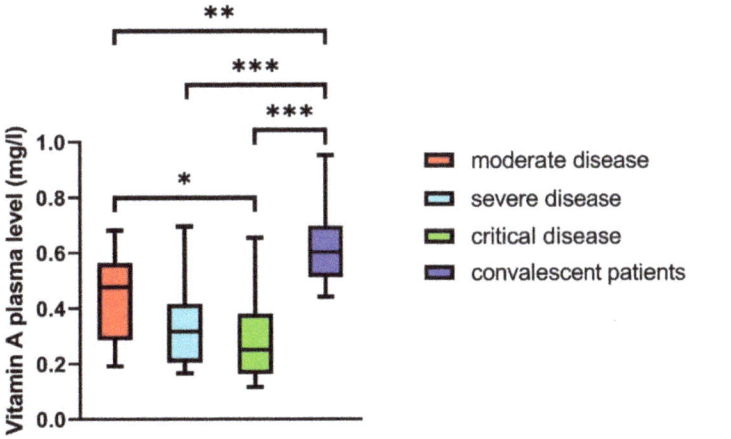

Figure 2. Vitamin A plasma levels in patients with moderate, severe, and critical disease, and in convalescent patients; the Wilcoxon rank test showed significant differences ($p < 0.001$). Subgroups were tested for differences in the Bonferroni correction (* $p < 0.05$, ** $p < 0.01$, *** $p < 0.001$). Mann–Whitney U test was used to compare groups (* $p < 0.05$, ** $p < 0.01$, *** $p < 0.001$).

3.4. Association of Severely Reduced Vitamin A Plasma Levels with the Development of ARDS and Mortality

As described in the methods section, Vitamin A plasma levels <0.2 mg/L were considered clinically relevant reduced. In the overall study group, 14% ($n = 11/87$) of participants revealed clinically relevant reduced vitamin A plasma levels. Looking at different patient groups, 41% ($n = 9/22$) of critically ill, 11% ($n = 1/9$) of moderately ill, and 11% ($n = 1/9$) of severely ill patients had vitamin A plasma levels <2 mg/L, while none of the participants in the convalescent group had clinically relevant reduced vitamin A levels (0/47) (Figure 3).

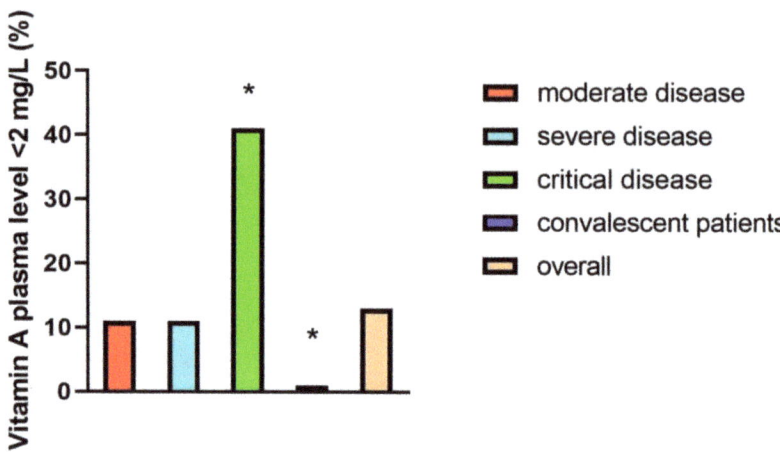

Figure 3. Percentages of patients with vitamin A plasma levels <2 mg/L in different patient groups: moderate disease ($n = 9$), severe disease ($n = 9$), critical disease ($n = 22$), and convalescent patients ($n = 47$). Representation of significances according to Bonferroni correction (* $p < 0.05$).

After dividing the hospitalized patients into two groups (Group 1: Vitamin A < 2 mg/L; Group 2: Vitamin A $\geq$ 2 mg/L), Group 1 patients ($n = 11$) revealed significantly higher C-reactive protein levels (median 13.9 vs. 6 mg/dL, $p = 0.03$), lower absolute lymphocyte counts (median 0.69 Tsd/µL vs. 1.13 Tsd/µL, $p = 0.01$), and lower relative lymphocyte counts (median 9.4% vs. 15.2%, $p = 0.049$) compared to Group 2 ($n = 29$). Patients in Group 1 developed ARDS much more frequently ($p = 0.038$), and mortality was significantly higher ($p = 0.047$) (Table 2). Logistic regression analysis revealed significant associations of clinically relevant reduced vitamin A plasma levels with the development of ARDS (OR = 5.54 [1.01–30.26] $p = 0.048$) and with mortality (OR 5.21 [1.06–25.5], $p = 0.042$) in the hospitalized patient group ($n = 40$).

Table 2. Clinical outcomes and inflammation parameters based on vitamin A plasma levels; differences were calculated using the Mann–Whitney U test or Fisher's exact test (both 2-tailed); SAPS II = Simplified Acute Physiology Score II; BMI = body mass index; ARDS = acute respiratory distress syndrome; IQR = interquartile range; LDH = lactate dehydrogenase; PCHe = pseudocholinesterase, ALT = alanine aminotransferase.

	Vitamin A < 2 mg/L (n = 11)	Vitamin A $\geq$ 2 mg/L (n = 29)	p-Value
Age, median (min–max)	52.6 (30–66)	57.1 (33–82)	0.52
Gender, male (%)	91	90	0.56
BMI, median (IQR)	25 (24–28)	25 (23–28)	0.51
Interval from first symptom to acquisition of blood sample in days, median (IQR)	11 (9–12)	13 (8–17.5)	0.42
Preexisting disease (%)	45	48	0.45
ARDS (abs.)	9	13	0.038
Death (abs.)	5	4	0.047

Table 2. Cont.

	Vitamin A < 2 mg/L (n = 11)	Vitamin A ≥ 2 mg/L (n = 29)	p-Value
SAPS II score, median (IQR)	43 (22–61)	28 (15.5–55.5)	0.39
Leukocytes × 10^9/L, median (IQR)	5.99 (2.67–11.9)	6.97 (4.56–9.89)	0.56
Lymphocytes (rel., %), median (IQR)	9.4 (7.2–16.9)	15.2 (9.35–22.1)	0.049
Lymphocytes (abs., Tsd/μL), median (IQR)	0.69 (0.47–1.01)	1.13 (0.79–1.38)	0.01
D-Dimer (mg/L), median (IQR)	2.01 (0.78–4.25)	1.78 (0.65–3.57)	0.84
Creatinine mg/dL, median (IQR)			0.15
Ferritin (μg/L), median (IQR)	917 (554–1788)	738 (465–1008)	0.39
Interleukin-6 (pg/mL), median (IQR)	88 (37–199)	33 (16–95)	0.05
Procalcitonin (ng/mL), median (IQR)	0.31 (0.12–0.80)	0.13 (0.08–0.7)	0.3
C-reactive protein (mg/dL), median (IQR)	13.9 (8.5–26.9)	6 (1.95–13.7)	0.03
PCHe (U/L), median (IQR)	4082 (3012–5643)	5555 (3566–7814)	0.15
Gamma-GT (U/L), median (IQR)	116 (40–211)	55 (34–130)	0.13
ALT (U/L), median (IQR)	44 (39–70)	31 (26–48)	0.11
Albumin g/dL, median (IQR)	2.7 (2.2–3.3)	3.1 (2.2–4.0)	0.25
Vitamin A (mg/L), median (IQR)	0.17 (0.16–0.19)	0.38 (0.28–0.52)	<0.0001

4. Discussion

This study analyzed associations of vitamin A plasma levels with inflammatory parameters, disease severity, and outcomes in moderately, severely, and critically ill COVID-19 patients during the acute phase of the disease and in comparison to convalescent patients.

Age, gender, and time from disease onset to collection of blood sample adequately matched and did not differ significantly between hospitalized groups in the acute phase of the disease. Our cohort characteristics showed significantly higher levels of inflammatory markers (CRP, IL-6, ferritin) and lower lymphocyte counts in patients with critical disease cases compared to moderately and severely ill and convalescent patients. These data are in line with other studies as both increased inflammatory parameters and decreased lymphocyte counts are well-defined markers of active disease and predictive of a severe course of COVID-19 [21]. D-Dimer is also an established predictive marker [22] and its levels were found to be significantly increased along with disease severity in our study cohort.

This study revealed significantly decreased vitamin A plasma levels in the acute phase of moderately, severely, and critically ill patients compared to convalescent patients after recovery from acute disease. In the acute phase, critically ill patients had significantly lower vitamin A plasma levels compared to moderately ill patients. In the overall study cohort, correlation analysis provided evidence that higher inflammatory parameters such as C-reactive protein, ferritin, and albumin significantly correlated with reduced vitamin A plasma levels. This finding supports existing data showing reduced vitamin A plasma levels due to several mechanisms such as urinary loss [15], decreased hepatic mobilization [16], and reduced absorption [17] during infection and acute inflammatory conditions. Moreover, lymphopenia, an established disease activity marker and predictor of worse outcomes in COVID-19 patients [21], significantly correlated with reduced vitamin A plasma levels. Reduced serum albumin levels [23] and elevated LDH levels [24], also established predictors of severe disease and worse outcome, were both significantly correlated with lower vitamin A plasma levels. Liver damage is often found in severely ill COVID-19 patients [25]. Elevated levels of liver enzymes also correlated significantly with reduced vitamin A levels. Interestingly, a reduction in the levels of pseudocholinesterase (PChE), a parameter for liver synthetic capacity, correlated with reduced vitamin A levels. The association with decreased hepatic vitamin A mobilization during acute inflammation remains speculative but conceivable and needs further analysis.

Clinically relevant decreased vitamin A plasma levels (defined as <2 mg/L following the WHO definition for vitamin A deficiency [19]) were almost exclusively found in the acute phase of disease in critically ill patients. To analyze the correlation of severely reduced vitamin A plasma levels with disease outcome, we divided the hospitalized patient cohort in two groups (patients with vitamin A levels ≥ 2 and <2 mg/L). This subgroup analysis showed that patients with vitamin A plasma levels <2 mg/L developed ARDS at a significantly higher rate ($p < 0.05$), and mortality was also much higher in this group ($p < 0.05$). Levels of C-reactive protein were higher and lymphopenia more distinctive, indicating a more severe disease course [21]. These results provide evidence that the reduction of vitamin A plasma levels in COVID-19 is dependent on disease severity and that plasma levels are reduced due to acute infection and inflammation rather than preexisting vitamin A deficiency and malnutrition, as convalescent patients had normal levels of vitamin A in plasma. Furthermore, malnutrition and vitamin A deficiency are rare in Germany. Nonetheless, vitamin A deficiency due to malnutrition is still one of the most prevalent micronutrient deficiencies worldwide, affecting approximately one-third of preschool-age children, especially in underdeveloped countries. Vitamin A deficiency is associated with increased mortality in children and pregnant women due to severe gastrointestinal and respiratory infections [19,26]. Several studies have highlighted the importance of vitamin A for lung function and development [27]. Other studies confirmed that vitamin A has immune-modulating properties and plays an important role in the immune response to infections, mainly through retinoic acid, its main metabolite. Early randomized clinical trials studying the effect of vitamin A supplementation showed it resulted in a significant reduction of mortality and less severe manifestations of several infectious diseases in cases of vitamin A deficiency due to malnutrition [12,28]. On the contrary, the consequences of reduced vitamin A levels that are due to acute inflammation are not well understood.

Vitamin A influences cellular immunity in a wide variety. A number of studies have shown that vitamin A has a central function in the development and differentiation of dendritic cells (DCs), the most important antigen-presenting cells for activating naive T-cells. DCs express three isotypes of RA receptor and, therefore, directly respond to vitamin A [29]. After receptor activation, DCs drive T-cell differentiation into either anti-inflammatory regulating T-cells (Treg) or proinflammatory effector T-cells, and through this, they maintain homeostasis between anti-inflammatory and proinflammatory stimuli [30]. To resolve infection, vitamin A leads to the migration of effector T-cells to the inflammatory site via the induction of leukocyte-homing receptors such as CCR9 and $\alpha 4\beta 7$ integrin [31]. Vitamin A initiates the production of proinflammatory cytokines such as interferon-gamma to resolve viral infection [32]. Vitamin A also drives the humoral immune response, as it crucially promotes B-cell maturation and antibody responses in viral clearance [33,34]. To limit proinflammatory stimuli, vitamin A promotes the differentiation and extravasation of anti-inflammatory Treg cells to the site of inflammation [35]. Taken together, vitamin A can promote both proinflammatory and anti-inflammatory cellular immune responses.

In COVID-19, immune imbalance and the disruption of T-cell responses may be important drivers of severe disease. Real-world data suggest a strong antiviral T-cell response after infection with SARS-CoV-2. The majority of SARS-CoV-2-specific T-cells show an effector phenotype with the dominant production of antiviral proteins, such as interferon-gamma, to terminate infection [36]. However, in patients with severe and critical disease, T-cells exhibit lower levels of antiviral interferon-gamma compared to patients with mild disease [37]. This is known as COVID-19-associated "T-cell exhaustion" and may lead to impaired viral clearance. The resulting massive replication of SARS-CoV-2 and viral infection of cells and organs and subsequent viral release from dying cells is considered as an initial driver of cytokine storming, leading to uncontrolled immune reactions and often fatal outcomes due to multiple organ failure [38]. Furthermore, levels of anti-inflammatory

Treg cells in critically ill COVID-19 patients are lower than those in patients with mild disease [39], possibly leading to further uncontrolled immune reactions. As described above, vitamin A influences the production of interferon-gamma through effector T-cells as well as the differentiation of anti-inflammatory Treg cells. Our study results show a significant reduction of vitamin A levels in critically ill COVID-19 patients. Owing to these study results, vitamin A should be considered a relevant agent in maintaining immune balance in mild and moderate COVID-19. Immune imbalance and disruption of antiviral T-cell responses in cases of severe and critical COVID-19 may, in part, be driven by decreased vitamin A plasma levels during the acute phase.

This study has some limitations. First, this study can only reveal descriptive data and does not prove causality. Further studies are needed to clarify whether COVID-19 disease course worsens as a result of Vitamin A reduction in patients serum, or Vitamin A levels decrease as a consequence of severe COVID-19 and whether this reduction itself has an impact on disease course. Second, it has to be pointed out that in this study both unbound vitamin A and vitamin A bound to retinol binding protein (RBP) were measured. It is known that hepatic synthesis of RBP is reduced following acute phase reactions in terms of prioritization of the liver for synthesis of acute phase proteins such as CRP and ferritin [40]. Further studies including analysis of free (unbound) vitamin A in plasma are needed to clarify whether vitamin A reduction in plasma in COVID-19 patients is a consequence of reduced RBD synthesis or free (unbound) vitamin A is reduced as well. Third, the sample size in cohort subgroups is small, which can lead to bias especially in analyses for associations between Vitamin A levels and ARDS/mortality. The small number of events in univariate analyses could possibly lead to confounding factors and lead to misinterpretation. Taking these limitations into account the consequences of reduced vitamin A plasma levels in COVID-19 patients require further research to investigate possible therapeutic approaches of vitamin A supplementation during acute infection. Finally, controlled prospective studies are needed to investigate the therapeutic effect of vitamin A supplementation in cases of acute COVID-19.

Supplementary Materials: The following are available online at https://www.mdpi.com/article/10.3390/nu13072173/s1, Supplementary Figure S1: Study flowchart Vitamin A plasma levels in COVID-19 patients: A prospective multicenter study and hypothesis. COVID-19, coronavirus disease 2019, Supplementary Figure S2: Representation of the percentage symptom expression of the convalescent COVID-19 patient cohort during acute phase of disease. At the time of blood sampling after recovery from disease, the patients were all free of symptoms, Supplementary Figure S3: Presentation of important laboratory parameters. Classification into moderate, severe and ciritical disease and convalescent patients (* $p < 0.05$, ** $p < 0.01$, *** $p < 0.001$).

Author Contributions: Conceptualization, P.-R.T., R.V. and A.H.-K.; Investigation, P.-R.T., R.V. and T.N.; Methodology, M.F. and A.H.-K.; Software, J.A.M.; Supervision, I.K. and H.S.; Validation, J.A.M.; Visualization, P.-R.T. and J.A.M.; Writing—original draft, P.-R.T. and R.V.; Writing—review & editing, P.-R.T., I.K. and A.H.-K. All authors have read and agreed to the published version of the manuscript.

Funding: This research received no external funding.

Institutional Review Board Statement: The study was conducted according to the guidelines of the Declaration of Helsinki and approved by the local Ethics Committee of the University of Münster (AZ 2020-220-f-S and AZ 2020-210-f-S).

Informed Consent Statement: Informed consent was obtained from all subjects involved in the study.

Data Availability Statement: Data cannot be made public as personal patient data are included.

Conflicts of Interest: The authors declare no conflict of interest.

References

1. Coronaviridae Study Group of the International Committee on Taxonomy of Viruses. The species Severe acute respiratory syndrome-related coronavirus: Classifying 2019-nCoV and naming it SARS-CoV-2. *Nat. Microbiol.* **2020**, *5*, 536–544. [CrossRef] [PubMed]
2. Cummings, M.J.; Baldwin, M.R.; Abrams, D.; Jacobson, S.D.; Meyer, B.J.; Balough, E.M.; Aaron, J.G.; Claassen, J.; Rabbani, L.E.; Hastie, J.; et al. Epidemiology, clinical course, and outcomes of critically ill adults with COVID-19 in New York City: A prospective cohort study. *Lancet* **2020**. [CrossRef]
3. Jose, R.J.; Manuel, A. COVID-19 cytokine storm: The interplay between inflammation and coagulation. *Lancet Respir. Med.* **2020**. [CrossRef]
4. Beigel, J.H.; Tomashek, K.M.; Dodd, L.E.; Mehta, A.K.; Zingman, B.S.; Kalil, A.C.; Hohmann, E.; Chu, H.Y.; Luetkemeyer, A.; Kline, S.; et al. Remdesivir for the Treatment of Covid-19—Preliminary Report. *N. Engl. J. Med.* **2020**. [CrossRef]
5. Group, R.C.; Horby, P.; Lim, W.S.; Emberson, J.R.; Mafham, M.; Bell, J.L.; Linsell, L.; Staplin, N.; Brightling, C.; Ustianowski, A.; et al. Dexamethasone in Hospitalized Patients with Covid-19—Preliminary Report. *N. Engl. J. Med.* **2020**. [CrossRef]
6. Karagiannidis, C.; Mostert, C.; Hentschker, C.; Voshaar, T.; Malzahn, J.; Schillinger, G.; Klauber, J.; Janssens, U.; Marx, G.; Weber-Carstens, S.; et al. Case characteristics, resource use, and outcomes of 10 021 patients with COVID-19 admitted to 920 German hospitals: An observational study. *Lancet Respir. Med.* **2020**, *8*, 853–862. [CrossRef]
7. Timoneda, J.; Rodriguez-Fernandez, L.; Zaragoza, R.; Marin, M.P.; Cabezuelo, M.T.; Torres, L.; Vina, J.R.; Barber, T. Vitamin A Deficiency and the Lung. *Nutrients* **2018**, *10*, 1132. [CrossRef]
8. Chew, B.P.; Park, J.S. Carotenoid action on the immune response. *J. Nutr.* **2004**, *134*, 257S–261S. [CrossRef] [PubMed]
9. Huang, Z.; Liu, Y.; Qi, G.; Brand, D.; Zheng, S.G. Role of Vitamin A in the Immune System. *J. Clin. Med.* **2018**, *7*, 258. [CrossRef] [PubMed]
10. Raverdeau, M.; Mills, K.H. Modulation of T cell and innate immune responses by retinoic Acid. *J. Immunol.* **2014**, *192*, 2953–2958. [CrossRef]
11. Surman, S.L.; Rudraraju, R.; Sealy, R.; Jones, B.; Hurwitz, J.L. Vitamin A deficiency disrupts vaccine-induced antibody-forming cells and the balance of IgA/IgG isotypes in the upper and lower respiratory tract. *Viral Immunol.* **2012**, *25*, 341–344. [CrossRef]
12. Glasziou, P.P.; Mackerras, D.E. Vitamin A supplementation in infectious diseases: A meta-analysis. *BMJ* **1993**, *306*, 366–370. [CrossRef]
13. Hussey, G.D.; Klein, M. A randomized, controlled trial of vitamin A in children with severe measles. *N. Engl. J. Med.* **1990**, *323*, 160–164. [CrossRef]
14. Penkert, R.R.; Smith, A.P.; Hrincius, E.R.; McCullers, J.A.; Vogel, P.; Smith, A.M.; Hurwitz, J.L. Vitamin A deficiency dysregulates immune responses toward influenza virus and increases mortality after bacterial coinfections. *J. Infect. Dis.* **2020**. [CrossRef]
15. Stephensen, C.B. Vitamin A, infection, and immune function. *Annu. Rev. Nutr.* **2001**, *21*, 167–192. [CrossRef]
16. Gieng, S.H.; Green, M.H.; Green, J.B.; Rosales, F.J. Model-based compartmental analysis indicates a reduced mobilization of hepatic vitamin A during inflammation in rats. *J. Lipid Res.* **2007**, *48*, 904–913. [CrossRef]
17. Aklamati, E.K.; Mulenga, M.; Dueker, S.R.; Buchholz, B.A.; Peerson, J.M.; Kafwembe, E.; Brown, K.H.; Haskell, M.J. Accelerator mass spectrometry can be used to assess vitamin A metabolism quantitatively in boys in a community setting. *J. Nutr.* **2010**, *140*, 1588–1594. [CrossRef]
18. Force, A.D.T.; Ranieri, V.M.; Rubenfeld, G.D.; Thompson, B.T.; Ferguson, N.D.; Caldwell, E.; Fan, E.; Camporota, L.; Slutsky, A.S. Acute respiratory distress syndrome: The Berlin Definition. *JAMA* **2012**, *307*, 2526–2533. [CrossRef]
19. WHO. Global prevalence of vitamin A deficiency in populations at risk 1995–2005. In *WHO Global Database on Vitamin A Deficiency*; World Health Organization: Geneva, Switzerland, 2009.
20. Lucena, J.F.; Alegre, F.; Martinez-Urbistondo, D.; Landecho, M.F.; Huerta, A.; Garcia-Mouriz, A.; Garcia, N.; Quiroga, J. Performance of SAPS II and SAPS 3 in intermediate care. *PLoS ONE* **2013**, *8*, e77229. [CrossRef]
21. Zhao, Q.; Meng, M.; Kumar, R.; Wu, Y.; Huang, J.; Deng, Y.; Weng, Z.; Yang, L. Lymphopenia is associated with severe coronavirus disease 2019 (COVID-19) infections: A systemic review and meta-analysis. *Int. J. Infect. Dis.* **2020**, *96*, 131–135. [CrossRef]
22. Zhang, L.; Yan, X.; Fan, Q.; Liu, H.; Liu, X.; Liu, Z.; Zhang, Z. D-dimer levels on admission to predict in-hospital mortality in patients with Covid-19. *J. Thromb. Haemost.* **2020**, *18*, 1324–1329. [CrossRef]
23. Aziz, M.; Fatima, R.; Lee-Smith, W.; Assaly, R. The association of low serum albumin level with severe COVID-19: A systematic review and meta-analysis. *Crit. Care* **2020**, *24*, 255. [CrossRef]
24. Zhang, J.J.Y.; Lee, K.S.; Ang, L.W.; Leo, Y.S.; Young, B.E. Risk Factors for Severe Disease and Efficacy of Treatment in Patients Infected With COVID-19: A Systematic Review, Meta-Analysis, and Meta-Regression Analysis. *Clin. Infect. Dis.* **2020**, *71*, 2199–2206. [CrossRef]
25. Wang, Y.; Liu, S.; Liu, H.; Li, W.; Lin, F.; Jiang, L.; Li, X.; Xu, P.; Zhang, L.; Zhao, L.; et al. SARS-CoV-2 infection of the liver directly contributes to hepatic impairment in patients with COVID-19. *J. Hepatol.* **2020**, *73*, 807–816. [CrossRef]
26. Sommer, A.; Tarwotjo, I.; Hussaini, G.; Susanto, D. Increased mortality in children with mild vitamin A deficiency. *Lancet* **1983**, *2*, 585–588. [CrossRef]
27. Biesalski, H.K.; Nohr, D. Importance of vitamin-A for lung function and development. *Mol. Aspects Med.* **2003**, *24*, 431–440. [CrossRef]

28. Sommer, A. Vitamin a deficiency and clinical disease: An historical overview. *J. Nutr.* **2008**, *138*, 1835–1839. [CrossRef]
29. Manicassamy, S.; Ravindran, R.; Deng, J.; Oluoch, H.; Denning, T.L.; Kasturi, S.P.; Rosenthal, K.M.; Evavold, B.D.; Pulendran, B. Toll-like receptor 2-dependent induction of vitamin A-metabolizing enzymes in dendritic cells promotes T regulatory responses and inhibits autoimmunity. *Nat. Med.* **2009**, *15*, 401–409. [CrossRef]
30. Ruane, D.; Brane, L.; Reis, B.S.; Cheong, C.; Poles, J.; Do, Y.; Zhu, H.; Velinzon, K.; Choi, J.H.; Studt, N.; et al. Lung dendritic cells induce migration of protective T cells to the gastrointestinal tract. *J. Exp. Med.* **2013**, *210*, 1871–1888. [CrossRef]
31. Iwata, M.; Hirakiyama, A.; Eshima, Y.; Kagechika, H.; Kato, C.; Song, S.Y. Retinoic acid imprints gut-homing specificity on T cells. *Immunity* **2004**, *21*, 527–538. [CrossRef]
32. Hall, J.A.; Cannons, J.L.; Grainger, J.R.; Dos Santos, L.M.; Hand, T.W.; Naik, S.; Wohlfert, E.A.; Chou, D.B.; Oldenhove, G.; Robinson, M.; et al. Essential role for retinoic acid in the promotion of CD4(+) T cell effector responses via retinoic acid receptor alpha. *Immunity* **2011**, *34*, 435–447. [CrossRef] [PubMed]
33. Chen, Q.; Ross, A.C. Retinoic acid promotes mouse splenic B cell surface IgG expression and maturation stimulated by CD40 and IL-4. *Cell Immunol.* **2007**, *249*, 37–45. [CrossRef] [PubMed]
34. Ma, Y.; Chen, Q.; Ross, A.C. Retinoic acid and polyriboinosinic:polyribocytidylic acid stimulate robust anti-tetanus antibody production while differentially regulating type 1/type 2 cytokines and lymphocyte populations. *J. Immunol.* **2005**, *174*, 7961–7969. [CrossRef] [PubMed]
35. Kang, S.G.; Lim, H.W.; Andrisani, O.M.; Broxmeyer, H.E.; Kim, C.H. Vitamin A metabolites induce gut-homing FoxP3+ regulatory T cells. *J. Immunol.* **2007**, *179*, 3724–3733. [CrossRef]
36. Weiskopf, D.; Schmitz, K.S.; Raadsen, M.P.; Grifoni, A.; Okba, N.M.A.; Endeman, H.; van den Akker, J.P.C.; Molenkamp, R.; Koopmans, M.P.G.; van Gorp, E.C.M.; et al. Phenotype and kinetics of SARS-CoV-2-specific T cells in COVID-19 patients with acute respiratory distress syndrome. *Sci. Immunol.* **2020**, *5*. [CrossRef]
37. Zheng, H.Y.; Zhang, M.; Yang, C.X.; Zhang, N.; Wang, X.C.; Yang, X.P.; Dong, X.Q.; Zheng, Y.T. Elevated exhaustion levels and reduced functional diversity of T cells in peripheral blood may predict severe progression in COVID-19 patients. *Cell Mol. Immunol.* **2020**, *17*, 541–543. [CrossRef]
38. McGonagle, D.; Sharif, K.; O'Regan, A.; Bridgewood, C. The Role of Cytokines including Interleukin-6 in COVID-19 induced Pneumonia and Macrophage Activation Syndrome-Like Disease. *Autoimmun. Rev.* **2020**, *19*, 102537. [CrossRef]
39. Tan, M.; Liu, Y.; Zhou, R.; Deng, X.; Li, F.; Liang, K.; Shi, Y. Immunopathological characteristics of coronavirus disease 2019 cases in Guangzhou, China. *Immunology* **2020**, *160*, 261–268. [CrossRef]
40. Biolo, G.; Toigo, G.; Ciocchi, B.; Situlin, R.; Iscra, F.; Gullo, A.; Guarnieri, G. Metabolic response to injury and sepsis: Changes in protein metabolism. *Nutrition* **1997**, *13*, 52S–57S. [CrossRef]

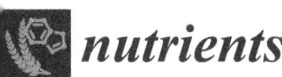 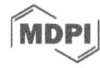

Article

Adherence to COVID-19 Nutrition Guidelines Is Associated with Better Nutritional Management Behaviors of Hospitalized COVID-19 Patients

Amelia Faradina [1], Sung-Hui Tseng [2,3], Dang Khanh Ngan Ho [1], Esti Nurwanti [4], Hamam Hadi [5,6,7], Sintha Dewi Purnamasari [5,6,7], Imaning Yulia Rochmah [8] and Jung-Su Chang [1,9,10,11,*]

1. School of Nutrition and Health Sciences, College of Nutrition, Taipei Medical University, Taipei 110, Taiwan; amelia.faradinaa@gmail.com (A.F.); nganhdk91@gmail.com (D.K.N.H.)
2. Department of Physical Medicine and Rehabilitation, Taipei Medical University Hospital, Taipei 110, Taiwan; d301091012@tmu.edu.tw
3. Department of Physical Medicine and Rehabilitation, School of Medicine, College of Medicine, Taipei Medical University, Taipei 110, Taiwan
4. Department of Nutrition, Faculty of Health Sciences, University of Pembangunan Nasional Veteran, Jakarta 12450, Indonesia; estinurwanti@upnvj.ac.id
5. Department of Nutrition, Faculty of Health Sciences, Alma Ata University, Yogyakarta 55183, Indonesia; hhadi@almaata.ac.id (H.H.); sinthadewips@almaata.ac.id (S.D.P.)
6. Department of Public Health, Faculty of Health Sciences, Alma Ata University, Yogyakarta 55183, Indonesia
7. Alma Ata Center for Healthy Life and Foods (ACHEAF), Alma Ata University, Yogyakarta 55183, Indonesia
8. Nutrition Department, Hermina Tangkubanprahu Hospital, Malang 651194, Indonesia; rochmah.imaning@gmail.com
9. Graduate Institute of Metabolism and Obesity Sciences, College of Nutrition, Taipei Medical University, Taipei 110, Taiwan
10. Nutrition Research Center, Taipei Medical University Hospital, Taipei 110, Taiwan
11. Chinese Taipei Society for the Study of Obesity (CTSSO), Taipei 110, Taiwan
* Correspondence: susanchang@tmu.edu.tw; Tel.: +886-(2)-27361661 (ext. 6542); Fax: +886-(2)-2737-3112

Abstract: Good nutritional support is crucial for the immune system to fight against coronavirus disease 2019 (COVID-19). However, in the context of a pandemic with a highly transmissible coronavirus, implementation of nutrition practice may be difficult. A multicenter electronic survey involving 62 dieticians was conducted, in order to understand barriers associated with dieticians' adherence to nutrition guidelines for hospitalized COVID-19 patients in Indonesia. 69% of dieticians felt under stress when performing nutrition care, and 90% took supplements to boost their own immunity against the coronavirus. The concerns related to clinical practice included a lack of clear guidelines (74%), a lack of access to medical records (55%), inadequate experience or knowledge (48%), and a lack of self-efficacy/confidence (29%) in performing nutritional care. Half (52%) of the dieticians had performed nutrition education/counseling, 47% had monitored a patient's body weight, and 76% had monitored a patient's dietary intake. An adjusted linear regression showed that guideline adherence independently predicted the dieticians' nutrition care behaviors of nutrition counselling (ß: 0.24 (0.002, 0.08); $p = 0.04$), and monitoring of body weight (ß: 0.43 (0.04, 0.11); $p = 0.001$) and dietary intake (ß: 0.47(0.03, 0.10); $p = 0.001$) of COVID-19 patients. Overall, adherence to COVID-19 nutrition guidelines is associated with better nutritional management behaviors in hospitalized COVID-19 patients.

Keywords: COVID-19; nutrition care; guidelines adherence; length of stay; mortality; Indonesia

1. Introduction

Indonesia is among the 20 countries currently most severely affected by coronavirus disease 2019 (COVID-19) worldwide, with the fifth highest observed case–fatality ratio (3.0% per 100 confirmed cases) [1]. The clinical characteristics of COVID-19 are diverse, and symptoms range from asymptomatic, mild with nonspecific symptoms (e.g., fever, cough, sore throat, and headaches), moderate/severe pneumonia with acute respiratory distress syndrome (ARDS) demanding mechanical ventilation, and multi-organ failure to death [2]. Currently, remdesivir is the only antiviral drug approved by the U.S. Food and Drug Administration (FDA) for treating COVID-19. Since there are limited effective antiviral drugs, supportive care with good nutritional support is crucial for the immune system to fight against coronavirus infection in hospitalized COVID-19 patients [2–5].

Dieticians are an integral part of healthcare systems, and are responsible for assessing the nutritional needs of hospitalized COVID-19 patients. However, one of the practical challenges of nutritional management with COVID-19 is the lack of clear guidelines, as the emerging coronavirus and its impacts on health are constantly evolving [2–5]. Although nutritional management of COVID-19 disease is, in principle, similar to that of hospitalized patients or patients in intensive care units (ICUs) [6], implementation of nutrition guidelines into clinical practice is a great challenge in the context of this pandemic with the highly transmissible coronavirus [7]. For example, dieticians might not be allowed to meet patients or perform nutritional assessments due to the risk of contracting or transmitting COVID-19. Frequently, some instruments for evaluating nutritional status are not readily available in most settings dedicated to COVID-19 patients. Indeed, dieticians should rely on rapid/alternative measures [8]. With the ongoing pandemic, health workers are burned out and are suffering from psychological symptoms (e.g., depression, anxiety, and insomnia), and these may also affect their motivation to implement nutrition guidelines [9,10]. Currently, little is known about the challenges and barriers that affect dieticians' implementation of COVID-19 nutritional guidelines. The broad aim of this study was to investigate barriers to dieticians' adherence to nutritional guidelines in hospitalized COVID-19 patients in Indonesia. Specific aims were: (1) to understand the practical challenges and concerns associated with nutritional care, and (2) to understand barriers (guideline knowledge, attitudes, and environmental factors) associated with nutritional management behaviors of dieticians (as indicated by monitoring a patient's body weight (BW) and dietary intake, as well as performing nutrition counseling/education).

2. Materials and Methods

2.1. Study Participants

This study was a multicenter electronic survey designed to understand the barriers associated with dieticians' adherence to clinical practice of nutrition care for hospitalized COVID-19 patients in Indonesia. This study was conducted during November 2020–January 2021. The link of the questionnaire (as a Google Form) was sent to social media groups of Indonesian dietetic association networks, where an estimated number of 210 of the group members were working as dieticians in a hospital. In total, 62 dieticians from 44 hospitals completed the online questionnaire, giving a response rate of 29.5%. Out of the 44 participating hospitals, 39 (88.6%) were located in Jakarta and Java Island, and had higher COVID-19 cases compared to other regions in Indonesia. In addition, 20 participating hospitals (45%) were hospitals designated for COVID-19 by the Indonesia Ministry of Health. The study was conducted anonymously, and no personal data were collected (e.g., name or contact address). Participants were informed of the purpose of the online survey, and their consent to participate in the study was assumed if they completed the online survey. Each participant was allowed to complete the online survey only once. Participants were included if they were of Indonesian nationality, were employed as a dietician in a hospital, had performed nutritional care for hospitalized COVID-19 patients, and completed the online surveys. Exclusion criteria were a non-Indonesian nationality, dieticians who never performed nutritional care for hospitalized COVID-19 patients, and those who did not complete the online survey questionnaires. The study was approved by the Research Ethic Committee of Alma Alta University, Indonesia (KE/AA/XI/10323/EC/2020).

2.2. Survey Questionnaire: Barriers to Dietician Adherence to Nutrition Care for Hospitalized COVID-19 Patients

The questionnaire was developed based on the framework of "barriers to physician adherence to practice guidelines in relation to behavior change", which was proposed by Cabana et al. and published in the Journal of the American Medical Association (JAMA) in 1999 [11]. The questionnaire consisted of four domains: knowledge (12 questions), attitudes (six questions), environmental factors (seven questions), and behaviors (three questions) (Supplementary Table S1). Depending on a participant's answers, each question was awarded 1 or 0 points, with a maximum of 28 points in total (Supplementary Table S1). For example, 1 point was awarded to a participant if they know "ESPEN guidelines on clinical nutrition in the intensive care unit" [6] or if they had "monitored the body weight of hospitalized COVID-19 patients". A higher total score of guideline knowledge, attitudes, environment, and behavior indicates better dietician adherence to clinical nutrition practices for hospitalized COVID-19 patients.

The "guideline knowledge section" (12 questions in total) included awareness of the guidelines (four questions) and familiarity with clinical nutrition practice of the guidelines (eight questions). The four guidelines were published between February 2019 and July 2020, and included the Coronavirus Disease 2019 (COVID-19) Treatment Guidelines (National Institutes of Health, USA) [2], ESPEN guidelines on clinical nutrition care in the intensive care unit (ICU) [6], ESPEN expert statements and practical guidance for nutritional management of individuals with SARS-CoV-2-infection [3], and Nutrition Therapy in the Patient with COVID-19 Disease Requiring ICU Care (reviewed and approved by the Society of Critical Care Medicine and the American Society for Parenteral and Enteral Nutrition) [5]. Familiarity with clinical practice associated with the guidelines included questions such as "is it important to conduct nutritional screening and nutritional assessment for hospitalized COVID-19 patients?" and "must the nutritional assessment and early nutritional care management of COVID-19 patients be integrated into the overall therapeutic strategy?" Respondents answered with "agree" or "disagree".

The "attitude section" (six question in total) consisted of two parts: self-efficacy or confidence (three questions) and motivation (three questions) in performing nutritional care for hospitalized COVID-19 patients. Examples of the statements included: "lack of self-efficacy or confidence in performing nutrition care for hospitalized COVID-19 patients?", and "feel stress when performing nutrition care for hospitalized COVID-19 patients?" Respondents answered with "agree" or "disagree". "Environmental factors" included seven questions including "lack of time, lack of resources, limited budget, limited food supply, lack of access to meet hospitalized COVID-19 patients, lack of access to medical records, and inadequate authority to perform nutritional care for hospitalized COVID-19 patients". "Dieticians' behavior" mainly focused on three nutrition care behaviors: (1) "Do you give nutrition education/counseling to hospitalized COVID-19 patients? If yes, how do you give nutrition education/counseling: educational video, educational leaflet, phone call, or text message?"; (2) "Do you monitor COVID-19 patient's body weight change? If yes, who monitors body weight and how do you do it?"; and (3) "Do you monitor dietary intake of hospitalized COVID-19 patients? If yes, who monitors it and how do you do it?" Total guidelines adherence score (maximum 28 points) was defined as knowledge (12 points), attitudes (six points), environmental factors (seven points), and dieticians' nutrition practice behaviors (three points). A high total score indicated a better adherence to nutrition guidelines for hospitalized COVID-19 patients.

2.3. Primary Outcome

The primary outcomes were dieticians' behaviors of nutrition care and self-efficacy or confidence in providing nutrition care for hospitalized COVID-19 patients. The dieticians' behaviors of nutrition care included: (1) conducting nutrition counseling/education, (2) monitoring patients' weight changes, and (3) monitoring patients' dietary intake.

2.4. Data Analysis

Statistical analyses were conducted using SPSS 19 (IBM, Armonk, NY, USA). Continuous data are presented as the mean and standard deviation (SD), and categorical data are presented as the number (n) and percentage (%). Differences between two groups were analyzed by an unpaired t-test. Chi-squared or Fisher's exact test was employed to compare proportions. An age, gender, years of practice, and type of hospital-adjusted multivariate linear regression model was employed to examine relationships between dependent variables (dieticians' nutrition practice behaviors) and potential variables related to guideline adherence (total adherence score and its individual components: knowledge, attitude, and environmental factors). $p < 0.05$ was considered statistically significant.

3. Results

3.1. Participant Characteristics

Table 1 shows baseline characteristics of study participants. In total, 62 Indonesian dieticians participated in the survey; 89% were female and 56% had ≤5 years of clinical experience. Most participants worked in hospitals located in Jakarta (40%), East Java (21%), and Central Java (16%). All participants (100%) had experience in performing nutritional therapy for hospitalized COVID-19 patients, with 48% conducting nutritional therapy for severely and critically ill patients, 40% for patients with mild and moderate illness, and 12% for asymptomatic patients. However, 69% of dieticians felt stress when performing nutritional therapy for hospitalized COVID-19 patients. Ninety percent of participants took supplements or herbal remedies to boost their own immunity against COVID-19, with 63% taking vitamin C, 45% taking vitamin B complex, 30% taking multivitamins and minerals, and 25% consuming ginger (Table 1).

3.2. Concerns Related to Nutritional Practices of COVID-19

Table 2 shows concerns related to clinical practices of nutrition care of COVID-19 patients. The most commonly used nutritional screening tools were malnutrition universal screening tools (MUST) (34%) and malnutrition screening tools (MST) (34%), and nutrition assessments were mainly performed by nurses (58%) and dieticians (40%) (Table 2). Seventy-six percent of participants had monitored a patient's dietary intake; however, only half had monitored a patient's weight change (47%) or had provided nutrition education or counseling (52%). Ninety-seven percent of participants had recommended supplements for hospitalized COVID-19 patients, of which vitamin C (61%), vitamin B complex (60%), multivitamins/minerals (48%), zinc (40%), and omega 3 fatty acids (27%) were the most frequently recommended supplements. Sixty-eight percent of participants had experience in designing individual diets for hospitalized COVID-19 patients, with 68% modifying the protein content and 63% modifying the total energy. Concerns related to nutritional practices of hospitalized COVID-19 patients included a lack of clear guidelines (74%), a lack of access to meet COVID-19 patients (55%), inadequate experience or knowledge (48%), a lack of self-efficacy or confidence in performing nutrition care (29%), a lack of resources (29%), a limited food supply (29%), and a limited budget (26%) (Table 2).

3.3. Barriers to Dieticians' Adherence to Nutrition Guidelines for COVID-19

Next, we evaluated barriers to dieticians' adherence to clinical guidelines (Table 3). More than half of the dieticians were aware of "COVID-19 treatment guidelines" (total: 65%; among those with >5 years of experience: 74%; and among those with ≤5 years of experience: 57%) and "ESPEN guideline on clinical nutrition in the intensive care unit" (total: 58%; among those with >5 years of experience: 48%; and among those with ≤5 years of experience: 66%), but to a lesser extent, "nutrition therapy in the patient with COVID-19 disease requiring ICU care" (total: 35%; among those with >5 years of experience: 37%; and among those with ≤5 years of experience: 34%), and "ESPEN expert statements and practical guidance for nutritional management of individuals with SARS-CoV-2 infection" (total: 24%; among those with >5 years of experience: 26%; and among those with ≤5 years of experience: 23%). Most participants were familiar with knowledge of nutrition practice (95–100%) (Table 3). However, 74% of participants thought that there was a lack of clear guidelines for COVID-19, and this rate was slightly higher among junior dieticians (those with ≤5 years of experience: 83%) than senior (those with >5 years of experience: 63%) ($p = 0.076$) (Table 3: Knowledge: Familiarity with clinical practice). Junior dieticians also had lower agreement rates on questions of "I am knowledgeable about the role of nutrition therapy for hospitalized COVID-19 patients" (junior: 43% vs. senior: 81%, $p = 0.004$) and "self-efficacy or confidence in performing nutrition care for hospitalized COVID-19 patients" (junior: 57% vs. senior: 89%, $p = 0.006$), but had a higher rate of "feeling stress when performing nutrition care for hospitalized COVID-19 patients" (junior: 83% vs. senior: 52%, $p = 0.009$). Although 95% of participants agreed that "nutrition counseling is important for hospitalized COVID-19 patients" (Table 3: Knowledge: Familiarity of the guidelines), only half of dieticians (total: 52%) had conducted nutrition education/counseling for hospitalized COVID-19 patients, and this rate was much higher among junior dieticians (junior: 71% vs. senior: 26%; $p < 0.0001$). Only 47% (junior: 54% vs. senior: 37%, $p = 0.177$) had monitored BW changes and 76% (junior: 74% vs. senior: 78%) had monitored dietary intake of hospitalized COVID-19 patients (Table 3: Behavior)

Table 1. Characteristics of the study participants ($N = 62$).

Characteristic	Responses
Hospital Characteristic	
Type of hospital (*n*, %)	
Government hospital	23 (52%)
Private hospital	21 (48%)
Region of hospital (*n*, %)	
Yogyakarta and Central Java	10 (23%)
East Java	11 (25%)
Jakarta	12 (27%)
West Java	5 (11%)
Bali and others	6 (14%)
Number of hospitalized COVID-19 patients	14,898.69 ± 23,441.78
Mortality rate (n, ratio)	1186 (0.02)
Average length of stay of COVID-19 patients (day)	19.58 ± 1.61
Asymptomatic	N/A
Mild Illness	12.58 ± 1.61
Moderate Illness	16.04 ± 1.55
Severe Illness	21.50 ± 2.13
Critical Illness	27.54 ± 2.64
Dieticians' characteristics	
Age (years)	29.27 ± 6.10
Female (*n*, %)	55 (89%)
Years of practice	
<1 year	16 (26%)
1~5 years	19 (31%)
5~10 years	14 (23%)
>10 years	13 (21%)
Have you ever performed nutrition therapy for COVID-19 patients? (yes)	62 (100%)
Stages of COVID-19 patients treated? (*n*, %)	
Asymptomatic	4 (6%)
Mild and moderate illness	20 (32%)
Severe and critical illness	38 (61%)
Feel stress when performing nutritional therapy for COVID-19 patients?	43 (69%)
Take supplements to boost your own immunity against COVID-19?	56 (90%)
B complex	25 (45%)
Vitamin C	35 (63%)
Multivitamins and minerals	17 (30%)
Ginger	14 (25%)

Continuous variables are presented as the mean ± standard deviation (SD), and categorical data as the number (*n*) (percentage). Mortality rate (case fatality rate) was defined as the number of deaths divided by the number of confirmed cases.

Table 2. Nutrition practice and concerns related to hospitalized COVID-19 patients ($N = 62$).

Nutritional Practice	Responses
Nutritional screening tools used?	
Nutrition Risk Screening-2002 (NRS-2002)	7 (11%)
Mini Nutritional Assessment (MNA)	12 (19%)
Malnutrition Universal Screening Tools (MUST)	21 (34%)
Subjective Global Assessment (SGA)	4 (6%)
Malnutrition Screening Tools (MST)	21 (34%)
Who performs nutritional screening for COVID-19 patients?	
Dietitian	25 (40%)
Doctor	1 (2%)
Nurse	36 (58%)
Monitor weight change in COVID-19 patients? (yes: n, %)	29 (47%)
If yes, who monitors it?	
Dietitian	21 (34%)
Nurse	6 (20%)
Self-reported by patient	2 (3%)
Monitor dietary intake of COVID-19 patients? (yes: n, %)	47 (76%)
If yes, who monitors it?	
Dietitian	28 (35%)
Nurse	13 (27%)
Health care	4 (8%)
Reported by patient	6 (10%)
Performed nutritional counseling for COVID-19 patients? (yes: n, %)	32 (52%)
If yes, how do you do it?	
Educational leaflet	8 (13%)
Phone call	19 (31%)
Text message	10 (16%)
Meet the patient in person	4 (6%)
Video call	1 (2%)
Give education to the family	1 (2%)
Recommend supplements for COVID-19 patients? (yes: n, %)	60 (97%)
B complex	37 (60%)
Vitamin C	38 (61%)
Multivitamins and minerals	30 (48%)
Zinc	25 (40%)
Omega-3 fatty acids	17 (27%)
Designed individual diets for hospitalized COVID-19 patients? (yes: n, %)	42 (68%)
Modify total energy	39 (63%)
Modify carbohydrate content	15 (24%)
Modify protein content	42 (68%)
Modify lipid content	10 (16%)
Modify fruits and vegetables	20 (32%)
Give supplements	13 (21%)
No differences	7 (11%)
Confidence in performing nutritional support for COVID-19 patients with poly-comorbidities (5: very confident; 3: slightly confident; 1: not confident)	3.37 ± 0.96
Concerns related to nutrition care for COVID-19 patients	
Lack of clear guidelines	46 (74%)
Lack of self-efficacy or confidence in performing nutritional care	18 (29%)
Inadequate experience or knowledge	30 (48%)
Limited budget	16 (26%)
Lack of time	7 (11%)
Lack of resources	18 (29%)
Limited food supply	18 (29%)
Lack of access to meet COVID-19 patients	34 (55%)
Lack of access to medical records	9 (15%)

Continuous variables are presented as the mean ± standard deviation (SD). Categorical variables are presented as number (n) (percentage).

Table 3. Barriers to dietician adherence to nutritional guidelines in relation to nutritional practice behaviors of hospitalized COVID-19 patients.

Barriers	Total (N = 62)	Years of Practice ≤5 Years (N = 35)	Years of Practice >5 Years (N = 27)	p Value *
Knowledge				
Awareness of guidelines				
ESPEN guidelines on clinical nutrition in the intensive care unit [6]	36 (58%)	23 (66%)	13 (48%)	0.165
ESPEN expert statements and practical guidance for nutritional management of individuals with SARS-CoV-2-infection (Europe) [3]	15 (24%)	8 (23%)	7 (26%)	0.780
Nutrition Therapy in Patients with COVID-19 Disease Requiring ICU Care (reviewed and approved by the Society of Critical Care Medicine and the American Society for Parenteral and Enteral Nutrition) [5]	22 (35%)	12 (34%)	10 (37%)	0.822
Coronavirus Disease 2019 (COVID-19) Treatment Guidelines (National Institutes of Health, USA) [2]	40 (65%)	20 (57%)	20 (74%)	0.167
Familiarity with the guidelines				
The nutritional assessment and early nutritional care management of COVID-19 patients must be integrated into the overall therapeutic strategy	62 (100%)	35 (100%)	27 (100%)	NA
It is important to conduct nutritional screening and nutritional assessment of hospitalized Covid-19 patients	61 (98%)	34 (97%)	27 (100%)	0.376
It is important to monitor the body weight change in hospitalized COVID-19 patients	48 (77%)	27 (77%)	21 (78%)	0.953
It is important to monitor the dietary intake of hospitalized COVID-19 patients	62 (100%)	35 (100%)	27 (100%)	NA
Nutrition therapy plays an important role in the outcomes of COVID-19 treatment	62 (100%)	35 (100%)	27 (100%)	NA
Nutrition supplementation is useful for treating COVID-19 patients	60 (97%)	33 (94%)	27 (100%)	0.207
Nutrition counseling is important for COVID-19 patients	59 (95%)	32 (91%)	27 (100%)	0.119
Lack of clear guidelines	46 (74%)	29 (83%)	17 (63%)	0.076
Attitudes				
Self-efficacy/confidence in performing nutritional care				
I am knowledgeable about the role of nutrition therapy for COVID-19 patients	37 (60%)	15 (43%)	22 (81%)	0.004
Self-efficacy or confidence in performing nutrition care for hospitalized COVID-19 patients	44 (71%)	20 (45%)	24 (89%)	0.006
I have adequate knowledge to design meals for hospitalized COVID-19 patients	32 (52%)	16 (50%)	16 (50%)	0.290
Motivation in performing nutritional care				
I regularly make decisions regarding nutrition therapy as part of the management of COVID-19 patients	50 (81%)	28 (80%)	22 (81%)	0.884
I have an obligation to improve the health of COVID-19 patients by discussing nutrition with them	59 (95%)	33 (94%)	26 (96%)	0.715
I feel stress when performing nutrition care for hospitalized COVID-19 patients	43 (69%)	29 (83%)	14 (52%)	0.009
Environmental factors				
Lack of time	7 (11%)	4 (11%)	3 (11%)	0.969
Lack of resources	18 (29%)	11 (31%)	7 (26%)	0.636
Limited budget	16 (26%)	8 (23%)	8 (30%)	0.546
Limited food supplies	18 (29%)	13 (37%)	5 (19%)	0.109
Lack of access to meet hospitalized COVID-19 patients	34 (55%)	16 (46%)	18 (67%)	0.100
Lack of access to medical records	9 (15%)	4 (11%)	5 (19%)	0.432
Inadequate authority to perform nutritional care for hospitalized COVID-19 patients	4 (6%)	3 (9%)	1 (4%)	0.439
Nutritional practice behaviors				
Perform nutrition education or counseling for hospitalized COVID-19 patients	32 (52%)	25 (71%)	7 (26%)	<0.0001
Monitor body weight of hospitalized COVID-19 patients	29 (47%)	19 (54%)	10 (37%)	0.177
Monitor dietary intake of hospitalized COVID-19 patients	47 (76%)	26 (74%)	21 (78%)	0.502

All variables are expressed as the number (n), percentage (%). * The p value was analyzed using unpaired Student's t-test for continuous variables or Chi-squared test for categorical variables.

3.4. Factors Predicting Nutrition Care Behaviors of COVID-19 Patients

3.4.1. Self-Efficacy or Confidence in Providing Nutrition Care

Next, we performed a multivariate linear regression analysis to identify factors associated with behaviors of nutrition care for hospitalized COVID-19 patients (Table 4). Age, gender and years of practice-adjusted regression showed that nutrition guideline adherence score (ß: −0.25 (−0.07, −0.01); $p = 0.03$) was negatively correlated with lack of self-efficacy, and, to a lesser extent, disease severity (ß: 0.22 (−0.01, 0.33); $p = 0.057$) (Table 4).

Table 4. Adjusted multivariate regression coefficient (ß) and 95% confidence intervals (CIs) of barriers of nutrition practice behaviors of COVID-19 patients.

Variables	Lack of Self-Efficacy *	p-Value	Nutrition Counseling *	p-Value	Monitor Body Weight *	p-Value	Monitor Dietary Intake *	p-Value
Disease severity	0.22 (−0.01, 0.33)	0.057	0.24 (−0.02, 0.41)	0.077	0.05 (−0.17, 0.25)	0.690	0.15 (−0.09, 0.28)	0.286
Type of hospital	−0.07 (−0.29, 0.15)	0.527	0.05 (−0.20, 0.30)	0.674	0.03 (−0.29, 0.24)	0.844	0.11 (−0.32, 0.14)	0.435
Total adherence score	−0.25 (−0.07, −0.01)	0.030	0.24 (0.01, 0.08)	0.040	0.43 (0.04, 0.11)	0.001	0.47 (0.03, 0.10)	0.001
Knowledge (total score)	−0.15 (−0.12, 0.03)	0.209	0.19 (−0.03, 0.15)	0.157	0.13 (−0.04, 0.13)	0.287	0.05 (−0.06, 0.09)	0.708
Guideline awareness	−0.01 (−0.08, 0.08)	0.969	0.70 (0.18, 0.31)	<0.0001	0.15 (−0.04, 0.15)	0.273	0.35 (0.03, 0.19)	0.010
Guideline Familiarity	−0.05 (−0.22, 0.14)	0.666	0.11 (0.13, 0.33)	0.402	0.01 (−0.19, 0.18)	0.936	0.03 (−0.22, 0.17)	0.173
Attitude (total score)	NA		0.07 (−0.08, 0.14)	0.584	0.15 (−0.30, 0.13)	0.210	0.03 (0.02, 0.15)	0.012
Self-efficacy or confidence	NA		0.05 (−0.45, 0.03)	0.660	0.08 (−0.10, 0.19)	0.643	0.31 (0.03, 0.26)	0.013
Motivation	−0.18 (−0.04, 0.35)	0.112	0.03 (−0.26, 0.20)	0.800	0.07 (−0.17, 0.30)	0.568	0.23 (0.02, 0.39)	0.040
Feel stress	0.23 (−0.48, 0.31)	0.080	−0.37 (−0.67, −0.12)	0.006	−0.24 (−0.57, 0.04)	0.091	−0.21 (−0.46, 0.08)	0.172
Environmental factor (total score)	−0.15 (−0.15, 0.03)	0.186	0.08 (−0.15, 0.08)	0.535	0.15 (−0.04, 0.18)	0.217	0.12 (−0.06, 0.14)	0.384

Total adherence score (maximum 28 points) was defined as knowledge (12 questions), attitudes (six questions), environmental factors (seven questions), and behaviors (three questions). * Results were adjusted for age, gender, years of practice, and type of hospital.

3.4.2. Nutrition Care Behaviors: Nutrition Counseling, and Monitoring of BW and Dietary Intake

A regression analysis adjusted for age, gender and years of practice showed that guideline adherence scores also independently predicted dieticians' nutrition care behaviors of nutrition counselling (ß: 0.24 (0.002, 0.08); $p = 0.04$), and monitoring of BW (ß: 0.43 (0.04, 0.11); $p = 0.001$) and dietary intake (ß: 0.47(0.03, 0.10); $p = 0.001$) of hospitalized COVID-19 patients (Table 4). Detail analysis of barriers to dieticians' adherence to nutrition guidelines found that awareness of guidelines was positively correlated with nutrition counselling (ß: 0.70 (0.18, 0.31); $p < 0.0001$), and monitoring patient's dietary intake (ß: 0.35 (0.03, 0.19); $p = 0.01$). Those dieticians who had better attitude (total score) (ß: 0.03 (0.02, 0.15); $p = 0.012$), self-efficacy or confidence (ß: 0.31 (0.03, 0.26); $p = 0.013$) or motivation (ß: 0.23 (0.02, 0.39); $p = 0.04$) in performing nutrition care were more likely to monitor a patient's BW (Table 4: adjusted for age, gender, years of practice, and type of hospital).

Next, we investigated the relationship between dieticians' adherence to nutrition guidelines, length of stay and COVID-19 mortality. Adjusted linear regression analysis showed that guideline awareness was negatively correlated with the length of stay for moderate symptoms (ß: −0.51 (−1.22, −0.14); $p = 0.017$), severe symptoms (ß: −0.31 (−1.48, −0.26); $p = 0.04$) and critical illness (ß: −0.46 (−1.45, −0.16); $p = 0.029$), but not mild symptoms. Guideline familiarity also independently predicted COVID-19 mortality (ß: −40.95 (−63.95, −17.95); $p = 0.001$) (Supplementary Table S2).

4. Discussion

Our study results indicated that adherence to COVID-19 nutrition guidelines is associated with better nutritional management and, possibly, related to clinical outcome. Studies showed that adherence to nutrition guidelines in critically ill patients is associated with better survival outcomes [12,13]. Currently, Indonesia is not only facing capacity constraints in the health care sector (e.g., man power, funding and facility) but also the unprecedented economic burden of the direct medical cost of COVID-19. It is estimated that median lengths of stay of hospitalized COVID-19 patients were 4~53 days in China and 4~21 days outside of China [14]. In the United States, a single symptomatic COVID-19 infection would cost a direct medical cost of USD 3,045 and one hospitalized case would cost a median of USD 14,366, which only covers costs during the course of the infection and not the follow-up care [15]. The importance of appropriate nutritional assessments and treatments cannot be overstated. The health of COVID-19 patients may rapidly deteriorate after being hospitalized, and patients may develop progressive hypermetabolism 1 week after being intubated in the ICU, which may require 1.6~1.8-times higher energy inputs by the third week post-intubation [16]. Screening and monitoring of a patient's BW and dietary intake can help doctors and dieticians identify patients at risk of poor outcomes, and also allow planning of individualized nutrition care to support a patient's immune system in fighting the coronavirus [17]. This is of particular importance for COVID-19, since supportive care is the major treatment method for hospitalized COVID-19 patients, and most severe and critically ill COVID-19 patients are at risk of malnutrition [18,19].

Awareness of guidelines also predicts a dietician's adherence to nutrition guidelines for COVID-19. In the context of a constantly evolving and highly contagious coronavirus, implementation of nutrition guidelines might not be straightforward. Dieticians need to quickly adapt to a wide range of work environments and upgrade their nutrition care programs through training, self-study, or discussing practical problems in real-time through online social networks with fellow dieticians to provide optimal service to COVID-19 patients. Our study found that major concerns related to the nutrition care of COVID-19 patients were a lack of clear guidelines (74%), a lack of self-efficacy (29%), and inadequate experience or knowledge (48%). Dissemination of COVID-19 guidelines with their management algorithm may improve dieticians' knowledge and promote adherence to guidelines. However, passive dissemination of guidelines might not be effective in the context of the ever-changing COVID-19 pandemic, as the guidelines need to be adapted to local healthcare environments. It is likely that active dissemination or targeted approaches together with supportive networks would improve awareness of, and adherence to, guidelines. For example, Canadian dieticians launched a "COVID-19 response group" on Facebook for dieticians and nutrition students to discuss nutrition care issues, share experiences, and seek advice. Online supportive networks may be particularly important for junior dieticians as our study showed that they had lower self-efficacy/confidence and knowledge than senior dieticians.

Currently, Indonesian hospitals are overwhelmed by COVID-19 and our study found that most Indonesia dieticians, in particularly junior dieticians, are suffering from psychological stress when performing nutritional care for hospitalized COVID-19 patients. Increased psychological stress among junior dieticians is likely due to the combination factors of a higher rate of performing nutritional counseling and a lack of self-efficacy/confidence in performing nutritional care for hospitalized COVID-19 patients. The current study found that psychological stress not only predicted dieticians' self-efficacy/confidence but also their behaviors of nutrition care of COVID-19. Lu and Dollahite showed that years of nutrition counselling experience significantly predicted self-efficacy scores [20]. Currently, we do not know why Indonesian junior dieticians had a higher rate of performing nutritional counseling for hospitalized COVID-19 patients than senior dieticians, despite the lack of clinical experience. Another interesting finding is that most of dieticians (90%) took supplements as well as recommending supplements (Vitamins C and B complex, multivitamins and zinc) to COVID-19 patients, despite the fact that the COVID-19 Treatment Guidelines stated that there are insufficient data for the panel to recommend the use of vitamins or minerals for the treatment of COVID-19 [2]. Using Google Trends to analyze worldwide concerns with immune-boosting nutrients/herbs during the COVID-19 pandemic, our previous study found that vitamin C, D, E and zinc were the most searched nutrients during the first wave of COVID-19 pandemic [21]. Vitamins and minerals have anti-inflammatory and antioxidant properties, which may support a healthy immune system against coronavirus infection. However, the effects of vitamin and mineral supplementation on COVID-19 remain inconclusive [22,23]. It is very important to prevent or treat nutritional deficiencies. However, supplementation with a supraphysiologic or supratherapeutic amount of micronutrients has not been recommended in the prevention or improvement of clinical outcomes of COVID-19 infection. Therefore, the provision of daily allowances for vitamins and trace elements has been suggested [3,24].

Our study found that environmental factors such as a lack of access to meet COVID-19 patients in person was not a barrier to nutrition care practice. To overcome physical barriers, Indonesian dieticians have employed telemedicine to perform nutrition counseling and monitor patients' food intake and weight changes. However, feeling stress when independently performing nutrition care predicts the behavior of monitoring a patient's BW. This suggests that, even when upgrading one's skills through telehealth channels, dieticians still suffer from psychological stress when dealing with COVID-19. Health organizations need to identify sources of stress and adapt their clinical practice to support nutrition care. Another barrier that predicts the behavior of monitoring a patient's food intake is the lack of access to medical records. Nutrition care might not be considered a priority in the COVID-19 pandemic, as acknowledged by Thibault and colleagues [7]. Based on their experiences with the COVID-19 pandemic in France, those authors emphasized the need to adapt protocols of nutrition care that are simple and easily applied [7]. Overall, our study results suggest that dieticians need to upgrade their skills in telemedicine and adapt to the local healthcare environment in order to strategize plans for performing individualized nutrition care during the ever-changing COVID-19 pandemic.

The strength of this study includes its novelty, as it is the first to investigate barriers affecting COVID-19 nutrition care, as well as being a multicenter survey with all participants having experience in nutrition care of hospitalized COVID-19 patients. The present study also has several limitations. Firstly, there was a relatively small sample size ($n = 62$) with only one country surveyed (Indonesia) and a low response rate (29.5%). We recognized that a regional study with small sample size may not provide a complete picture of dietetic practice in Indonesia and other countries during the COVID-19 outbreak. The low response rate in our study is due, in part, to the exclusion of dieticians who never performed nutritional care for hospitalized COVID-19 patients in Indonesia. The COVID-19 outbreak itself may also contribute to the low response rate. A recent study in UK also found a limited number of dietitians was able to participate in the online survey due to COVID-19 outbreak, though no response rate was reported [25]. Secondly, information was collected online and not through face-to face interviews. Limitations of online surveys have been noted and intensively discussed [26]. The major strengths of the online survey were its cost effectiveness and the ability to be conducted in a short period of time with no regional restrictions; however, there were concerns about internet accessibility, a lack of control of the sampling or response rate, and ethical issues (e.g., consent, anonymity, and confidentiality) [26]. Nonetheless, it was performed in the context of social distancing during the COVID-19 pandemic, and consent was obtained through participation in the online survey, and all responses were anonymous; the research ethics committee in Indonesia approved the current study. Other limitations include the fact that more confounding factors are needed for the linear regression model when analyzing the relationship between the predictive effect of dieticians' adherence to nutrition guidelines and the clinical outcomes (survival and length of stay).

5. Conclusions

Our study results indicate that adherence to COVID-19 nutrition guidelines is associated with better nutritional management and, possibly, better clinical outcomes. A further validation study is needed in order to provide some definitive guidance on how to implement nutrition guidelines, as well as how the adherence to COVID-19 nutrition guidelines may affect medical cost and economy during the ever-changing COVID-19 pandemic.

Supplementary Materials: The following are available online at https://www.mdpi.com/article/10.3390/nu13061918/s1, Supplementary Table S1: Barriers to dietician adherence to clinical practice of nutrition guidelines for hospitalized COVID-19 patients. Supplementary Table S2: Adjusted multivariate regression coefficient (β) and 95% Confidence Intervals (95% CI) for length of stay and mortality of hospitalized COVID-19 patients in Indonesia.

Author Contributions: A.F., D.K.N.H., S.-H.T., H.H. and J.-S.C. designed the study and conducted the initial searches. A.F., E.N., S.D.P. and I.Y.R. contributed to recruitment of dieticians. Data were analyzed by A.F. and J.-S.C. drafted the paper. All authors have read and agreed to the published version of the manuscript.

Funding: Jung-Su Chang was supported by grants from Taipei Medical University Hospital (110TMU-TMUH-09) and the Ministry of Science and Technology, Taiwan (MOST 107-2320-B-038-010-MY3 and MOST 109-2923-B-038-001-MY3).

Institutional Review Board Statement: The study was approved by the Research Ethic Committee of Alma Alta University, Indonesia (KE/AA/XI/10323/EC/2020).

Informed Consent Statement: Informed consent was obtained from all subjects involved in the study.

Data Availability Statement: The data are not publicly available due to participant confidentiality.

Acknowledgments: We thank all Indonesian dieticians who participated in the survey.

Conflicts of Interest: The authors declare that no competing interest exists.

References

1. John Hopkins University and Medicine Coronavirus Resource Center. Mortality in the Most Affected Countries. Available online: https://coronavirus.jhu.edu/data/mortality (accessed on 5 January 2021).
2. National Institutes of Health USA. COVID-19 Treatment Guidelines Panel. Coronavirus Disease 2019 (COVID-19) Treatment Guidelines. National Institutes of Health. Available online: https://www.covid19treatmentguidelines.nih.gov/ (accessed on 4 January 2021).
3. Barazzoni, R.; Bischoff, S.C.; Breda, J.; Wickramasinghe, K.; Krznaric, Z.; Nitzan, D.; Pirlich, M.; Singer, P. Espen expert statements and practical guidance for nutritional management of individuals with sars-cov-2 infection. *Clin. Nutr.* **2020**, *39*, 1631–1638. [CrossRef]
4. Thibault, R.; Seguin, P.; Tamion, F.; Pichard, C.; Singer, P. Nutrition of the covid-19 patient in the intensive care unit (icu): A practical guidance. *Crit. Care* **2020**, *24*, 1–8. [CrossRef] [PubMed]
5. Martindale, R.; Patel, J.J.; Taylor, B.; Warren, M.; McClave, S.A. Nutrition therapy in the patient with covid-19 disease requiring icu care. *Soc. Crit. Care Med.* **2020**, 1–8.
6. Singer, P.; Blaser, A.R.; Berger, M.M.; Alhazzani, W.; Calder, P.C.; Casaer, M.P.; Hiesmayr, M.; Mayer, K.; Montejo, J.C.; Pichard, C.; et al. Espen guideline on clinical nutrition in the intensive care unit. *Clin. Nutr.* **2019**, *38*, 48–79. [CrossRef] [PubMed]
7. Thibault, R.; Coeffier, M.; Joly, F.; Bohe, J.; Schneider, S.M.; Dechelotte, P. How the covid-19 epidemic is challenging our practice in clinical nutrition-feedback from the field. *Eur. J. Clin. Nutr.* **2021**, *75*, 407–416. [CrossRef]
8. Azzolino, D.; Passarelli, P.C.; D'Addona, A.; Cesari, M. Nutritional strategies for the rehabilitation of covid-19 patients. *Eur. J. Clin. Nutr.* **2021**, *75*, 728–730. [CrossRef]
9. Shanafelt, T.; Ripp, J.; Trockel, M. Understanding and addressing sources of anxiety among health care professionals during the covid-19 pandemic. *JAMA* **2020**, *323*, 2133–2134. [CrossRef]
10. Lai, J.; Ma, S.; Wang, Y.; Cai, Z.; Hu, J.; Wei, N.; Wu, J.; Du, H.; Chen, T.; Li, R.; et al. Factors associated with mental health outcomes among health care workers exposed to coronavirus disease 2019. *JAMA Netw. Open* **2020**, *3*, e203976. [CrossRef] [PubMed]
11. Cabana, M.D.; Rand, C.S.; Powe, N.R.; Wu, A.W.; Wilson, M.H.; Abboud, P.A.; Rubin, H.R. Why don't physicians follow clinical practice guidelines? A framework for improvement. *JAMA* **1999**, *282*, 1458–1465. [CrossRef]
12. Briassoulis, G.; Briassoulis, P.; Ilia, S. Nutrition is more than the sum of its parts. *Pediatri. Crit. Care Med. J. Soc. Crit. Care Med. World Fed. Pediatri. Intensive Crit. Care Soc.* **2018**, *19*, 1087–1089. [CrossRef]
13. Briassoulis, G.; Briassoulis, P.; Ilia, S. If you get good nutrition, you will become happy; if you get a bad one, you will become an icu philosopher. *Pediatr. Crit. Care Med. J. Soc. Crit. Care Med. World Fed. Pediatri. Intensive Crit. Care Soc.* **2019**, *20*, 89–90. [CrossRef]
14. Rees, E.M.; Nightingale, E.S.; Jafari, Y.; Waterlow, N.R.; Clifford, S.; CA, B.P.; Group, C.W.; Jombart, T.; Procter, S.R.; Knight, G.M. Covid-19 length of hospital stay: A systematic review and data synthesis. *BMC Med.* **2020**, *18*, 270. [CrossRef]
15. Bartsch, S.M.; Ferguson, M.C.; McKinnell, J.A.; O'Shea, K.J.; Wedlock, P.T.; Siegmund, S.S.; Lee, B.Y. The potential health care costs and resource use associated with covid-19 in the united states. *Health Aff.* **2020**, *39*, 927–935. [CrossRef]
16. Whittle, J.; Molinger, J.; MacLeod, D.; Haines, K.; Wischmeyer, P.E.; Group, L.-C.S. Persistent hypermetabolism and longitudinal energy expenditure in critically ill patients with covid-19. *Crit. Care* **2020**, *24*, 581. [CrossRef]
17. Arkin, N.; Krishnan, K.; Chang, M.G.; Bittner, E.A. Nutrition in critically ill patients with covid-19: Challenges and special considerations. *Clin. Nutr.* **2020**, *39*, 2327–2328. [CrossRef]

18. Zhao, X.; Li, Y.; Ge, Y.; Shi, Y.; Lv, P.; Zhang, J.; Fu, G.; Zhou, Y.; Jiang, K.; Lin, N.; et al. Evaluation of nutrition risk and its association with mortality risk in severely and critically ill covid-19 patients. *JPEN J. Parenter. Enter. Nutr.* **2021**, *45*, 32–42. [CrossRef]
19. Haraj, N.E.; El Aziz, S.; Chadli, A.; Dafir, A.; Mjabber, A.; Aissaoui, O.; Barrou, L.; El Kettani El Hamidi, C.; Nsiri, A.; Al Harrar, R.; et al. Nutritional status assessment in patients with covid-19 after discharge from the intensive care unit. *Clin. Nutr. ESPEN* **2021**, *41*, 423–428. [CrossRef]
20. Lu, A.H.; Dollahite, J. Assessment of dietitians' nutrition counselling self-efficacy and its positive relationship with reported skill usage. *J. Hum. Nutr. Diet. Off. J. Br. Diet. Assoc.* **2010**, *23*, 144–153. [CrossRef] [PubMed]
21. Mayasari, N.R.; Ho, D.K.N.; Lundy, D.J.; Skalny, A.V.; Tinkov, A.A.; Teng, I.-C.; Wu, M.-C.; Faradina, A.; Mohammed, A.Z.M.; Park, J.M.; et al. Impacts of the covid-19 pandemic on food security and diet-related lifestyle behaviors: An analytical study of google trends-based query volumes. *Nutrients* **2020**, *12*, 3103. [CrossRef] [PubMed]
22. Zhang, J.; Rao, X.; Li, Y.; Zhu, Y.; Liu, F.; Guo, G.; Luo, G.; Meng, Z.; De Backer, D.; Xiang, H.; et al. Pilot trial of high-dose vitamin c in critically ill covid-19 patients. *Ann. Intensive Care* **2021**, *11*, 5. [CrossRef] [PubMed]
23. Hiedra, R.; Lo, K.B.; Elbashabsheh, M.; Gul, F.; Wright, R.M.; Albano, J.; Azmaiparashvili, Z.; Patarroyo Aponte, G. The use of iv vitamin c for patients with covid-19: A case series. *Expert Rev. Anti-Infect. Ther.* **2020**, *18*, 1259–1261. [CrossRef]
24. Azzolino, D.; Saporiti, E.; Proietti, M.; Cesari, M. Nutritional considerations in frail older patients with covid-19. *J. Nutr. Health Aging* **2020**, *24*, 696–698. [CrossRef] [PubMed]
25. Lawrence, V.; Hickson, M.; Weekes, C.E.; Julian, A.; Frost, G.; Murphy, J. A uk survey of nutritional care pathways for patients with covid-19 prior to and post-hospital stay. *J. Hum. Nutr. Diet. Off. J. Br. Diet. Assoc.* **2021**. [CrossRef] [PubMed]
26. Buchanan, E.A.; Hvsizdak, E.E. Online survey tools: Ethical and methodological concerns of human research ethics committees. *J. Empir. Res. Hum. Res. Ethics* **2009**, *4*, 37–48. [CrossRef] [PubMed]

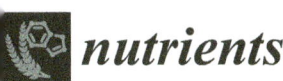

Review

The Complex Interplay between Immunonutrition, Mast Cells, and Histamine Signaling in COVID-19

Sotirios Kakavas [1], Dimitrios Karayiannis [2,*] and Zafeiria Mastora [3]

1. Critical Care Department, "Sotiria" General Hospital of Chest Diseases, 152 Mesogeion Avenue, 11527 Athens, Greece; sotikaka@yahoo.com
2. Department of Clinical Nutrition, Evangelismos General Hospital of Athens, Ypsilantou 45-47, 10676 Athens, Greece
3. First Department of Critical Care Medicine and Pulmonary Services, Evangelismos General Hospital, National and Kapodistrian University of Athens, 11527 Athens, Greece; zafimast@yahoo.gr
* Correspondence: dkarag@hua.gr; Tel.: +30-213-2045035; Fax: +30-213-2041385

Abstract: There is an ongoing need for new therapeutic modalities against SARS-CoV-2 infection. Mast cell histamine has been implicated in the pathophysiology of COVID-19 as a regulator of proinflammatory, fibrotic, and thrombogenic processes. Consequently, mast cell histamine and its receptors represent promising pharmacological targets. At the same time, nutritional modulation of immune system function has been proposed and is being investigated for the prevention of COVID-19 or as an adjunctive strategy combined with conventional therapy. Several studies indicate that several immunonutrients can regulate mast cell activity to reduce the de novo synthesis and/or release of histamine and other mediators that are considered to mediate, at least in part, the complex pathophysiology present in COVID-19. This review summarizes the effects on mast cell histamine of common immunonutrients that have been investigated for use in COVID-19.

Keywords: immunonutrition; COVID-19; histamine

1. Introduction

Severe acute respiratory syndrome coronavirus 2 (SARS-CoV-2) is an enveloped single-stranded positive-sense ribonucleic acid (RNA) virus that was first detected in China and has caused an ongoing global pandemic [1]. SARS-CoV-2 comprises four identified structural proteins, namely, spike (S), membrane (M), envelope (E), and nucleocapsid (N) [2]. In general, the virus infects by binding its S protein to the host's angiotensin-converting enzyme 2 (ACE2) receptors, then entering by endocytosis into airway epithelium cells, lung macrophages, alveolar epithelial cells, and vascular endothelial cells [3,4]. Patients may remain asymptomatic or develop symptoms of varying severity [5,6]. In the resulting coronavirus disease 2019 (COVID-19), activation of the innate immunity, specific antibodies, and activated T cells represent basic defensive factors, while in more severe cases, lung injury progresses and leads to respiratory failure [5,7]. Severe lung injury in SARS-CoV-2 patients is considered the result of immune hyperreaction that involves both innate and adaptive immune responses [6,8]. Briefly, coronavirus infection activates antigen-presenting cells, such as macrophages, that display viral antigens to T and B cells resulting in antibody production and increased cytokine secretion in the form of a cytokine storm. Other immune cells are also implicated, including mast cells, which are important coordinators for both innate and adaptive immunity [9]. Endothelial injury and microthromboses ensue in the lungs and other organs of COVID-19 patients [10,11]. Patients may require mechanical ventilation and develop multiple organ failure [5,6].

Histamine is an endogenous biogenic amine that functions as a neurotransmitter and an immunoregulatory factor. In the immune system, histamine is mainly stored in cytoplasmic granules of mast cells and basophils and is released upon triggering along with other mediators such as serotonin, proteases (e.g., tryptase and chymase), heparin, a variety of cytokines, and angiogenic factors [12]. Histamine release can be activated by numerous innate signals or exogenous triggers [13] including allergens, toxins, and viruses [14]. The high-affinity immunoglobulin (Ig)E receptor, FcepsilonRI (FcɛRI), is the primary receptor in mast cells that mediates IgE-dependent (allergic) reactions [12]. Yet, it is apparent that non-IgE-mediated mechanisms of mast cell activation also exist [13]. Histamine exerts its biological actions through four types of G protein-coupled histamine receptors (i.e., H1 receptor, H2 receptor, H3 receptor, and H4 receptor) [15]. It also activates acute immune-mediated reactions and enhances vascular smooth muscle contraction and the migration of other immune cells, antibodies, and mediators to the site of insult [7]. The release of histamine by perivascular mast cells may also affect adjacent lymphatic vessel function inducing immune cell trafficking through its lumen, which potentially contribute to acute inflammatory stimulus [16]. In the lungs, this may cause bronchoconstriction, increased mucus production, increased vasopermeability with edema, microthrombosis, and infiltration by leukocytes, predominantly neutrophils [17]. Histamine can regulate the balance between Th1 and Th2 effector cells [18]. During histamine-mediated lung inflammation, secretion of Th2 cytokines is enhanced, while production of Th1 cytokines is suppressed [19]. This response may increase susceptibility to viral and bacterial infections of the respiratory tract [5]. In addition, viral remnants may prolong and exaggerate the inflammatory process, causing a histamine-induced release of more pro-inflammatory Th2 cytokines through an IgE-mediated positive feedback vicious cycle [5].

A growing body of evidence has implicated histamine and mast cells in COVID-19 [20–22]. In animal models of COVID-19, mast cells detected in the lungs were chymase positive [23]. Mast cells are shown to express histamine receptors by themselves which, in an autocrine fashion, can potentially ensue a feedback regulation further enhancing inflammatory response [16,24]. The SARS-CoV 2 infection has been shown to activate mast cells leading to histamine release that increases IL-1 levels, causing hyper-inflammation and cytokine storm [25]. Mast cell degranulation has been reported in alveolar septa of deceased patients with COVID-19 and in SARS-CoV-2-infected mice and non-human primates [23,26]. Furthermore, this mast cell activation was associated with interstitial edema and immunothrombosis [27], while the levels of the mast cell-specific protease, chymase, correlated significantly with disease severity [23]. Moreover, studies have reported that H1 as well as H2 receptor antagonists, such as famotidine, are associated with a reduced risk of infection and deterioration leading to intubation or death from COVID-19 [28,29]. These agents are considered to improve pulmonary symptoms of SARS-CoV-2 infection by blocking the histamine-mediated cytokine storm [30]. Nevertheless, these observational findings need further validation by the ongoing randomized clinical trials.

Given that limited therapeutic modalities are available for the treatment of COVID-19, nutritional modulation of the immune system function has been proposed and is being investigated [31–34]. It is widely accepted that normal nutritional status is vital for immune homeostasis [35], while a number of recently published key studies suggest promising effects of immunonutrition on acute respiratory infections [36,37]. Briefly, immunonutrition can be defined as modulation of either the activity of the immune system or modulation of the consequences of activation of the immune system by nutrients or specific food items fed in amounts above those normally encountered in the diet [38]. Until now, specific immunonutrients have been proposed as effective for the prevention of COVID-19 or as an adjunctive strategy combined with conventional therapy [39]. At the same time, these nutraceuticals have been reported to modulate mast cell activation and histamine release with similar potency to pharmacological interventions [40,41]. This review summarizes the effects on mast cell and histamine signaling of common immunonutrients that have been investigated for use in COVID-19.

2. Vitamins

2.1. Vitamin D

Vitamin D has been linked to the susceptibility to SARS-CoV-2 infection and the prognosis of COVID-19 based on a series of data [32]. There is evidence that vitamin D inhibits the entry and replication of SARS-CoV-2 and suppresses the levels of pro-inflammatory cytokines while enhancing the production of anti-inflammatory cytokines and antimicrobial peptides [42]. According to epidemiological observations, vitamin D deficiency has been associated with a higher risk, severity, and mortality rate of COVID-19 [43,44]. However, conflicting results have been reported concerning the effects of vitamin D supplementation in outpatients and hospitalized patients after COVID-19 diagnosis in terms of disease severity, hospital length of stay, ICU admission, or mortality rate [45–48]. Although, no official guidelines exist, it has been proposed to aim for adequate serum 25(OH)D levels of at least 30 ng/mL (75 nmol/L) during the pandemic [49]. Further results are pending ongoing clinical trials [50].

Vitamin D seems to preserve the stability of mast cells, possibly by maintaining the expression of vitamin D receptors. In a vitamin D-deficient environment, mast cell activation occurs automatically, even in the absence of specific triggering [51]. In addition, it has been shown that vitamin D inhibits histamine release from mast cell activation including IgE-mediated activation [52]. Likewise, decreased levels of serum histamine have been found after the antigenic challenging of sensitized mice previously receiving a vitamin D supplemented diet [51]. According to this study, vitamin D receptor binding inhibits mast cell activation by blocking the non-receptor tyrosine kinase Lyn. Lyn is recruited immediately during mast cell activation following the crosslinking of FcεRI–IgE complexes by multivalent antigens or exposure to the bacterial lipopolysaccharide [53,54]. Furthermore, the phosphorylation of the Syk tyrosine kinase was also suppressed by vitamin D receptor binding to the β chain of FcεRI. Syk activation can be triggered by Lyn and is involved in mast cell degranulation [55]. Recent data also indicate a positive effect of vitamin D supplementation on functional humoral immunity levels as determined by IgG levels [56].

2.2. Vitamin E

Vitamin E is a lipid-soluble vitamin with antioxidant and immunomodulatory properties. In addition to scavenging free radicals, vitamin E can affect immune function by modulating signal transduction and gene expression [57–59]. In this way, vitamin E has been found to reduce susceptibility to respiratory infections as well as allergy-related diseases such as asthma [59]. Vitamin E has been implicated in the treatment of SARS-CoV-2 infection in an effort to minimize oxidative damage in these patients [33]. However, limited evidence exists on the use of vitamin E as an adjuvant agent for the treatment of COVID-19 patients, and information resulting from clinical trials is wanted [60].

Vitamin E has been shown to have an inhibitory effect on the proliferation, secretion, and survival of mast cells [61]. This effect originates from the modulation of protein kinase C, protein phosphatase 2A, and protein kinase B in mast cells. Furthermore, in vitro studies in various mast cell lines have shown that vitamin E affects mast cell activation, resulting in a decreased release of proinflammatory mediators including histamine [62,63]. The effects of vitamin E on mast cell function could be related with the antioxidative properties of the vitamin [61]. Interestingly, oxidative stress and mast cells interact and participate in acute lung injury. Reactive oxygen species generation promotes pulmonary mast cell degranulation which, in turn, can increase oxidative stress and inflammation during acute lung injury [64].

2.3. Vitamin C

Vitamin C or ascorbic acid is a water-soluble antioxidant vitamin that possesses anti-inflammatory and immunomodulatory properties [5]. Although the value of vitamin C has not yet been demonstrated in COVID-19, it has gained interest in this context because of its antiviral action [65] and beneficial effects in oxidative damage and inflammation [66]. Vitamin C has previously been implicated in sepsis and ARDS, both of which represent major complications of COVID-19 [67]. Although low levels of vitamin C have been reported in sepsis, conflicting results have been produced by studies evaluating vitamin C supplementation in septic shock and ARDS [68,69]. At present, we are awaiting the results of several ongoing trials evaluating the value of oral or intravenous vitamin C supplementation in the treatment of COVID-19. A daily oral dosage of 1–2 g/day of vitamin C has been proposed as beneficial for the prevention or treatment of COVID-19, while higher doses of intravenous vitamin C, up to 24 gm/day, are being evaluated in critically ill patients with COVID-19. Proposed mechanisms for the ability of vitamin C to benefit patients with COVID-19 point to the prevention of IL-6 increase in several (pro)inflammatory conditions and the inhibition of increases for a range of inflammatory cytokines [70,71].

Previous studies have shown that vitamin C administration attenuates a robust immune response [72]. In fact, mast cell-mediated bronchial hypersensitivity caused by the common cold was inhibited by the administration of vitamin C [73]. These patients exhibited decreased bronchial hypersensitivity to histamine and bronchoconstriction after vitamin C administration [40]. Both preclinical [74–76] and clinical studies [76–78] have evaluated histamine blood levels after vitamin C administration. In a recent study, 7.5 g of vitamin C administered intravenously in 89 patients with allergies or upper respiratory infections caused a significant reduction in serum histamine [79]. Several mechanisms may be responsible for the inhibitory effect of vitamin C on histamine [79,80]; vitamin C may inhibit mast cell activation, increase histamine degradation by diamine oxidase or, alternatively, decrease histamine production by inhibiting histidine decarboxylase [81].

3. Minerals
3.1. Zinc

Zinc is the second most abundant essential trace element that plays important roles in the development, differentiation, and function of immune cells [33]. The perceived antiviral properties of zinc against upper respiratory tract viral infections derive from its participation in metallothioneins [82]. In this context, zinc may interfere with viral infection in many ways [83,84]. First, zinc may prevent viral attachment to nasopharyngeal mucous as well as fusion with the host's membrane and virus entry into cells. In particular, zinc has been shown to decrease the activity of the ACE2 receptor, which is essential for SARS-CoV-2 binding and the provocation of cytokine storm. Moreover, this trace element has been shown to hinder SARS-CoV-1 viral replication by inhibiting SARS-CoV RNA polymerase [85]. Further antiviral effects of zinc include the impairment of viral protein translation and the blockade of viral particle release [86]. Zinc deficiency is common in COVID-19 patients and is associated with more complications and increased mortality [42]. In older adults, supplementation with 45 mg elemental zinc per day has been shown to reduce the risk of infection [31]. In summary, it has been proposed that zinc supplementation may be beneficial in the prevention and treatment of SARS-CoV-2 infection and the associated inflammation [87–89]. At present, a series of clinical trials have been registered to test the efficacy of various regimens containing zinc against COVID-19.

Zinc deficiency has been demonstrated to affect the function of various types of immune cells including mast cells [90,91]. Zinc seems to be essential for mast cell activation. In an in vitro study, the release of histamine from human basophils and lung mast cells was inhibited from physiological concentrations of zinc [92]. A possible mechanism may include the blockade of Ca^{2+} influx induced by the IgE-mediated activation of mast cells [6]. On the other hand, a zinc chelator (N,N,N,N-tetrakis (2-pyridylmethyl) ethylenediamine) has been recently shown to contribute to the inhibition of histamine release from mast cells and this effect was reversed by zinc supplementation [93]. Zinc may regulate mast cell activation and function by modulating the PKC/NF-κB signaling pathway [90]. Various mechanisms have been suggested, but modulation of the NF-kB pathway could be the result of the inhibition of cyclic nucleotide phosphodiesterase, cross activation of protein kinase

A, and inhibitory phosphorylation of protein kinase Raf-1 [94]. In addition, activation of NF-kB can also activate mast cells thereby releasing histamine secretion and an ensuing inflammatory response along with cytokine secretion [95].

3.2. Selenium

Selenium is a trace element that serves as an essential component of antioxidant enzymes. In this way, it exhibits a protective effect against respiratory infections including viral infections [96,97] (33, 97, 98). It has been suggested that selenium deficiency might be implicated in the evolution of SARS-CoV-2 [87]. Moreover, a number of studies have linked selenium with SARS-CoV2 infection and recovery rates [98–100]. Selenium may halt oxidative stress in patients with COVID-19 [33,39]. Interestingly, oxidative stress and mast cells show a bidirectional interaction. Intracellular reactive oxygen species production is the result of mast cells by various triggers [101], while mast cell degranulation can be controlled via the decrease in reactive oxygen species generation using antioxidants [62]. In accordance with this, an in vitro study showed that selenium can suppress the IgE-mediated release of inflammatory mediators in a murine mast cell line, although histamine release only slightly decreased [102]. The regulation of redox-sensitive transcription factors is considered the responsible mechanism by which selenium affects mast cell histamine release [103]. Published data also highlight the important role of biological functions that occur via incorporation of selenium into selenoproteins in the form of selenocysteine amino acid residue. Selenocysteine (Sec-Cys) is involved in a variety of prostanoid metabolism processes and, therefore, have an impact on immunity [104].

4. Omega-3 Fatty Acids

Omega-3 fatty acids are polyunsaturated fatty acids (PUFAs) obtained mainly from two dietary sources: marine and plant oils. These fatty acids incorporate into the bi-phospholipid layer of the cell membrane and result in the reduced production of pro-inflammatory mediators [105]. To date, sparse evidence has implicated omega-3 fatty acids in the prevention and treatment of COVID-19 [106,107]. Nevertheless, it has been shown that the omega-3 PUFAs inactivate enveloped viruses like SARS-CoV2 and inhibit ACE2-mediated binding and cellular entry of SARS-CoV-2 [108]. Furthermore, beneficial reports of omega-3 PUFAs have been reported in patients with sepsis and sepsis-induced ARDS [109,110]. Several clinical trials assessing the effect of omega-3 PUFAs in COVID-19 management are currently registered (ZPD37). In a recent double-blind, randomized clinical trial, enteral supplementation with omega-3 PUFAs significantly improved respiratory and renal function indices as well as one-month survival rates in critically ill patients with COVID-19 [111].

Similar to other immune cells, fatty acids are incorporated into mast cell membranes and can differentially influence mast cell secretive properties [62,112,113]. Collectively, the actions of omega-3 PUFAs on mast cells are mainly inhibitory. A series of studies in animal models and in human cells has demonstrated the inhibitory effect of omega-3 PUFAs on IgE-mediated activation of mast cells [26,114,115]. This effect is mediated by the inhibition of GATA transcription factors in mast cells and leads to suppressed Th2 cytokine expression [116]. As expected, this action of omega-3 PUFAs was tested to ameliorate the severity of mast cell-associated diseases [117,118]. In a canine atopic dermatitis model mast cell histamine release was reduced after treatment by γ-linolenic acid or α-linolenic acid. On the other hand, linoleic acid or arachidonic acid enhanced histamine release [113,119]. However, in a model of stress-induced visceral hypersensitivity in maternally separated rats, neither mast cell degranulation nor hypersensitivity were affected by the administration of an omega-3 PUFA-enriched diet [120]. Clinical trials of the dietary omega-3 supplementation in asthma patients have reported beneficial effects on airway inflammation but inconsistent clinical benefits in terms of lung function indices [121]. Nonetheless, it should be noted that two of these studies reported clinical benefits of dietary supplementation with omega-3 PUFAs in asthma patients without an accompanying decrease in mast cell activation and histamine release [122,123].

5. Phytochemicals

5.1. Flavonoids

Flavonoids are a group of naturally occurring polyphenolic substances with antioxidative and anti-inflammatory actions in various disease states [124]. They may also have antiviral properties and several representatives of this family, such as quercetin, have been proposed as a potential treatment of COVID-19 [125,126]. Luteolin from Veronica linariifolia may also be beneficial, since it has been shown to prevent viral entry into the host cell by inhibiting the binding of the SARS-CoV spike protein [127]. A potential antiviral activity via the inhibition of the SARS-CoV helicase has been reported for luteolin, myricetin (from Myricanagi), and scutellarin (from Scutellaria barbata) [128]. Finally, the antiviral activity of kaempferol has been suggested to derive from the inhibition of the 3a-channel protein of SARS-CoV [129].

Several flavonoids inhibit in vitro the expression and/or release of mediators, such as histamine, by human and rodent mast cells [130–132]. More specifically, quercetin inhibits mast cell activation and release of histamine and may modulate airway inflammation [133,134]. Likewise, luteolin or a structural analog of luteolin inhibit mast cell activation and histamine release from animal and human mast cells [135–137]. The modulatory action of flavonoids on mast cell secretory function affects both IgE-dependent and independent processes and appears to be selective [130]. Some flavonoids, such as caffeic acid, inhibit selective histamine release, while others, such as luteolin and myricetin, inhibit both histamine and β-hexosaminidase release [138]. This inhibitory action may involve the suppression of NF-κB activation [137,139]. The inhibition of calcium influx and protein kinase C translocation and activity mediate the actions of luteolin and quercetin on histamine release from murine bone marrow-derived mast cells, rat peritoneal mast cells, and human cultured cord blood-derived mast cells [131,140,141]. Similarly, quercetin, kaempferol, and myricetin suppressed IgE-mediated activation and histamine release from human umbilical cord blood-derived cultured mast cells. The proposed mechanism includes the decrease of intracellular calcium influx and the inhibition of protein kinase C-theta isoenzyme signaling [140]. Finally, luteolin inhibits neuropeptide (non-IgE mediated) stimulation of mast cells via the mammalian target of rapamycin (mTOR) signaling [142].

5.2. Curcumin

Curcumin is a natural yellow constituent of turmeric or curry powder that is derived from the rhizome of Curcuma longa plants [143]. Curcumin has been reported as a pleiotropic molecule with various biological actions including antioxidant and anti-inflammatory effects [144]. The oral or intranasal administration of curcumin has been shown to suppress airway inflammation and remodeling and to inhibit airway hyperreactivity to histamine and bronchoconstriction in animal models of asthma [145,146]. Curcumin may also exhibit antiviral activities and has been shown to hamper the replication and proliferation of SARS-CoV-1, the first beta-coronavirus that caused the 2003 SARS outbreak and shares a substantial genetic similarity with SARS-CoV-2 [147]. Moreover, in a rat experimental model, curcumin administration resulted in the attenuation of myocardial fibrosis by modulating angiotensin receptors and ACE2 [4,148]. A similar role could be proposed in the fibrotic process that emerges as a secondary event in severe COVID-19 [148]. Along with its well-known anti-inflammatory effects, curcumin has been reported to inhibit mast cell degranulation and histamine release in vitro and in vivo [149–151]. A possible mechanism may include the in vivo suppression of the Syk-dependent phosphorylations, which are critical for mast cell activation. Although the phosphorylation of Syk itself was not affected, curcumin directly inhibited Syk kinase activity in vitro [149]. Curcumin also inhibited the phosphorylation of additional down-stream signaling molecules including Akt, p38, and JNK [149].

6. Conclusions

There is an ongoing need for new therapeutic modalities against SARS-CoV-2 infection that continues to spread rapidly around the world. Mounting evidence shows that hyper-inflammation is the hallmark of COVID-19 pathophysiology leading to significant morbidity and mortality. The majority of the histamine secreted by mast cells may play an important role in the pathophysiology of COVID-19 and is regarded as a promising pharmacological target. The activation of pulmonary mast cells releases mediators with proinflammatory, fibrotic, and thrombogenic properties. Moreover, observational studies have shown the potential benefits of H2 receptor antagonists in patients with COVID-19. However, given the relative paucity of agents targeting mast cells, it may be rational to consider alternative treatments with pleiotropic properties including the modulation of histamine release. Mast cell-derived histamine can regulate not only adaptive and immune system responses but also vasodilatation by binding to endothelial H1 receptors and enhancing NO production. In an inverse way, histamine-induced NO can negatively modulate mast cell activation, mediator expression, and secretion, thus creating an autocrine loop [152]. In this context, several in vivo and in vitro studies indicate that mast cell activity can be regulated by various nutraceuticals that have gained interest for the treatment of COVID-19. In this way, immunonutrition could lead to a reduction in the de novo synthesis and/or release of histamine and other mast cell mediators that are considered to mediate, at least in part, the immune and microvascular alterations present in COVID-19 (Figure 1). These regimens could be used prophylactically or adjunctively to the conventional treatment of patients infected with SARS-CoV-2. We should point out that for other nutrients, such as glutamine and arginine that have been extensively studied for their immune modifying effect, there are no data available regarding their role on mast cells and histamine during SARS-CoV-2 infection. Nevertheless, the clinical evidence is still limited, and further investigations are necessary to validate the efficacy of nutraceuticals in managing the immune response in COVID-19, and, in particular, modulating mast cell activity.

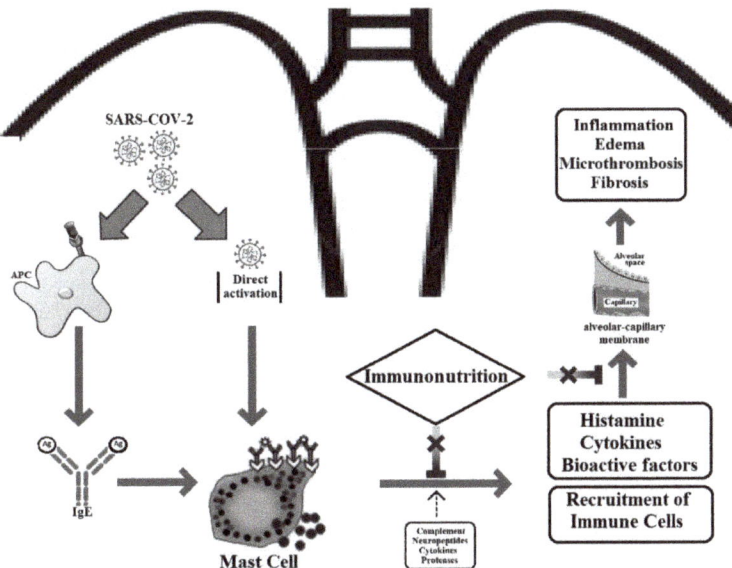

Figure 1. Schematic representation of the modulatory activity of immunonutrients with potential use in COVID-19 on mast cells and histamine during SARS-CoV-2 infection. APC: antigen-producing cells (macrophages or dendritic cells).

Author Contributions: D.K. and S.K. contributed equally to this work. S.K. drafted the manuscript and D.K. and Z.M. revised it. All authors have read and agreed to the published version of the manuscript.

Funding: This research received no external funding.

Institutional Review Board Statement: Not applicable.

Informed Consent Statement: Not applicable.

Data Availability Statement: Not applicable.

Conflicts of Interest: The authors declare no conflict of interest.

Abbreviations

SARS-CoV-2	severe acute respiratory syndrome coronavirus 2
COVID-19	coronavirus disease 2019
ACE2	angiotensin-converting enzyme 2
ARDS	acute respiratory distress syndrome

References

1. Poon, L.L.M.; Peiris, M. Emergence of a novel human coronavirus threatening human health. *Nat. Med.* **2020**, *26*, 317–319. [CrossRef] [PubMed]
2. Naqvi, A.A.T.; Fatima, K.; Mohammad, T.; Fatima, U.; Singh, I.K.; Singh, A.; Atif, S.M.; Hariprasad, G.; Hasan, G.M.; Hassan, M.I. Insights into SARS-CoV-2 genome, structure, evolution, pathogenesis and therapies: Structural genomics approach. *Biochim. Biophys. Acta Mol. Basis Dis.* **2020**, *1866*, 165878. [CrossRef]
3. Tai, W.; He, L.; Zhang, X.; Pu, J.; Voronin, D.; Jiang, S.; Zhou, Y.; Du, L. Characterization of the receptor-binding domain (RBD) of 2019 novel coronavirus: Implication for development of RBD protein as a viral attachment inhibitor and vaccine. *Cell. Mol. Immunol.* **2020**, *17*, 613–620. [CrossRef] [PubMed]
4. Liu, Z.; Xiao, X.; Wei, X.; Li, J.; Yang, J.; Tan, H.; Zhu, J.; Zhang, Q.; Wu, J.; Liu, L. Composition and divergence of coronavirus spike proteins and host ACE2 receptors predict potential intermediate hosts of SARS-CoV-2. *J. Med. Virol.* **2020**, *92*, 595–601. [CrossRef] [PubMed]
5. Chen, G.; Wu, D.; Guo, W.; Cao, Y.; Huang, D.; Wang, H.; Wang, T.; Zhang, X.; Chen, H.; Yu, H.; et al. Clinical and immunological features of severe and moderate coronavirus disease 2019. *J. Clin. Investig.* **2020**, *130*, 2620–2629. [CrossRef] [PubMed]
6. Huang, C.; Wang, Y.; Li, X.; Ren, L.; Zhao, J.; Hu, Y.; Zhang, L.; Fan, G.; Xu, J.; Gu, X.; et al. Clinical features of patients infected with 2019 novel coronavirus in Wuhan, China. *Lancet* **2020**, *395*, 497–506. [CrossRef]
7. Peddapalli, A.; Gehani, M.; Kalle, A.M.; Peddapalli, S.R.; Peter, A.E.; Sharad, S. Demystifying Excess Immune Response in COVID-19 to Reposition an Orphan Drug for Down-Regulation of NF-κB: A Systematic Review. *Viruses* **2021**, *13*, 378. [CrossRef]
8. Ye, Q.; Wang, B.; Mao, J. The pathogenesis and treatment of the 'Cytokine Storm' in COVID-19. *J. Infect.* **2020**, *80*, 607–613. [CrossRef]
9. Tete, S.; Tripodi, D.; Rosati, M.; Conti, F.; Maccauro, G.; Saggini, A.; Salini, V.; Cianchetti, E.; Caraffa, A.; Antinolfi, P.; et al. Role of mast cells in innate and adaptive immunity. *J. Biol. Regul. Homeost. Agents* **2012**, *26*, 193–201.
10. McFadyen, J.D.; Stevens, H.; Peter, K. The Emerging Threat of (Micro)Thrombosis in COVID-19 and Its Therapeutic Implications. *Circ. Res.* **2020**, *127*, 571–587. [CrossRef]
11. Ackermann, M.; Verleden, S.E.; Kuehnel, M.; Haverich, A.; Welte, T.; Laenger, F.; Vanstapel, A.; Werlein, C.; Stark, H.; Tzankov, A.; et al. Pulmonary Vascular Endothelialitis, Thrombosis, and Angiogenesis in Covid-19. *N. Engl. J. Med.* **2020**, *383*, 120–128. [CrossRef]
12. Thangam, E.B.; Jemima, E.A.; Singh, H.; Baig, M.S.; Khan, M.; Mathias, C.B.; Church, M.K.; Saluja, R. The Role of Histamine and Histamine Receptors in Mast Cell-Mediated Allergy and Inflammation: The Hunt for New Therapeutic Targets. *Front. Immunol.* **2018**, *9*, 1873. [CrossRef]
13. Yu, Y.; Blokhuis, B.R.; Garssen, J.; Redegeld, F.A. Non-IgE mediated mast cell activation. *Eur. J. Pharmacol.* **2016**, *778*, 33–43. [CrossRef]
14. Marshall, J.S.; Portales-Cervantes, L.; Leong, E. Mast Cell Responses to Viruses and Pathogen Products. *Int. J. Mol. Sci.* **2019**, *20*, 4241. [CrossRef]
15. Thurmond, R.L.; Gelfand, E.W.; Dunford, P.J. The role of histamine H1 and H4 receptors in allergic inflammation: The search for new antihistamines. *Nat. Rev. Drug Discov.* **2008**, *7*, 41–53. [CrossRef] [PubMed]
16. Pal, S.; Gasheva, O.Y.; Zawieja, D.C.; Meininger, C.J.; Gashev, A.A. Histamine-mediated autocrine signaling in mesenteric perilymphatic mast cells. *Am. J. Physiol. Regul. Integr. Comp. Physiol.* **2020**, *318*, R590–R604. [CrossRef] [PubMed]
17. Movat, H.Z. The role of histamine and other mediators in microvascular changes in acute inflammation. *Can. J. Physiol. Pharmacol.* **1987**, *65*, 451–457. [CrossRef]

18. Jutel, M.; Watanabe, T.; Klunker, S.; Akdis, M.; Thomet, O.A.; Malolepszy, J.; Zak-Nejmark, T.; Koga, R.; Kobayashi, T.; Blaser, K.; et al. Histamine regulates T-cell and antibody responses by differential expression of H1 and H2 receptors. *Nature* **2001**, *413*, 420–425. [CrossRef]
19. Branco, A.; Yoshikawa, F.S.Y.; Pietrobon, A.J.; Sato, M.N. Role of Histamine in Modulating the Immune Response and Inflammation. *Mediat. Inflamm.* **2018**, *2018*, 9524075. [CrossRef] [PubMed]
20. Theoharides, T.C. COVID-19, pulmonary mast cells, cytokine storms, and beneficial actions of luteolin. *Biofactors* **2020**, *46*, 306–308. [CrossRef]
21. Theoharides, T.C. Potential association of mast cells with coronavirus disease 2019. *Ann. Allergy Asthma Immunol.* **2021**, *126*, 217–218. [CrossRef]
22. Ennis, M.; Tiligada, K. Histamine receptors and COVID-19. *Inflamm. Res.* **2021**, *70*, 67–75. [CrossRef]
23. Tan, J.A.D.; Rathore, A.P.S.; O'Neill, A.; Mantri, C.K.; Saron, W.A.A.; Lee, C.; Cui, C.W.; Kang, A.E.Z.; Foo, R.; Kalimuddin, S.; et al. Signatures of mast cell activation are associated with severe COVID-19. *medRxiv* **2021**. [CrossRef]
24. Carlos, D.; Sá-Nunes, A.; de Paula, L.; Matias-Peres, C.; Jamur, M.C.; Oliver, C.; Serra, M.F.; Martins, M.A.; Faccioli, L.H. Histamine modulates mast cell degranulation through an indirect mechanism in a model IgE-mediated reaction. *Eur. J. Immunol.* **2006**, *36*, 1494–1503. [CrossRef]
25. Conti, P.; Caraffa, A.; Tetè, G.; Gallenga, C.E.; Ross, R.; Kritas, S.K.; Frydas, I.; Younes, A.; di Emidio, P.; Ronconi, G. Mast cells activated by SARS-CoV-2 release histamine which increases IL-1 levels causing cytokine storm and inflammatory reaction in COVID-19. *J. Biol. Regul. Homeost. Agents* **2020**, *34*, 1629–1632. [CrossRef]
26. Abdel Latif, M.; Abdul-Hamid, M.; Galaly, S.R. Effect of diethylcarbamazine citrate and omega-3 fatty acids on trimellitic anhydride-induced rat skin allergy. *Asian Pac. J. Allergy Immunol.* **2015**, *33*, 33–41. [CrossRef]
27. Motta Junior, J.D.S.; Miggiolaro, A.; Nagashima, S.; de Paula, C.B.V.; Baena, C.P.; Scharfstein, J.; de Noronha, L. Mast Cells in Alveolar Septa of COVID-19 Patients: A Pathogenic Pathway That May Link Interstitial Edema to Immunothrombosis. *Front. Immunol.* **2020**, *11*, 574862. [CrossRef]
28. Vila-Córcoles, A.; Ochoa-Gondar, O.; Satué-Gracia, E.M.; Torrente-Fraga, C.; Gomez-Bertomeu, F.; Vila-Rovira, A.; Hospital-Guardiola, I.; de Diego-Cabanes, C.; Bejarano-Romero, F.; Basora-Gallisà, J. Influence of prior comorbidities and chronic medications use on the risk of COVID-19 in adults: A population-based cohort study in Tarragona, Spain. *BMJ Open* **2020**, *10*, e041577. [CrossRef] [PubMed]
29. Qu, C.; Fuhler, G.M.; Pan, Y. Could Histamine H1 Receptor Antagonists Be Used for Treating COVID-19? *Int. J. Mol. Sci.* **2021**, *22*, 5672. [CrossRef] [PubMed]
30. Hogan Ii, R.B.; Hogan Iii, R.B.; Cannon, T.; Rappai, M.; Studdard, J.; Paul, D.; Dooley, T.P. Dual-histamine receptor blockade with cetirizine—Famotidine reduces pulmonary symptoms in COVID-19 patients. *Pulm. Pharmacol. Ther.* **2020**, *63*, 101942. [CrossRef] [PubMed]
31. Subedi, L.; Tchen, S.; Gaire, B.P.; Hu, B.; Hu, K. Adjunctive Nutraceutical Therapies for COVID-19. *Int. J. Mol. Sci.* **2021**, *22*, 1963. [CrossRef]
32. Story, M.J. Essential sufficiency of zinc, ω-3 polyunsaturated fatty acids, vitamin D and magnesium for prevention and treatment of COVID-19, diabetes, cardiovascular diseases, lung diseases and cancer. *Biochimie* **2021**, *187*, 94–109. [CrossRef] [PubMed]
33. Shakoor, H.; Feehan, J.; Al Dhaheri, A.S.; Ali, H.I.; Platat, C.; Ismail, L.C.; Apostolopoulos, V.; Stojanovska, L. Immune-boosting role of vitamins D, C, E, zinc, selenium and omega-3 fatty acids: Could they help against COVID-19? *Maturitas* **2021**, *143*, 1–9. [CrossRef] [PubMed]
34. Hamulka, J.; Jeruszka-Bielak, M.; Górnicka, M.; Drywień, M.E.; Zielinska-Pukos, M.A. Dietary Supplements during COVID-19 Outbreak. Results of Google Trends Analysis Supported by PLifeCOVID-19 Online Studies. *Nutrients* **2020**, *13*, 54. [CrossRef] [PubMed]
35. Minnelli, N.; Gibbs, L.; Larrivee, J.; Sahu, K.K. Challenges of Maintaining Optimal Nutrition Status in COVID-19 Patients in Intensive Care Settings. *JPEN J. Parenter. Enter. Nutr.* **2020**, *44*, 1439–1446. [CrossRef]
36. Derbyshire, E.; Delange, J. COVID-19: Is there a role for immunonutrition, particularly in the over 65s? *BMJ Nutr. Prev. Health* **2020**, *3*, 100–105. [CrossRef]
37. Jovic, T.H.; Ali, S.R.; Ibrahim, N.; Jessop, Z.M.; Tarassoli, S.P.; Dobbs, T.D.; Holford, P.; Thornton, C.A.; Whitaker, I.S. Could Vitamins Help in the Fight Against COVID-19? *Nutrients* **2020**, *12*, 2550. [CrossRef]
38. Grimble, R.F. Basics in clinical nutrition: Immunonutrition—Nutrients which influence immunity: Effect and mechanism of action. *Eur. E-J. Clin. Nutr. Metab.* **2009**, *4*, e10–e13. [CrossRef]
39. Bae, M.; Kim, H. Mini-Review on the Roles of Vitamin C, Vitamin D, and Selenium in the Immune System against COVID-19. *Molecules* **2020**, *25*, 5346. [CrossRef]
40. Yazdani, S.C.P. Relationship between Vitamin C, Mast Cells and Inflammation. *J. Nutr. Food Sci.* **2016**, *6*, 1–3. [CrossRef]
41. Weng, Z.; Zhang, B.; Asadi, S.; Sismanopoulos, N.; Butcher, A.; Fu, X.; Katsarou-Katsari, A.; Antoniou, C.; Theoharides, T.C. Quercetin is more effective than cromolyn in blocking human mast cell cytokine release and inhibits contact dermatitis and photosensitivity in humans. *PLoS ONE* **2012**, *7*, e33805. [CrossRef]
42. Jothimani, D.; Kailasam, E.; Danielraj, S.; Nallathambi, B.; Ramachandran, H.; Sekar, P.; Manoharan, S.; Ramani, V.; Narasimhan, G.; Kaliamoorthy, I.; et al. COVID-19: Poor outcomes in patients with zinc deficiency. *Int. J. Infect. Dis.* **2020**, *100*, 343–349. [CrossRef]

43. Yisak, H.; Ewunetei, A.; Kefale, B.; Mamuye, M.; Teshome, F.; Ambaw, B.; Yideg Yitbarek, G. Effects of Vitamin D on COVID-19 Infection and Prognosis: A Systematic Review. *Risk Manag. Healthc. Policy* **2021**, *14*, 31–38. [CrossRef]
44. Mitchell, F. Vitamin-D and COVID-19: Do deficient risk a poorer outcome? *Lancet Diabetes Endocrinol.* **2020**, *8*, 570. [CrossRef]
45. Ohaegbulam, K.C.; Swalih, M.; Patel, P.; Smith, M.A.; Perrin, R. Vitamin D Supplementation in COVID-19 Patients: A Clinical Case Series. *Am. J. Ther.* **2020**, *27*, e485–e490. [CrossRef] [PubMed]
46. Annweiler, G.; Corvaisier, M.; Gautier, J.; Dubée, V.; Legrand, E.; Sacco, G.; Annweiler, C. Vitamin D Supplementation Associated to Better Survival in Hospitalized Frail Elderly COVID-19 Patients: The GERIA-COVID Quasi-Experimental Study. *Nutrients* **2020**, *12*, 3377. [CrossRef]
47. Murai, I.H.; Fernandes, A.L.; Sales, L.P.; Pinto, A.J.; Goessler, K.F.; Duran, C.S.C.; Silva, C.B.R.; Franco, A.S.; Macedo, M.B.; Dalmolin, H.H.H.; et al. Effect of a Single High Dose of Vitamin D3 on Hospital Length of Stay in Patients with Moderate to Severe COVID-19: A Randomized Clinical Trial. *JAMA* **2021**, *325*, 1053–1060. [CrossRef] [PubMed]
48. Cereda, E.; Bogliolo, L.; Lobascio, F.; Barichella, M.; Zecchinelli, A.L.; Pezzoli, G.; Caccialanza, R. Vitamin D supplementation and outcomes in coronavirus disease 2019 (COVID-19) patients from the outbreak area of Lombardy, Italy. *Nutrition* **2021**, *82*, 111055. [CrossRef]
49. Maghbooli, Z.; Sahraian, M.A.; Ebrahimi, M.; Pazoki, M.; Kafan, S.; Tabriz, H.M.; Hadadi, A.; Montazeri, M.; Nasiri, M.; Shirvani, A.; et al. Vitamin D sufficiency, a serum 25-hydroxyvitamin D at least 30 ng/mL reduced risk for adverse clinical outcomes in patients with COVID-19 infection. *PLoS ONE* **2020**, *15*, e0239799. [CrossRef]
50. ClinicalTrials. Available online: https://clinicaltrials.gov/ct2/home (accessed on 27 June 2021).
51. Liu, Z.Q.; Li, X.X.; Qiu, S.Q.; Yu, Y.; Li, M.G.; Yang, L.T.; Li, L.J.; Wang, S.; Zheng, P.Y.; Liu, Z.G.; et al. Vitamin D contributes to mast cell stabilization. *Allergy* **2017**, *72*, 1184–1192. [CrossRef]
52. Yip, K.H.; Kolesnikoff, N.; Yu, C.; Hauschild, N.; Taing, H.; Biggs, L.; Goltzman, D.; Gregory, P.A.; Anderson, P.H.; Samuel, M.S.; et al. 3 metabolite repression of IgE-dependent mast cell activation. *J. Allergy Clin. Immunol.* **2014**, *133*, 1356–1364. [CrossRef]
53. Lin, S.; Cicala, C.; Scharenberg, A.M.; Kinet, J.P. The Fc(epsilon)RIbeta subunit functions as an amplifier of Fc(epsilon)RIgamma-mediated cell activation signals. *Cell* **1996**, *85*, 985–995. [CrossRef]
54. Ban, T.; Sato, G.R.; Nishiyama, A.; Akiyama, A.; Takasuna, M.; Umehara, M.; Suzuki, S.; Ichino, M.; Matsunaga, S.; Kimura, A.; et al. Lyn Kinase Suppresses the Transcriptional Activity of IRF5 in the TLR-MyD88 Pathway to Restrain the Development of Autoimmunity. *Immunity* **2016**, *45*, 319–332. [CrossRef]
55. Amir-Moazami, O.; Alexia, C.; Charles, N.; Launay, P.; Monteiro, R.C.; Benhamou, M. Phospholipid scramblase 1 modulates a selected set of IgE receptor-mediated mast cell responses through LAT-dependent pathway. *J. Biol. Chem.* **2008**, *283*, 25514–25523. [CrossRef]
56. Luciani, F.; Caroleo, M.C.; Cannataro, R.; Mirra, D.; D'Agostino, B.; Gallelli, L.; Cione, E. Immunological Response to SARS-CoV-2 Is Sustained by Vitamin D: A Case Presentation of One-Year Follow-Up. *Reports* **2021**, *4*, 18. [CrossRef]
57. Tanaka, J.; Fujiwara, H.; Torisu, M. Vitamin E and immune response. I. Enhancement of helper T cell activity by dietary supplementation of vitamin E in mice. *Immunology* **1979**, *38*, 727–734. [PubMed]
58. Lewis, E.D.; Meydani, S.N.; Wu, D. Regulatory role of vitamin E in the immune system and inflammation. *IUBMB Life* **2019**, *71*, 487–494. [CrossRef] [PubMed]
59. Lee, G.Y.; Han, S.N. The Role of Vitamin E in Immunity. *Nutrients* **2018**, *10*, 1614. [CrossRef] [PubMed]
60. Beigmohammadi, M.T.; Bitarafan, S.; Hoseindokht, A.; Abdollahi, A.; Amoozadeh, L.; Mahmoodi Ali Abadi, M.; Foroumandi, M. Impact of vitamins A, B, C, D, and E supplementation on improvement and mortality rate in ICU patients with coronavirus-19: A structured summary of a study protocol for a randomized controlled trial. *Trials* **2020**, *21*, 614. [CrossRef]
61. Zingg, J.M. Vitamin E and mast cells. *Vitam. Horm.* **2007**, *76*, 393–418. [CrossRef]
62. Gueck, T.; Aschenbach, J.R.; Fuhrmann, H. Influence of vitamin E on mast cell mediator release. *Vet. Dermatol.* **2002**, *13*, 301–305. [CrossRef] [PubMed]
63. Ranadive, N.S.; Lewis, R. Differential effects of antioxidants and indomethacin on compound 48/80 induced histamine release and Ca^{2+} uptake in rat mast cells. *Immunol. Lett.* **1982**, *5*, 145–150. [CrossRef]
64. Zhao, W.; Gan, X.; Su, G.; Wanling, G.; Li, S.; Hei, Z.; Yang, C.; Wang, H. The interaction between oxidative stress and mast cell activation plays a role in acute lung injuries induced by intestinal ischemia-reperfusion. *J. Surg. Res.* **2014**, *187*, 542–552. [CrossRef]
65. Colunga Biancatelli, R.M.L.; Berrill, M.; Marik, P.E. The antiviral properties of vitamin C. *Expert Rev. Anti Infect. Ther.* **2020**, *18*, 99–101. [CrossRef] [PubMed]
66. Mandl, J.; Szarka, A.; Bánhegyi, G. Vitamin C: Update on physiology and pharmacology. *Br. J. Pharmacol.* **2009**, *157*, 1097–1110. [CrossRef] [PubMed]
67. Kuhn, S.O.; Meissner, K.; Mayes, L.M.; Bartels, K. Vitamin C in sepsis. *Curr. Opin. Anaesthesiol.* **2018**, *31*, 55–60. [CrossRef]
68. Marik, P.E.; Khangoora, V.; Rivera, R.; Hooper, M.H.; Catravas, J. Hydrocortisone, Vitamin C, and Thiamine for the Treatment of Severe Sepsis and Septic Shock: A Retrospective Before-After Study. *Chest* **2017**, *151*, 1229–1238. [CrossRef]
69. Fowler, A.A., 3rd; Truwit, J.D.; Hite, R.D.; Morris, P.E.; DeWilde, C.; Priday, A.; Fisher, B.; Thacker, L.R., 2nd; Natarajan, R.; Brophy, D.F.; et al. Effect of Vitamin C Infusion on Organ Failure and Biomarkers of Inflammation and Vascular Injury in Patients with Sepsis and Severe Acute Respiratory Failure: The CITRIS-ALI Randomized Clinical Trial. *JAMA* **2019**, *322*, 1261–1270. [CrossRef]

70. Liu, F.; Zhu, Y.; Zhang, J.; Li, Y.; Peng, Z. Intravenous high-dose vitamin C for the treatment of severe COVID-19: Study protocol for a multicentre randomised controlled trial. *BMJ Open* **2020**, *10*, e039519. [CrossRef]
71. Feyaerts, A.F.; Luyten, W. Vitamin C as prophylaxis and adjunctive medical treatment for COVID-19? *Nutrition* **2020**, *79–80*, 110948. [CrossRef] [PubMed]
72. Ellulu, M.S.; Rahmat, A.; Patimah, I.; Khaza'ai, H.; Abed, Y. Effect of vitamin C on inflammation and metabolic markers in hypertensive and/or diabetic obese adults: A randomized controlled trial. *Drug Des. Devel. Ther.* **2015**, *9*, 3405–3412. [CrossRef]
73. Hemilä, H. Vitamin C and common cold-induced asthma: A systematic review and statistical analysis. *Allergy Asthma Clin. Immunol.* **2013**, *9*, 46. [CrossRef]
74. Nandi, B.K.; Subramanian, N.; Majumder, A.K.; Chatterjee, I.B. Effect of ascorbic acid on detoxification of histamine under stress conditions. *Biochem. Pharmacol.* **1974**, *23*, 643–647. [CrossRef]
75. Subramanian, N.; Nandi, B.K.; Majumder, A.K.; Chatterjee, I.B. Effect of ascorbic acid on detoxification of histamine in rats and guinea pigs under drug treated conditions. *Biochem. Pharmacol.* **1974**, *23*, 637–641. [CrossRef]
76. Johnston, C.S.; Martin, L.J.; Cai, X. Antihistamine effect of supplemental ascorbic acid and neutrophil chemotaxis. *J. Am. Coll. Nutr.* **1992**, *11*, 172–176. [CrossRef]
77. Clemetson, C.A. Histamine and ascorbic acid in human blood. *J. Nutr.* **1980**, *110*, 662–668. [CrossRef]
78. Johnston, C.S.; Solomon, R.E.; Corte, C. Vitamin C depletion is associated with alterations in blood histamine and plasma free carnitine in adults. *J. Am. Coll. Nutr.* **1996**, *15*, 586–591. [CrossRef]
79. Hagel, A.F.; Layritz, C.M.; Hagel, W.H.; Hagel, H.J.; Hagel, E.; Dauth, W.; Kressel, J.; Regnet, T.; Rosenberg, A.; Neurath, M.F.; et al. Intravenous infusion of ascorbic acid decreases serum histamine concentrations in patients with allergic and non-allergic diseases. *Naunyn Schmiedebergs Arch. Pharmacol.* **2013**, *386*, 789–793. [CrossRef] [PubMed]
80. Mio, M.; Yabuta, M.; Kamei, C. Ultraviolet B (UVB) light-induced histamine release from rat peritoneal mast cells and its augmentation by certain phenothiazine compounds. *Immunopharmacology* **1999**, *41*, 55–63. [CrossRef]
81. Maintz, L.; Novak, N. Histamine and histamine intolerance. *Am. J. Clin. Nutr.* **2007**, *85*, 1185–1196. [CrossRef]
82. Ibs, K.H.; Rink, L. Zinc-altered immune function. *J. Nutr.* **2003**, *133*, 1452s–1456s. [CrossRef] [PubMed]
83. Skalny, A.V.; Rink, L.; Ajsuvakova, O.P.; Aschner, M.; Gritsenko, V.A.; Alekseenko, S.I.; Svistunov, A.A.; Petrakis, D.; Spandidos, D.A.; Aaseth, J.; et al. Zinc and respiratory tract infections: Perspectives for COVID-19 (Review). *Int. J. Mol. Med.* **2020**, *46*, 17–26. [CrossRef] [PubMed]
84. Mayor-Ibarguren, A.; Busca-Arenzana, C.; Robles-Marhuenda, Á. A Hypothesis for the Possible Role of Zinc in the Immunological Pathways Related to COVID-19 Infection. *Front. Immunol.* **2020**, *11*, 1736. [CrossRef] [PubMed]
85. Te Velthuis, A.J.; van den Worm, S.H.; Sims, A.C.; Baric, R.S.; Snijder, E.J.; van Hemert, M.J. $Zn^{(2+)}$ inhibits coronavirus and arterivirus RNA polymerase activity in vitro and zinc ionophores block the replication of these viruses in cell culture. *PLoS Pathog.* **2010**, *6*, e1001176. [CrossRef] [PubMed]
86. Wessels, I.; Rolles, B.; Rink, L. The Potential Impact of Zinc Supplementation on COVID-19 Pathogenesis. *Front. Immunol.* **2020**, *11*, 1712. [CrossRef] [PubMed]
87. Zhang, J.; Taylor, E.W.; Bennett, K.; Saad, R.; Rayman, M.P. Association between regional selenium status and reported outcome of COVID-19 cases in China. *Am. J. Clin. Nutr.* **2020**, *111*, 1297–1299. [CrossRef] [PubMed]
88. Finzi, E. Treatment of SARS-CoV-2 with high dose oral zinc salts: A report on four patients. *Int. J. Infect. Dis.* **2020**, *99*, 307–309. [CrossRef]
89. Carlucci, P.M.; Ahuja, T.; Petrilli, C.; Rajagopalan, H.; Jones, S.; Rahimian, J. Zinc sulfate in combination with a zinc ionophore may improve outcomes in hospitalized COVID-19 patients. *J. Med. Microbiol.* **2020**, *69*, 1228–1234. [CrossRef]
90. Nishida, K.; Uchida, R. Role of Zinc Signaling in the Regulation of Mast Cell-, Basophil-, and T Cell-Mediated Allergic Responses. *J. Immunol. Res.* **2018**, *2018*, 5749120. [CrossRef]
91. Haase, H.; Rink, L. Zinc signals and immune function. *Biofactors* **2014**, *40*, 27–40. [CrossRef]
92. Marone, G.; Columbo, M.; de Paulis, A.; Cirillo, R.; Giugliano, R.; Condorelli, M. Physiological concentrations of zinc inhibit the release of histamine from human basophils and lung mast cells. *Agents Actions* **1986**, *18*, 103–106. [CrossRef]
93. Kabu, K.; Yamasaki, S.; Kamimura, D.; Ito, Y.; Hasegawa, A.; Sato, E.; Kitamura, H.; Nishida, K.; Hirano, T. Zinc is required for Fc epsilon RI-mediated mast cell activation. *J. Immunol.* **2006**, *177*, 1296–1305. [CrossRef]
94. Jarosz, M.; Olbert, M.; Wyszogrodzka, G.; Młyniec, K.; Librowski, T. Antioxidant and anti-inflammatory effects of zinc. Zinc-dependent NF-κB signaling. *Inflammopharmacology* **2017**, *25*, 11–24. [CrossRef] [PubMed]
95. Nizamutdinova, I.T.; Dusio, G.F.; Gasheva, O.Y.; Skoog, H.; Tobin, R.; Peddaboina, C.; Meininger, C.J.; Zawieja, D.C.; Newell-Rogers, M.K.; Gashev, A.A. Mast cells and histamine are triggering the NF-κB-mediated reactions of adult and aged perilymphatic mesenteric tissues to acute inflammation. *Aging* **2016**, *8*, 3065–3090. [CrossRef]
96. Harthill, M. Review: Micronutrient selenium deficiency influences evolution of some viral infectious diseases. *Biol. Trace Elem. Res.* **2011**, *143*, 1325–1336. [CrossRef]
97. Avery, J.C.; Hoffmann, P.R. Selenium, Selenoproteins, and Immunity. *Nutrients* **2018**, *10*, 1203. [CrossRef] [PubMed]
98. Fakhrolmobasheri, M.; Nasr-Esfahany, Z.; Khanahmad, H.; Zeinalian, M. Selenium supplementation can relieve the clinical complications of COVID-19 and other similar viral infections. *Int. J. Vitam. Nutr. Res.* **2021**, *91*, 197–199. [CrossRef] [PubMed]
99. Kieliszek, M.; Lipinski, B. Selenium supplementation in the prevention of coronavirus infections (COVID-19). *Med. Hypotheses* **2020**, *143*, 109878. [CrossRef]

100. Seale, L.A.; Torres, D.J.; Berry, M.J.; Pitts, M.W. A role for selenium-dependent GPX1 in SARS-CoV-2 virulence. *Am. J. Clin. Nutr.* **2020**, *112*, 447–448. [CrossRef]
101. Brooks, A.C.; Whelan, C.J.; Purcell, W.M. Reactive oxygen species generation and histamine release by activated mast cells: Modulation by nitric oxide synthase inhibition. *Br. J. Pharmacol.* **1999**, *128*, 585–590. [CrossRef]
102. Safaralizadeh, R.; Nourizadeh, M.; Zare, A.; Kardar, G.A.; Pourpak, Z. Influence of selenium on mast cell mediator release. *Biol. Trace Elem. Res.* **2013**, *154*, 299–303. [CrossRef]
103. Wintergerst, E.S.; Maggini, S.; Hornig, D.H. Contribution of selected vitamins and trace elements to immune function. *Ann. Nutr. Metab.* **2007**, *51*, 301–323. [CrossRef] [PubMed]
104. Fenghua Qian, S.M.K.S.P. Selenium and selenoproteins in prostanoid metabolism and immunity. *Crit. Rev. Biochem. Mol. Biol.* **2019**, *54*, 484–516. [CrossRef] [PubMed]
105. Hathaway, D.; Pandav, K.; Patel, M.; Riva-Moscoso, A.; Singh, B.M.; Patel, A.; Min, Z.C.; Singh-Makkar, S.; Sana, M.K.; Sanchez-Dopazo, R.; et al. Omega 3 Fatty Acids and COVID-19: A Comprehensive Review. *Infect. Chemother.* **2020**, *52*, 478–495. [CrossRef] [PubMed]
106. Das, U.N. Can Bioactive Lipids Inactivate Coronavirus (COVID-19)? *Arch. Med. Res.* **2020**, *51*, 282–286. [CrossRef] [PubMed]
107. Weill, P.; Plissonneau, C.; Legrand, P.; Rioux, V.; Thibault, R. May omega-3 fatty acid dietary supplementation help reduce severe complications in Covid-19 patients? *Biochimie* **2020**, *179*, 275–280. [CrossRef]
108. Goc, A.; Niedzwiecki, A.; Rath, M. Polyunsaturated ω-3 fatty acids inhibit ACE2-controlled SARS-CoV-2 binding and cellular entry. *Sci. Rep.* **2021**, *11*, 5207. [CrossRef] [PubMed]
109. Chen, H.; Wang, S.; Zhao, Y.; Luo, Y.; Tong, H.; Su, L. Correlation analysis of omega-3 fatty acids and mortality of sepsis and sepsis-induced ARDS in adults: Data from previous randomized controlled trials. *Nutr. J.* **2018**, *17*, 57. [CrossRef]
110. Langlois, P.L.; D'Aragon, F.; Hardy, G.; Manzanares, W. Omega-3 polyunsaturated fatty acids in critically ill patients with acute respiratory distress syndrome: A systematic review and meta-analysis. *Nutrition* **2019**, *61*, 84–92. [CrossRef]
111. Doaei, S.; Gholami, S.; Rastgoo, S.; Gholamalizadeh, M.; Bourbour, F.; Bagheri, S.E.; Samipoor, F.; Akbari, M.E.; Shadnoush, M.; Ghorat, F.; et al. The effect of omega-3 fatty acid supplementation on clinical and biochemical parameters of critically ill patients with COVID-19: A randomized clinical trial. *J. Transl. Med.* **2021**, *19*, 128. [CrossRef]
112. Schumann, J.; Basiouni, S.; Gück, T.; Fuhrmann, H. Treating canine atopic dermatitis with unsaturated fatty acids: The role of mast cells and potential mechanisms of action. *J. Anim. Physiol. Anim. Nutr. (Berl.)* **2014**, *98*, 1013–1020. [CrossRef]
113. Gueck, T.; Seidel, A.; Baumann, D.; Meister, A.; Fuhrmann, H. Alterations of mast cell mediator production and release by gamma-linolenic and docosahexaenoic acid. *Vet. Dermatol.* **2004**, *15*, 309–314. [CrossRef] [PubMed]
114. Wang, X.; Ma, D.W.; Kang, J.X.; Kulka, M. n-3 Polyunsaturated fatty acids inhibit Fc ε receptor I-mediated mast cell activation. *J. Nutr. Biochem.* **2015**, *26*, 1580–1588. [CrossRef] [PubMed]
115. Van den Elsen, L.W.; Nusse, Y.; Balvers, M.; Redegeld, F.A.; Knol, E.F.; Garssen, J.; Willemsen, L.E. n-3 Long-chain PUFA reduce allergy-related mediator release by human mast cells in vitro via inhibition of reactive oxygen species. *Br. J. Nutr.* **2013**, *109*, 1821–1831. [CrossRef] [PubMed]
116. Park, B.K.; Park, S.; Park, J.B.; Park, M.C.; Min, T.S.; Jin, M. Omega-3 fatty acids suppress Th2-associated cytokine gene expressions and GATA transcription factors in mast cells. *J. Nutr. Biochem.* **2013**, *24*, 868–876. [CrossRef] [PubMed]
117. Jang, H.Y.; Koo, J.H.; Lee, S.M.; Park, B.H. Atopic dermatitis-like skin lesions are suppressed in fat-1 transgenic mice through the inhibition of inflammasomes. *Exp. Mol. Med.* **2018**, *50*, 1–9. [CrossRef] [PubMed]
118. Kim, T.H.; Kim, G.D.; Jin, Y.H.; Park, Y.S.; Park, C.S. Omega-3 fatty acid-derived mediator, Resolvin E1, ameliorates 2,4-dinitrofluorobenzene-induced atopic dermatitis in NC/Nga mice. *Int. Immunopharmacol.* **2012**, *14*, 384–391. [CrossRef] [PubMed]
119. Gueck, T.; Seidel, A.; Fuhrmann, H. Effects of essential fatty acids on mediators of mast cells in culture. *Prostaglandins Leukot. Essent. Fat. Acids* **2003**, *68*, 317–322. [CrossRef]
120. Van Diest, S.A.; van den Elsen, L.W.; Klok, A.J.; Welting, O.; Hilbers, F.W.; van de Heijning, B.J.; Gaemers, I.C.; Boeckxstaens, G.E.; Werner, M.F.; Willemsen, L.E.; et al. Dietary Marine n-3 PUFAs Do Not Affect Stress-Induced Visceral Hypersensitivity in a Rat Maternal Separation Model. *J. Nutr.* **2015**, *145*, 915–922. [CrossRef]
121. Willemsen, L.E.M. Dietary n-3 long chain polyunsaturated fatty acids in allergy prevention and asthma treatment. *Eur. J. Pharmacol.* **2016**, *785*, 174–186. [CrossRef]
122. Brannan, J.D.; Bood, J.; Alkhabaz, A.; Balgoma, D.; Otis, J.; Delin, I.; Dahlén, B.; Wheelock, C.E.; Nair, P.; Dahlén, S.E.; et al. The effect of omega-3 fatty acids on bronchial hyperresponsiveness, sputum eosinophilia, and mast cell mediators in asthma. *Chest* **2015**, *147*, 397–405. [CrossRef]
123. Arm, J.P.; Horton, C.E.; Spur, B.W.; Mencia-Huerta, J.M.; Lee, T.H. The effects of dietary supplementation with fish oil lipids on the airways response to inhaled allergen in bronchial asthma. *Am. Rev. Respir. Dis.* **1989**, *139*, 1395–1400. [CrossRef]
124. Cushnie, T.P.; Lamb, A.J. Antimicrobial activity of flavonoids. *Int. J. Antimicrob. Agents* **2005**, *26*, 343–356. [CrossRef]
125. Derosa, G.; Maffioli, P.; D'Angelo, A.; di Pierro, F. A role for quercetin in coronavirus disease 2019 (COVID-19). *Phytother. Res.* **2021**, *35*, 1230–1236. [CrossRef] [PubMed]
126. Colunga Biancatelli, R.M.L.; Berrill, M.; Catravas, J.D.; Marik, P.E. Quercetin and Vitamin C: An Experimental, Synergistic Therapy for the Prevention and Treatment of SARS-CoV-2 Related Disease (COVID-19). *Front. Immunol.* **2020**, *11*, 1451. [CrossRef] [PubMed]

27. Yi, L.; Li, Z.; Yuan, K.; Qu, X.; Chen, J.; Wang, G.; Zhang, H.; Luo, H.; Zhu, L.; Jiang, P.; et al. Small molecules blocking the entry of severe acute respiratory syndrome coronavirus into host cells. *J. Virol.* **2004**, *78*, 11334–11339. [CrossRef] [PubMed]
28. Yu, M.S.; Lee, J.; Lee, J.M.; Kim, Y.; Chin, Y.W.; Jee, J.G.; Keum, Y.S.; Jeong, Y.J. Identification of myricetin and scutellarein as novel chemical inhibitors of the SARS coronavirus helicase, nsP13. *Bioorg. Med. Chem. Lett.* **2012**, *22*, 4049–4054. [CrossRef] [PubMed]
29. Wen, C.C.; Shyur, L.F.; Jan, J.T.; Liang, P.H.; Kuo, C.J.; Arulselvan, P.; Wu, J.B.; Kuo, S.C.; Yang, N.S. Traditional Chinese medicine herbal extracts of Cibotium barometz, Gentiana scabra, Dioscorea batatas, Cassia tora, and Taxillus chinensis inhibit SARS-CoV replication. *J. Tradit. Complement. Med.* **2011**, *1*, 41–50. [CrossRef]
30. Alexandrakis, M.; Singh, L.; Boucher, W.; Letourneau, R.; Theofilopoulos, P.; Theoharides, T.C. Differential effect of flavonoids on inhibition of secretion and accumulation of secretory granules in rat basophilic leukemia cells. *Int. J. Immunopharmacol.* **1999**, *21*, 379–390. [CrossRef]
31. Kimata, M.; Inagaki, N.; Nagai, H. Effects of luteolin and other flavonoids on IgE-mediated allergic reactions. *Planta Med.* **2000**, *66*, 25–29. [CrossRef]
32. Yang, Y.; Oh, J.M.; Heo, P.; Shin, J.Y.; Kong, B.; Shin, J.; Lee, J.C.; Oh, J.S.; Park, K.W.; Lee, C.H.; et al. Polyphenols differentially inhibit degranulation of distinct subsets of vesicles in mast cells by specific interaction with granule-type-dependent SNARE complexes. *Biochem. J.* **2013**, *450*, 537–546. [CrossRef]
33. Pearce, F.L.; Befus, A.D.; Bienenstock, J. Mucosal mast cells. III. Effect of quercetin and other flavonoids on antigen-induced histamine secretion from rat intestinal mast cells. *J. Allergy Clin. Immunol.* **1984**, *73*, 819–823. [CrossRef]
34. Mlcek, J.; Jurikova, T.; Skrovankova, S.; Sochor, J. Quercetin and Its Anti-Allergic Immune Response. *Molecules* **2016**, *21*, 623. [CrossRef] [PubMed]
35. Seelinger, G.; Merfort, I.; Schempp, C.M. Anti-oxidant, anti-inflammatory and anti-allergic activities of luteolin. *Planta Med.* **2008**, *74*, 1667–1677. [CrossRef] [PubMed]
36. Weng, Z.; Patel, A.B.; Panagiotidou, S.; Theoharides, T.C. The novel flavone tetramethoxyluteolin is a potent inhibitor of human mast cells. *J. Allergy Clin. Immunol.* **2015**, *135*, 1044–1052. [CrossRef] [PubMed]
37. Bawazeer, M.A.; Theoharides, T.C. IL-33 stimulates human mast cell release of CCL5 and CCL2 via MAPK and NF-κB, inhibited by methoxyluteolin. *Eur. J. Pharmacol.* **2019**, *865*, 172760. [CrossRef]
38. Hagenlocher, Y.; Lorentz, A. Immunomodulation of mast cells by nutrients. *Mol. Immunol.* **2015**, *63*, 25–31. [CrossRef] [PubMed]
39. Park, H.H.; Lee, S.; Son, H.Y.; Park, S.B.; Kim, M.S.; Choi, E.J.; Singh, T.S.; Ha, J.H.; Lee, M.G.; Kim, J.E.; et al. Flavonoids inhibit histamine release and expression of proinflammatory cytokines in mast cells. *Arch. Pharm. Res.* **2008**, *31*, 1303–1311. [CrossRef]
40. Kempuraj, D.; Madhappan, B.; Christodoulou, S.; Boucher, W.; Cao, J.; Papadopoulou, N.; Cetrulo, C.L.; Theoharides, T.C. Flavonols inhibit proinflammatory mediator release, intracellular calcium ion levels and protein kinase C theta phosphorylation in human mast cells. *Br. J. Pharmacol.* **2005**, *145*, 934–944. [CrossRef]
41. Kimata, M.; Shichijo, M.; Miura, T.; Serizawa, I.; Inagaki, N.; Nagai, H. Effects of luteolin, quercetin and baicalein on immunoglobulin E-mediated mediator release from human cultured mast cells. *Clin. Exp. Allergy* **2000**, *30*, 501–508. [CrossRef]
42. Patel, A.B.; Theoharides, T.C. Methoxyluteolin Inhibits Neuropeptide-stimulated Proinflammatory Mediator Release via mTOR Activation from Human Mast Cells. *J. Pharmacol. Exp. Ther.* **2017**, *361*, 462–471. [CrossRef]
43. Gupta, S.C.; Kismali, G.; Aggarwal, B.B. Curcumin, a component of turmeric: From farm to pharmacy. *Biofactors* **2013**, *39*, 2–13. [CrossRef] [PubMed]
44. Kurup, V.P.; Barrios, C.S. Immunomodulatory effects of curcumin in allergy. *Mol. Nutr. Food Res.* **2008**, *52*, 1031–1039. [CrossRef] [PubMed]
45. Ram, A.; Das, M.; Ghosh, B. Curcumin attenuates allergen-induced airway hyperresponsiveness in sensitized guinea pigs. *Biol. Pharm. Bull.* **2003**, *26*, 1021–1024. [CrossRef] [PubMed]
46. Chauhan, P.S.; Subhashini; Dash, D.; Singh, R. Intranasal curcumin attenuates airway remodeling in murine model of chronic asthma. *Int. Immunopharmacol.* **2014**, *21*, 63–75. [CrossRef]
47. Wen, C.C.; Kuo, Y.H.; Jan, J.T.; Liang, P.H.; Wang, S.Y.; Liu, H.G.; Lee, C.K.; Chang, S.T.; Kuo, C.J.; Lee, S.S.; et al. Specific plant terpenoids and lignoids possess potent antiviral activities against severe acute respiratory syndrome coronavirus. *J. Med. Chem.* **2007**, *50*, 4087–4095. [CrossRef]
48. Spagnolo, P.; Balestro, E.; Aliberti, S.; Cocconcelli, E.; Biondini, D.; Casa, G.D.; Sverzellati, N.; Maher, T.M. Pulmonary fibrosis secondary to COVID-19: A call to arms? *Lancet Respir. Med.* **2020**, *8*, 750–752. [CrossRef]
49. Lee, J.H.; Kim, J.W.; Ko, N.Y.; Mun, S.H.; Her, E.; Kim, B.K.; Han, J.W.; Lee, H.Y.; Beaven, M.A.; Kim, Y.M.; et al. Curcumin, a constituent of curry, suppresses IgE-mediated allergic response and mast cell activation at the level of Syk. *J. Allergy Clin. Immunol.* **2008**, *121*, 1225–1231. [CrossRef]
50. Zhang, N.; Li, H.; Jia, J.; He, M. Anti-inflammatory effect of curcumin on mast cell-mediated allergic responses in ovalbumin-induced allergic rhinitis mouse. *Cell. Immunol.* **2015**, *298*, 88–95. [CrossRef]
51. Ju, H.R.; Wu, H.Y.; Nishizono, S.; Sakono, M.; Ikeda, I.; Sugano, M.; Imaizumi, K. Effects of dietary fats and curcumin on IgE-mediated degranulation of intestinal mast cells in brown Norway rats. *Biosci. Biotechnol. Biochem.* **1996**, *60*, 1856–1860. [CrossRef]
52. Galli, S.J.; Gaudenzio, N.; Tsai, M. Mast Cells in Inflammation and Disease: Recent Progress and Ongoing Concerns. *Annu. Rev. Immunol.* **2020**, *38*, 49–77. [CrossRef] [PubMed]

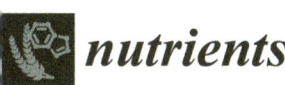

Review

Ketogenic Diet as a Preventive and Supportive Care for COVID-19 Patients

Elena Gangitano [1,*,†], Rossella Tozzi [2,†], Orietta Gandini [2], Mikiko Watanabe [1], Sabrina Basciani [1], Stefania Mariani [1], Andrea Lenzi [1], Lucio Gnessi [1] and Carla Lubrano [1,*]

1. Department of Experimental Medicine, Sapienza University of Rome, 00161 Rome, Italy; mikiko.watanabe@uniroma1.it (M.W.); sabrinabasciani@yahoo.it (S.B.); s.mariani@uniroma1.it (S.M.); andrea.lenzi@uniroma1.it (A.L.); lucio.gnessi@uniroma1.it (L.G.)
2. Department of Molecular Medicine, Sapienza University of Rome, 00161 Rome, Italy; rossella.tozzi@uniroma1.it (R.T.); orietta.gandini@uniroma1.it (O.G.)
* Correspondence: elena.gangitano@uniroma1.it (E.G.); carla.lubrano@uniroma1.it (C.L.)
† These authors contributed equally to the article.

Abstract: Severe obesity is associated with an increased risk of admission to intensive care units and need for invasive mechanical ventilation in patients with COVID-19. The association of obesity and COVID-19 prognosis may be related to many different factors, such as chronic systemic inflammation, the predisposition to severe respiratory conditions and viral infections. The ketogenic diet is an approach that can be extremely effective in reducing body weight and visceral fat in the short term, preserving the lean mass and reducing systemic inflammation. Therefore, it is a precious preventive measure for severely obese people and may be considered as an adjuvant therapy for patients with respiratory compromise.

Keywords: SARS-CoV-2; COVID-19; obesity; ketogenic diet; VLCKD; inflammation; viral infections; respiratory failure

1. Introduction

Coronavirus 2019 disease (COVID-19), caused by SARS-CoV-2 virus, has spread worldwide causing a pandemic since March 2020, now leading to new waves of infection. Overall fatality rate reached 2.3% [1] and, to date, 2,343,069 cases of COVID-19 and 80,253 (3.4%) deaths have been registered in Italy [2].

In most cases the clinical presentation is characterized by fever, dry cough, fatigue and mild pneumonia, although critical forms with desaturation and respiratory failure, septic shock, and/or multiple organ dysfunction can also occur; it has been estimated that moderate and severe forms can affect 14% and 5% of patients, respectively [1]. COVID-19 management consists of supportive therapy and preventing respiratory insufficiency through oxygen therapy or positive ventilation. The most widely adopted therapeutic protocol is based on the use of antibiotic prophylaxis, steroids and anticoagulant therapy, although there is no conclusive evidence supporting their role [3]. In order to limit the typical coagulative hyperactivation and the well-known condition of thrombosis susceptibility [4,5], heparin is now used in early stage COVID-19 patients; however, intensive care units are gradually filling up again, fearing the national health system collapse.

COVID-19 mortality is highly correlated to the severity of the inflammation-related cytokine storm and to the presence of multiple comorbidities (obesity, type 2 diabetes, hypertension, chronic obstructive pulmonary disease) increasing the risk of developing critical forms of infection [6]. In light of these considerations, it is therefore mandatory to pursue new strategies to reduce risk factors and to limit the development of the cytokine storm syndrome (CSS) in order to prevent patients' worsening and access to emergency rooms.

The nutritional approach to COVID-19 patients is extremely important to ensure the correct amount of nutrients, necessary to face the infection and the body's capacity to

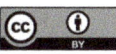

face and fight the virus. Current European Society for Clinical Nutrition and Metabolism (ESPEN) expert statements for COVID-19 patients recommend considering energy needs of 27–30 kcal per kg body weight and day, and 1–1.3 g per Kg of proteins, depending on disease status. Fat and carbohydrate ratio are currently suggested to be 30:70 for patients without respiratory deficiency and 50:50 for ventilated patients [7].

The ketogenic diet (KD), reducing carbohydrates oral intake, allows the hepatic production of ketone bodies and the onset of nutritional ketosis as a result of an increased utilization of fat as metabolic fuel when the availability of glucose is low. Ketone bodies are attracting more and more attention for their anti-inflammatory role and immune metabolism modulation [8]. Besides the well-known metabolic advantages (better hyperglycemia control, reduction of insulin resistance, improvement of hepatic steatosis), several "non-classical" beneficial effects have been attributed to KDs, including growth factors, leptin or IGF-1 modulation [9], together with the protection of renal, brain function and anti-viral effects [10].

KDs provide for a deprivation of carbohydrate content equal to 5–10% of total kcal daily intake, although the specific macronutrient composition may vary. As reported by Watanabe et al. [11], ketogenic diets differ mainly in calorie intake and protein content. High Fat Ketogenic Diets (HFKD) are characterized by a restriction of carbohydrates (CHO) < 50 g per day with unrestricted intake of fat, a relative increase of protein (0.8–1.2 g per day), and ad libitum caloric intake; very low-calorie ketogenic diets (VLCKD) are characterized by approximately the same amount of CHO and protein as in HFKDs, but significantly lower fat and therefore calorie intake, which goes as low as 600 kcal/daily. Very low-calorie diets (VLCD), providing a marked restriction of daily calorie intake, are characterized instead by a variable amount of carbohydrate intake which may or may not be able to induce ketosis [12] (Table 1).

Table 1. Main differences between ketogenic and low-carbohydrate diets (with the kind permission of Watanabe et al. [11]).

	Kcal/Day	CHO/Day	Fat/Day	Ketosis
High fat ketogenic diet (HFKD)	Usually unrestricted	<20–50 g	Unrestricted	Yes
Very low-calorie ketogenic diet (VLCKD)	<800 kcal	<20–50 g	Low	Yes
Very low-calorie diet (VLCD)	<800 kcal	<20–50 g	Low	Usually not
Low carbohydrate diet (LCD)	Variable	<130 g	Low	No

While HFKDs are still used in refractory epilepsy in children, VLCKD are now recommended in severe or sarcopenic obesity, prior to bariatric surgery, to improve glycemic control, dyslipidemia and for a rapid reduction of cardiovascular risk factors in obese patients, not responsive to standard diets [12].

Current contraindications to the VLCKD include type 1 diabetes mellitus, kidney or liver failure, heart failure, cardiac arrhythmias, recent stroke, myocardial infarction, pregnancy and breastfeeding. Of note, active/severe infections and respiratory failure are currently among the conditions not recommended for implementing a VLCKD regimen for a hypothesized immunosuppression and acidosis risk, respectively [13]. Nevertheless, studies conducted in the past have reported good results, also highlighting some benefits derived from ketosis [13]. As per HFKDs, patients with CVD, heart, liver or kidney disease need close medical supervision in order to safely undergo such regimen, and those with severe dyslipidemia or a history of hypertriglyceridemia associated pancreatitis are recommended against undergoing this dietary regimen [14].

The aim of this work is to highlight the potential role of KDs in the management and prevention of COVID-19, focusing on the beneficial effects that may exert on inflammation, immune system and respiratory function.

2. Low Chronic Inflammation, COVID-19 and Ketogenic Diet

As described above, severe forms of COVID-19 are characterized by an ineffective adaptive immune response that leads to a persistence in C-reactive protein (CRP) and interleukin (IL) -6 elevation [15]. This pattern falls within the so-called chronic low-grade inflammatory phenotype (CLIP), a phenomenon that underlies many of the diseases associated with more critical forms of COVID-19, such as diabetes, obesity, insulin-resistance, hypertension and atherosclerosis [16]. All these metabolic derangements are closely related to inflammation triggered by the abnormal expansion of visceral adipose tissue, which has been shown to predict poor COVID-19 prognosis as well as respiratory indicators [17]. Specifically, the white adipose tissue M1 macrophages secretion of pro-inflammatory cytokines including tumor necrosis factor (TNF) alpha, IL-6, CRP, IL-1, is increased, whereas a steep decline occurs in the production of anti-inflammatory cytokines like IL-10, the interleukin-1 receptor antagonist (IL-1RA), and adiponectin. Not only the adipose tissue, but also the immune cells, liver, brain, muscles and pancreas suffer from the inflammatory insult in subjects with obesity. Macrophage-like Kupffer cells initiate the inflammatory process in the liver preceding the inflammatory signals produced by the white adipose tissue, which may further lead to hepatic-necro-inflammation [18]. Moreover, role of P-loop domain belonging to the STAND class of NTPases with homology to the oligomerization module found in AAA+ ATPases (NACHT), Leucine-rich repeat (LRR), and NOD-like receptors (NLRs) Pyrin Domain-Containing 3 Protein (NLRP3) for maintenance of chronic inflammation is crucial. In fact, in response to activation of innate immune receptors by stimuli such as microbial ligands, transcription of pro-inflammatory genes, including those encoding NLRP3 and pro-IL1β, is induced [19].

KDs inhibit aerobic glycolysis, which has been proven to occur following inflammatory activation of cells from both myeloid and lymphoid lineage; in particular, KDs prevent the differentiation and effector functions of inflammatory cells, while promoting the differentiation of regulatory subsets. Moreover, the ketone body β- hydroxybutyrate blocks NLRP3 inflammasome activation [20].

3. Immune System, COVID-19 and Ketogenic Diet

SARS-CoV-2 infects lung cells and enters host epithelial cells through Transmembrane Serine Protease 2 (TMPRSS2) action and spike protein binding Angiotensin Converting Enzyme 2 (ACE-2) receptor. After alveolar epithelial cells pyroptosis-induced death and damage-associated molecular patterns (DAMPs) release, macrophages and monocytes are recruited and cytokines secreted. More specifically, in case of a dysfunctional immune response, we observe an abnormal monocytes, macrophages and T-cells infiltration favored by vascular permeability, a systemic cytokine storm (IL-6, IFN gamma, IL-2, IL-10, Granulocyte colony-stimulating factor G-CSF, TNF), clinical worsening (pulmonary oedema and pneumonia) and widespread inflammation and/or multiorgan damage due to excessive TNF and reactive oxygen species (ROS) production. On the contrary, in a healthy immune system, initial inflammation attracts virus specific T-cells to the site of infection, where they can eliminate the infected cells before the virus spreads. Neutralizing antibodies in these individuals can block viral infection resulting in early recovery [15]. Noteworthy, viral infection can also result in an aberrant cytokine production by the immune cells such as monocytes and macrophages. Elderly people seem to be more susceptible to critical forms of COVID-19 due to an ageing lung microenvironment causing altered dendritic cell maturation and migration to the lymphoid organs and to an inefficient IFN response [21].

Karagiannis et al. [22] demonstrated that restricting dietary glucose by feeding mice a HFKD (72% fat, 2.4% sugar) largely ablates lung-resident type 2 Innate Lymphoid Cells (ILC-2) and reduces airway inflammation by impairing fatty acid metabolism and the formation of lipid droplets. Chronic activation of ILCs, typical of allergenic airway inflammation, needs exogenous fatty acids which are transiently stored in lipid droplets and therefore converted into phospholipids to promote ILCs proliferation. This metabolic program, imprinted by IL-33 and regulated by the genes Peroxisome proliferator-activated receptor gamma (PPAR-γ) and Diacylglycerol O-Acyltransferase 1 (Dgat1), is controlled by glucose availability as well as mammalian target of rapamycin (mTOR) signaling. Moreover, Goldberg et al. reported that a HFKD allows for better survival and increased protective IL-17-secreting γδ T cells in the lungs of mice with influenza virus [10], while Ryu et al. have recently provided preclinical evidence that a HFKD is capable of providing a protective effect against the animal equivalent of COVID-19 in aged mice, with the maintenance of a better oxygen saturation and an increase in γδ T cells [23].

4. Obesity, Viral Infections and Respiratory Function

Weight excess is associated with a higher susceptibility to viral infections [3], as seasonal and H1N1 influenza [24,25], and a higher risk of hospitalization for these conditions [26–29]. In recent years, during the H1N1 influenza pandemic, obesity has been shown to be associated with hospitalization and death [29] and critically ill patients were frequently morbidly obese [25]. Similarly to other viral infections, severe obesity is associated with a high risk of COVID-19 complications [30]. Among obesity comorbidities, hypertension, dyslipidemia, prediabetes and insulin resistance might predispose individuals to cardiovascular events and increased susceptibility to infection via atherosclerosis. Resulting cardiac dysfunction and kidney failure can more easily lead to pneumonia-associated organ failures [31]. Moreover, visceral adipose tissue—a reliable and specific marker of insulin resistance—has been independently associated with the need of intensive care unit (ICU) resulting as the strongest predictor of worse prognosis in patients with COVID-19 [17]. Considered this, a nutritional approach that can break down insulin resistance such a HFKD, might have beneficial implications in COVID-19 prognosis likely without any detrimental effects.

Obese patients are predisposed to the development of chronic and acute respiratory illnesses [32,33], including respiratory tract infections [34]. The reasons for this susceptibility to respiratory disease are many and not completely elucidated yet [35,36]. Obese people have alterations in respiratory physiology [37] and immune response [24,33] and, consequently, develop a lower response to antiviral therapies and vaccinations [24]. The alterations in respiratory physiology consist in a decreased functional residual capacity and reduced expiratory reserve volume, hypoxemia and ventilation perfusion abnormalities [28,37]. The presence of Obstructive Sleep Apnea Syndrome (OSAS), which is common in obese people, may predispose the patients to COVID-19 complications [38].

Obesity is characterized by low-grade systemic inflammation, that may be related to the pathogenesis of respiratory conditions [33]. Fat tissue may accumulate within the lungs, as observed in the airways of obese humans [39] and in the alveolar interstitium of obese diabetic rats [40]. Adipose tissue accumulation in the outer wall of large airways positively correlated with inflammatory infiltrate of eosinophils and neutrophils in patients with fatal asthma [39].

Animal models of obesity showed that during influenza infection there is increased lung permeability, leading to protein leakage into the bronchoalveolar lavage fluid. For the resolution of the infection, the repair of the damaged epithelial surface is required, but wound repair is impaired. Increased lung oedema and oxidative stress have been observed as well [24].

There is evidence that immune system functioning is altered in obesity. T-cells diversity is reduced and this may be related to the T-cells poor response to influenza virus [24]. CD8+ T memory cells has been shown to be impaired, with consequent exacerbates lung complications and mortality [33]. These cells are responsible for an efficient immune response to vaccination [33], with consequent reduced response to vaccination in obese people [24]. Moreover, obesity may be a factor that exacerbates the aging of the immune system [24].

In addition, the high ACE-2 expression in adipose tissue may play a role in obese patients' susceptibility to COVID-19 infection, since SARS-CoV-2 shows high affinity for this enzyme [41].

Therefore, interventions aimed to weight loss in obese patients are warranted to prevent viral infection susceptibility and their complications and theoretically may ameliorate respiratory function.

5. Low-Carbohydrate Ketogenic Diets and Respiratory Function

VLCKDs are, to date, contraindicated for obese patients with respiratory failure [12]. However, some studies reported some beneficial effects from high-fat low-carbohydrate diets and detrimental effects of carbohydrate loads on respiratory parameters. These studies, anyway, often did not specify if patients were in ketosis, but used low amount of CHO, possibly leading to ketosis.

Two studies on a total of 40 healthy patients [42,43] reported that a VLCKD (848 kcal/day; protein: carbohydrate: fat = 43:14:43%) and a HFKD (10% calories from carbohydrate) diet reduced CO_2 output without modifying oxygen uptake. Moreover, Rubini et al. compared a VLCKD regimen to a hypocaloric Mediterranean diet showing that only the VLCKD significantly decreased respiratory exchange ratio ($p < 0.05$) in addition to higher fat mass loss in healthy patients. Therefore, these diets may be helpful in respiratory patients for reducing CO_2 body stores levels and dyspnea at rest. On the other hand, a study on 17 healthy women who were administered a HFKD (2400 kcal/day), reported earlier muscle fatigue during daily life activities [44].

Chronic Obstructive Pulmonary Disease (COPD) is often accompanied with hypercapnia and hypoxemia. A reduction in carbon dioxide production would reduce the workload of respiratory muscles and therefore be beneficial for these patients. Some studies focused on the administration of HFKD in COPD patients, and beneficial or, at least, neutral results were observed.

In twelve clinically stable COPD patients, the administration of a high-fat meal had a small effect on gas exchange parameters compared to 12 healthy controls, whereas a high-carbohydrate diet was detrimental on gas exchange parameters, especially in COPD patients [45]. No differences in pulmonary function were detected in 36 COPD patients comparing the administration of a moderate-fat meal with a high-fat meal [46]. On the other hand, the administration of a HFKD in COPD patients with hypercapnia led to an amelioration of respiratory parameters in an overall sample of 74 underweight patients [47,48].

In patients with respiratory failure, providing an adequate protein intake is extremely important to preserve skeletal muscle mass and function [7]. A high-fat low-carbohydrate diet has been reported as a potential useful tool to ameliorate respiratory failure [49–51].

In the literature, there are some evidences of a beneficial effect of a high-fat low-carbohydrate diet in mechanically ventilated patients [52–54], since it was able to reduce $PaCO_2$ levels [52,53,55] and the time of mechanical ventilation [52,53].

6. COVID-19, Lockdown and KDs

Both HFKD and VLCKD represent valuable treatments despite being characterized by the presence of contraindications and capable of causing side effects. Therefore, they should be followed under strict medical supervision and be considered similar to pharmacologic treatment. A concern may be that during the isolation imposed during the pandemic, it is difficult to monitor a patient on the ketogenic diet undergoing rehabilitation. Just a few studies reporting the administration of a ketogenic diet during this pandemic have been published, and to the best of our knowledge none published results on its use in COVID-19 infected and/or respiratory patients yet.

Kossof et al. [56] administered a HFKD to patients with uncontrolled seizures, mainly children, during the pandemic, using a combined approach with in person meetings and telemedicine. The authors and the other members of the International Ketogenic Diet Study Group, pediatric consensus group, reported no issues regarding the maintenance of ketosis and seizure control in their group, and raised no questions about the safety of the ketogenic diet in case of respiratory infection. A similar approach in similar setting was used by Ferraris et al. [57] and no major issues were reported, but they did not specify if any of their patients was infected by COVID-19.

Soliman et al. [58] proposed the use of a ketogenic diet and intermittent fasting, with administration of medium-chain triglycerides, as a prophylactic measure and an adjuvant therapy for COVID-19. In fact many viruses, as the varicella-zoster [59], the cytomegalovirus [60] and the hepatitis C [61], need the fatty acid metabolism pathway for their replication, therefore the diet-induced metabolic switch leading to a reduction in the fatty acid synthesis pathways may help in reducing viral replication [58].

7. Conclusion and Future Perspective

7.1. KDs in COVID-19 Prevention

Obesity, and in particular visceral abdominal fat, has been indicated as an independent risk factor for worse prognosis in COVID-19, often associated with the need for intensive care [17,30,41,62]. These may be due to the impaired respiratory mechanics, increased airway resistance and impaired gas exchange [25,28,54], as well as obesity-related comorbidities [63], which appear to be directly related to the onset of complications and severe course of COVID-19. In particular, OSAS [38], metabolic syndrome, hypertension, Non-Alcoholic Fatty Liver Disease (NAFLD) and diabetes or insulin resistance have all shown to affect COVID-19 outcome negatively [55–58]. Finally, it should not be overlooked that obesity is associated with low chronic inflammation within a state of immunological dysfunction that can lead to increased risk of allergies [64] or ineffective response against infections [35] and vaccines [65].

KDs, and specifically VLCKDs, demonstrated to induce weight loss and diabetes remission. VLCKDs are currently used in bariatric surgery preparation [12] thanks to the ability in reducing hepatic volume [11] with a subsequent improvement in intra and post-operative care. Recent findings underlined immune advantages derived from ketone bodies, such as blockage NLRP3 inflammasome [20], reduction in chronic activation of ILCs and induction of protective $\gamma\delta$ T-cells against infections [10]. Taken together, in addition to the benefit of airway inflammation prevention by impairing the formation of lipid droplets [22], KDs could be an excellent tool to prevent the infection and stem the damage induced by COVID-19 in the fragile population affected from obesity.

7.2. KDs in Supportive Care of COVID-19

Studies conducted in mice highlighted the beneficial effect of HFD- induced ketone bodies in COVID-19 models [10,23]. In humans, HFKDs has been experimented in Intensive Care Units (ICU) and good results have been reported in mechanically ventilated patients [52,55]. Moreover, telemedicine achieved good results in pediatric epileptic patients under HFKDs, either for safety and compliance, proving that it can be a valid tool to be adopted even in the event of quarantine and fiduciary isolation. On the basis of these considerations, several authors proposed KDs in COVID-19 management and some clinical trials are ongoing [66,67].

7.3. KDs during Rehabilitation Post SARS-CoV-2 Infection

Patients affected from COVID-19, especially elderly ones, often require ICU for a longer period (up to 20 days) than other more typical uses of ICU. Among Post Intensive Care Syndrome (PICS), impaired exercise tolerance, neuropathies, muscle weakness/paresis, severe fatigue are responsible for decreased exercise capacity, disability and compromised quality of life for months, even years after intensive care [68]. Muscle atrophy, as well as obesity and immune dysregulation, is associated with Growth Hormone/Insulin-like Growth Factor 1 (GH/IGF-1) impaired axis and might be a link between IGF-1 downregulation and COVID-19 severity [69]. Preserving muscle mass is essential in order to improve rehabilitation and to reduce costs for recovering people.

VLCKDs preserved muscle mass in obese patients [70,71] when a protein intake of at least 1.2 gr of protein/Kg was ensured; the same results have been confirmed when isocaloric KDs have been used in patients affected from multiple sclerosis, reporting a superiority compared to Mediterranean diet [72]. Furthermore, HFKD (75–80% calories from fat, carbohydrates <50 g per day and <10 g per meal) improves quality of life, lean mass and metabolic parameters (included IGF-1) in oncologic patients, compared to standard diet [73].

In conclusion, VLCKDs administration might be considered in severely obese patients as an effective adjuvant therapy for COVID-19, first of all as a preventive measure, to achieve a fast weight loss [67], and secondly as an adjuvant therapy during rehabilitation (see Figure 1). More challenging is the hypothesis of administering HFKD during hospitalization or even more in delicate settings such as an intensive care unit or during positive ventilation; although several data support the evidence that limiting carbohydrate intake and promoting ketone formation may be helpful in ameliorating respiratory parameters. Furthermore, as extensively discussed, HFKDs show a strong anti-inflammatory effect and some data suggest that they may be useful for reducing viral replication. However, many studies are old, the samples small, and the ketosis not specifically addressed, therefore new clinical trials are needed. Hoping that the promising results observed in animal studies can be passed on to humans, we herein suggest considering KDs as an option to be considered for COVID-19 management within the current indications.

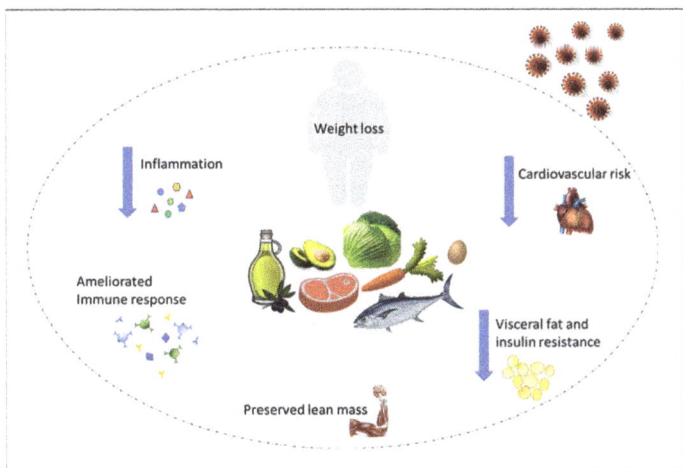

Figure 1. Mechanisms through which VLCKD with its consequent weight loss may reduce the susceptibility to severe SARS-CoV-2 infection and stem the damage induced by the virus.

Author Contributions: Conceptualization, L.G., A.L. and C.L.; writing—original draft preparation, E.G., R.T., M.W. and S.B.; writing—review and editing, O.G., S.M., L.G. and C.L.; supervision, L.G. and C.L. All authors have read and agreed to the published version of the manuscript.

Funding: This research received no external funding.

Data Availability Statement: Data sharing not applicable.

Conflicts of Interest: The authors declare no conflict of interest.

References

1. Wu, Z.; McGoogan, J.M. Characteristics of and Important Lessons from the Coronavirus Disease 2019 (COVID-19) Outbreak in China: Summary of a Report of 72314 Cases from the Chinese Center for Disease Control and Prevention. *JAMA J. Am. Med. Assoc.* **2020**, *323*, 1239–1242. [CrossRef]
2. Epicentro, Epidemiology for Public Health, Istituto Superiore di Sanità. *COVID-19 Integrated Surveillance Data in Italy*; Epicentro, Epidemiology for Public Health, Istituto Superiore di Sanità: Rome, Italy, 2021.
3. Pascarella, G.; Strumia, A.; Piliego, C.; Bruno, F.; del Buono, R.; Costa, F.; Scarlata, S.; Agrò, F.E. COVID-19 Diagnosis and Management: A Comprehensive Review. *J. Intern. Med.* **2020**, *288*, 192–206. [CrossRef]
4. Levi, M.; Thachil, J.; Iba, T.; Levy, J.H. Coagulation Abnormalities and Thrombosis in Patients with COVID-19. *Lancet Haematol.* **2020**, *7*, e438–e440. [CrossRef]
5. Spiezia, L.; Boscolo, A.; Poletto, F.; Cerruti, L.; Tiberio, I.; Campello, E.; Navalesi, P.; Simioni, P. COVID-19-Related Severe Hypercoagulability in Patients Admitted to Intensive Care Unit for Acute Respiratory Failure. *Thromb. Haemost.* **2020**, *120*, 998–1000. [CrossRef]
6. Yang, J.; Zheng, Y.; Gou, X.; Pu, K.; Chen, Z. Prevalence of Comorbidities and Its Effects in Patients Infected with SARS-CoV-2: A Systematic Review and Meta-Analysis. *Int. J. Infect. Dis.* **2020**, *94*, 91–95. [CrossRef] [PubMed]
7. Barazzoni, R.; Bischoff, S.C.; Breda, J.; Wickramasinghe, K.; Krznaric, Z.; Nitzan, D.; Pirlich, M.; Singer, P. ESPEN Expert Statements and Practical Guidance for Nutritional Management of Individuals with SARS-CoV-2 Infection. *Clin. Nutr.* **2020**, *39*, 1631–1638. [CrossRef] [PubMed]
8. Lee, A.K.; Kim, D.H.; Bang, E.; Choi, Y.J.; Chung, H.Y. β-Hydroxybutyrate Suppresses Lipid Accumulation in Aged Liver through GPR109A-mediated Signaling. *Aging Dis.* **2020**, *11*, 777–790. [CrossRef] [PubMed]
9. Vidali, S.; Aminzadeh, S.; Lambert, B.; Rutherford, T.; Sperl, W.; Kofler, B.; Feichtinger, R.G. Mitochondria: The Ketogenic Diet—A Metabolism-Based Therapy. *Int. J. Biochem. Cell Biol.* **2015**, *63*, 55–59. [CrossRef] [PubMed]
10. Goldberg, E.L.; Molony, R.D.; Kudo, E.; Sidorov, S.; Kong, Y.; Dixit, V.D.; Iwasaki, A. Ketogenic Diet Activates Protective γδ T Cell Responses against Influenza Virus Infection. *Sci. Immunol.* **2019**, *4*, eaav2026. [CrossRef] [PubMed]
11. Watanabe, M.; Tozzi, R.; Risi, R.; Tuccinardi, D.; Mariani, S.; Basciani, S.; Spera, G.; Lubrano, C.; Gnessi, L. Beneficial Effects of the Ketogenic Diet on Nonalcoholic Fatty Liver Disease: A Comprehensive Review of the Literature. *Obes. Rev.* **2020**, *21*, e13024. [CrossRef] [PubMed]
12. Caprio, M.; Infante, M.; Moriconi, E.; Armani, A.; Fabbri, A.; Mantovani, G.; Mariani, S.; Lubrano, C.; Poggiogalle, E.; Migliaccio, S.; et al. Very-Low-Calorie Ketogenic Diet (VLCKD) in the Management of Metabolic Diseases: Systematic Review and Consensus Statement from the Italian Society of Endocrinology (SIE). *J. Endocrinol. Investig.* **2019**, *42*, 1365–1386. [CrossRef] [PubMed]
13. Watanabe, M.; Tuccinardi, D.; Ernesti, I.; Basciani, S.; Mariani, S.; Genco, A.; Manfrini, S.; Lubrano, C.; Gnessi, L. Scientific Evidence Underlying Contraindications to the Ketogenic Diet: An Update. *Obes. Rev.* **2020**, *21*, e13053. [CrossRef] [PubMed]
14. Kirkpatrick, C.F.; Bolick, J.P.; Kris-Etherton, P.M.; Sikand, G.; Aspry, K.E.; Soffer, D.E.; Willard, K.-E.; Maki, K.C. Review of Current Evidence and Clinical Recommendations on the Effects of Low-Carbohydrate and Very-Low-Carbohydrate (Including Ketogenic) Diets for the Management of Body Weight and Other Cardiometabolic Risk Factors: A Scientific Statement from the National Lipid Association Nutrition and Lifestyle Task Force. *J. Clin. Lipidol.* **2019**, *13*, 689–711.e1. [CrossRef]
15. Tay, M.Z.; Poh, C.M.; Rénia, L.; MacAry, P.A.; Ng, L.F.P. The Trinity of COVID-19: Immunity, Inflammation and Intervention. *Nat. Rev. Immunol.* **2020**, *20*, 363–374. [CrossRef]
16. Chen, Y.; Liu, S.; Leng, S.X. Chronic Low-Grade Inflammatory Phenotype (CLIP) and Senescent Immune Dysregulation. *Clin. Ther.* **2019**, *41*, 400–409. [CrossRef] [PubMed]
17. Watanabe, M.; Caruso, D.; Tuccinardi, D.; Risi, R.; Zerunian, M.; Polici, M.; Pucciarelli, F.; Tarallo, M.; Strigari, L.; Manfrini, S.; et al. Visceral Fat Shows the Strongest Association with the Need of Intensive Care in Patients with COVID-19. *Metab. Clin. Exp.* **2020**, *111*, 1–8. [CrossRef]
18. Debnath, M.; Agrawal, S.; Agrawal, A.; Dubey, G.P. Metaflammatory Responses during Obesity: Pathomechanism and Treatment. *Obes. Res. Clin. Pract.* **2016**, *10*, 103–113. [CrossRef] [PubMed]
19. Levy, M.; Thaiss, C.A.; Elinav, E. Taming the Inflammasome. *Nat. Med.* **2015**, *21*, 213–215. [CrossRef] [PubMed]
20. Kornberg, M.D. The Immunologic Warburg Effect: Evidence and Therapeutic Opportunities in Autoimmunity. *Wiley Interdiscip. Rev. Syst. Biol. Med.* **2020**, *12*, 1–17. [CrossRef] [PubMed]
21. Pillai, P.S.; Molony, R.D.; Martinod, K.; Dong, H.; Pang, I.K.; Tal, M.C.; Solis, A.G.; Bielecki, P.; Mohanty, S.; Trentalange, M.; et al. Mx1 Reveals Innate Pathways to Antiviral Resistance and Lethal Influenza Disease. *Science* **2017**, *352*, 463–466. [CrossRef]
22. Karagiannis, F.; Masouleh, S.K.; Wunderling, K.; Surendar, J.; Schmitt, V.; Kazakov, A.; Michla, M.; Hölzel, M.; Thiele, C.; Wilhelm, C. Lipid-Droplet Formation Drives Pathogenic Group 2 Innate Lymphoid Cells in Airway Inflammation. *Immunity* **2020**, *52*, 620–634.e6. [CrossRef] [PubMed]
23. Ryu, S.; Shchukina, I.; Youm, Y.-H.; Qing, H.; Hilliard, B.K.; Dlugos, T.; Zhang, X.; Yasumoto, Y.; Booth, C.J.; Fernández-Hernando, C.; et al. Ketogenesis Restrains Aging-Induced Exacerbation of COVID in a Mouse Model. *bioRxiv* **2020**. [CrossRef]
24. Honce, R.; Schultz-Cherry, S. Impact of Obesity on Influenza A Virus Pathogenesis, Immune Response, and Evolution. *Front. Immunol.* **2019**, *10*, 1071. [CrossRef] [PubMed]
25. Kumar, A.; Zarychanski, R.; Pinto, R.; Cook, D.J.; Marshall, J.; Lacroix, J.; Stelfox, T.; Bagshaw, S.; Choong, K.; Lamontagne, F.; et al. Critically Ill Patients with 2009 Influenza A(H1N1) Infection in Canada. *JAMA* **2009**, *302*, 1872–1879. [CrossRef]

26. Kwong, J.C.; Campitelli, M.A.; Rosella, L.C. Obesity and Respiratory Hospitalizations During Influenza Seasons in Ontario, Canada: A Cohort Study. *Clin. Infect. Dis.* **2011**, *53*, 413–421. [CrossRef]
27. Moser, J.S.; Galindo-Fraga, A.; Ortiz-Hernández, A.A.; Gu, W.; Hunsberger, S.; Galán-Herrera, J.; Guerrero, M.L.; Ruiz-Palacios, G.M.; Beigel, J.H. The La Red ILI 002 Study Group Underweight, overweight, and obesity as independent risk factors for hospitalization in adults and children from influenza and other respiratory viruses. *Influenza Other Respir. Viruses* **2019**, *13*, 3–9. [CrossRef]
28. Kalligeros, M.; Shehadeh, F.; Mylona, E.K.; Benitez, G.; Beckwith, C.G.; Chan, P.A.; Mylonakis, E. Association of Obesity with Disease Severity Among Patients with Coronavirus Disease 2019. *Obesity* **2020**, *28*, 1200–1204. [CrossRef]
29. Morgan, O.W.; Bramley, A.; Fowlkes, A.; Freedman, D.S.; Taylor, T.H.; Belay, B.; Jain, S.; Cox, C.; Kamimoto, L.; Fiore, A.; et al. Morbid Obesity as a Risk Factor for Hospitalization and Death Due to 2009 Pandemic Influenza A (H1N1) Disease. *PLoS ONE* **2010**, *5*, 1–6. [CrossRef]
30. Simonnet, A.; Chetboun, M.; Poissy, J.; Raverdy, V.; Noulette, J.; Duhamel, A.; Labreuche, J.; Mathieu, D.; Pattou, F.; Jourdain, M.; et al. High Prevalence of Obesity in Severe Acute Respiratory Syndrome Coronavirus-2 (SARS-CoV-2) Requiring Invasive Mechanical Ventilation. *Obesity* **2020**, *28*, 1195–1199. [CrossRef]
31. Li, B.; Yang, J.; Zhao, F.; Zhi, L.; Wang, X.; Liu, L.; Bi, Z.; Zhao, Y. Prevalence and Impact of Cardiovascular Metabolic Diseases on COVID-19 in China. *Clin. Res. Cardiol.* **2020**, *109*, 531–538. [CrossRef]
32. Franssen, F.M.E.; Donnell, D.E.O.; Goossens, G.H.; Blaak, E.E.; Schols, A.M.W.J. Obesity and the Lung-Obesity and COPD. *Thorax* **2008**, *63*, 1110–1117. [CrossRef]
33. Mancuso, P. Obesity and lung inflammation. *J. Appl. Physiol.* **2010**, *108*, 722–728. [CrossRef]
34. Maccioni, L.; Weber, S.; Elgizouli, M.; Stoehlker, A.; Geist, I.; Peter, H.; Vach, W.; Nieters, A. Obesity and Risk of Respiratory Tract Infections: Results of an Infection-Diary Based Cohort Study. *BMC Public Health* **2018**, *18*, 1–13. [CrossRef]
35. Huttunen, R.; Syrja, J. Obesity and the Risk and Outcome of Infection. *Int. J. Obes.* **2013**, *37*, 333–340. [CrossRef]
36. Watanabe, M.; Risi, R.; Tuccinardi, D.; Baquero, C.J.; Manfrini, S.; Gnessi, L. Obesity and SARS-CoV-2: A Population to Safeguard. *Diabetes Metab. Res. Rev.* **2020**, *36*, e3325. [CrossRef] [PubMed]
37. Parameswaran, K.; Ctodd, D.; Soth, M. Altered Respiratory Physiology in Obesity. *Can. Respir. J.* **2006**, *13*, 203–210. [CrossRef] [PubMed]
38. Memtsoudis, S.G.; Ivascu, N.S.; Pryor, K.O.; Goldstein, P.A. Obesity as a Risk Factor for Poor Outcome in COVID-19-Induced Lung Injury: The Potential Role of Undiagnosed Obstructive Sleep Apnoea. *Br. J. Anaesth.* **2020**, *125*, e262–e263. [CrossRef] [PubMed]
39. Elliot, J.G.; Donovan, G.M.; Wang, K.C.W.; Green, F.H.Y.; James, A.L.; Noble, P.B. Fatty Airways: Implications for Obstructive Disease. *Eur. Respir. J.* **2019**, *54*, 1900857. [CrossRef] [PubMed]
40. Foster, D.J.; Ravikumar, P.; Bellotto, D.J.; Unger, R.H.; Hsia, C.C.W. Fatty Diabetic Lung: Altered Alveolar Structure and Surfactant Protein Expression. *Am. J. Physiol.* **2010**, *298*, L392–L403. [CrossRef]
41. Kassir, R. Risk of COVID-19 for Patients with Obesity. *Obes. Rev.* **2020**, *21*, e13034. [CrossRef]
42. Rubini, A.; Bosco, G.; Lodi, A.; Cenci, L.; Parmagnani, A.; Grimaldi, K.; Zhongjin, Y.; Paoli, A. Effects of Twenty Days of the Ketogenic Diet on Metabolic and Respiratory Parameters in Healthy Subjects. *Lung* **2015**, *193*, 939–945. [CrossRef]
43. Sue, Y.D.; Chung, M.M.; Grosvenor, M.; Wasserman, K. Effect of Altering the Proportion of Dietary Fat and Carbohydrate on Excercise Gas Exchange in Normal Subjects. *Am. Rev. Respir. Dis.* **1989**, *139*, 1430–1434. [CrossRef] [PubMed]
44. Sjödin, A.; Hellström, F.; Sehlstedt, E.; Svensson, M.; Burén, J. Effects of a Ketogenic Diet on Muscle Fatigue in Healthy, Young, Normal-Weight Women: A Randomized Controlled Feeding Trial. *Nutrients* **2020**, *12*, 955. [CrossRef] [PubMed]
45. Kuo, C.D.; Shiao, G.M.; Lee, J.D. The Effects of High-Fat and High-Carbohydrate Diet Loads on Gas Exchange and Ventilation in COPD Patients and Normal Subjects. *Chest* **1993**, *104*, 189–196. [CrossRef]
46. Akrabawi, S.S.; Mobarhan, S.; Stoltz, R.R.; Ferguson, P.W. Gastric Emptying, Pulmonary Function, Gas Exchange, and Respiratory Quotient after Feeding a Moderate versus High Fat Enteral Formula Meal in Chronic Obstructive Pulmonary Disease Patients. *Nutrition* **1996**, *12*, 366. [CrossRef]
47. Angelillo, A.V.; Sukhdarshan, B.; Durfee, D.; Dahl, J.; Patterson, A.J.; O'Donohue, W.J. Effects of Low and High Carbohydrate Feedings in Ambulatory Patients with Chronic Obstructive Pulmonary Disease and Chronic Hypercapnia. *Ann. Intern. Med.* **1985**, *103*, 883–885. [CrossRef] [PubMed]
48. Cai, B.; Zhu, Y.; Ma, Y.; Xu, Z.; Zao, Y.; Wang, J.; Lin, Y.; Comer, G.M. Effect of Supplementing a High-Fat, Low-Carbohydrate Enteral Formula in COPD Patients. *Nutrition* **2003**, *19*, 229–232. [CrossRef]
49. Kwan, R.M.F.; Thomas, S.; Mir, M.A. Effects of a Low Carbohydrate Isoenergetic Diet on Sleep Behavior and Pulmonary Functions in Healthy Female Adult Humans. *J. Nutr.* **1986**, *116*, 2393–2402. [CrossRef] [PubMed]
50. Tirlapur, V.G.; Mir, M.A. Effect of Low Calorie Intake on Abnormal Pulmonary Physiology in Patients with Chronic Hypercapneic Respiratory Failure. *Am. J. Med.* **1984**, *77*, 987–994. [CrossRef]
51. Kwan, R.; Mir, A. Beneficial Effects of Dietary Carbohydrate Restriction in Chronic Cor Pulmonale. *Am. J. Med.* **1987**, *82*, 751–758. [CrossRef]
52. Al-Saady, N.M.; Blackmore, C.M.; Bennett, E.D. High Fat, Low Carbohydrate, Enteral Feeding Lowers PaCO2 and Reduces the Period of Ventilation in Artificially Ventilated Patients. *Intensive Care Med.* **1989**, *15*, 290–295. [CrossRef]

53. Faramawy, M.A.E.S.; Allah, A.A.; El Batrawy, S.; Amer, H. Impact of High Fat Low Carbohydrate Enteral Feeding on Weaning from Mechanical Ventilation. *Egypt. J. Chest Dis. Tuberc.* **2014**, *63*, 931–938. [CrossRef]
54. Cook, D.; Meade, M.; Guyatt, G.; Butler, R.; Aldawood, A.; Epstein, S. Trials of Miscellaneous Interventions to Wean from Mechanical Ventilation. *Chest* **2001**, *120*, 438S–444S. [CrossRef]
55. Mohamed, N.; Koofy, E.; Rady, H.I.; Abdallah, S.M.; Bazaraa, H.M.; Rabie, A.; El-ayadi, A.A. The Effect of High Fat Dietary Modification and Nutritional Status on the Outcome of Critically Ill Ventilated Children: Single-Center Study. *Korean J. Pediatr.* **2019**, *62*, 344–352. [CrossRef]
56. Kossoff, E.H.; Turner, Z.; Adams, J.; Bessone, S.K.; Avallone, J.; Mcdonald, T.J.W.; Diaz-arias, L.; Barron, B.J.; Vizthum, D.; Cervenka, M.C. Ketogenic Diet Therapy Provision in the COVID-19 Pandemic: Dual-Center Experience and Recommendations. *Epilepsy Behav.* **2020**, *111*, 1–6. [CrossRef]
57. Ferraris, C.; Pasca, L.; Guglielmetti, M.; Marazzi, C.; Trentani, C.; Varesio, C.; Tagliabue, A.; de Giorgis, V. Comment on: Ketogenic Diet Therapy Provision in the COVID-19 Pandemic: Dual-Center Experience and Recommendations. *Epilepsy Behav.* **2020**, *112*, 1–2. [CrossRef]
58. Soliman, S.; Faris, M.A.I.E.; Ratemi, Z.; Halwani, R. Switching Host Metabolism as an Approach to Dampen SARS-CoV-2 Infection. *Ann. Nutr. Metab.* **2020**, *76*, 297–303. [CrossRef] [PubMed]
59. Namazue, J.; Kato, T.; Okuno, T.; Shiraki, K.; Yamanishi, K. Evidence for Attachment of Fatty Acid to Varicella-Zoster Virus Glycoproteins and Effect of Cerulenin on the Maturation of Varicella-Zoster Virus Glycoproteins. *Intervirology* **1989**, *30*, 268–277. [CrossRef] [PubMed]
60. Koyuncu, E.; Purdy, J.G.; Rabinowitz, J.D.; Shenk, T. Saturated Very Long Chain Fatty Acids Are Required for the Production of Infectious Human Cytomegalovirus Progeny. *PLoS Pathog.* **2013**, *9*, 1–15. [CrossRef] [PubMed]
61. Herker, E.; Ott, M. Unique Ties between Hepatitis C Virus Replication and Intracellular Lipids. *Trends Endocrinol. Metab.* **2011**, *22*, 241–248. [CrossRef]
62. Stefan, N.; Birkenfeld, A.L.; Schulze, M.B.; Ludwig, D.S. Obesity and Impaired Metabolic Health in Patients with COVID-19. *Nat. Rev. Endocrinol.* **2020**, *16*, 341–342. [CrossRef] [PubMed]
63. Campia, U.; Tesauro, M.; Di Daniele, N.; Cardillo, C. The Vascular Endothelin System in Obesity and Type 2 Diabetes: Pathophysiology and Therapeutic Implications. *Life Sci.* **2014**, *118*, 149–155. [CrossRef] [PubMed]
64. Watanabe, M.; Masieri, S.; Costantini, D.; Tozzi, R.; de Giorgi, F.; Gangitano, E.; Tuccinardi, D.; Poggiogalle, E.; Mariani, S.; Basciani, S.; et al. Overweight and Obese Patients with Nickel Allergy Have a Worse Metabolic Profile Compared to Weight Matched Non-Allergic Individuals. *PLoS ONE* **2018**, *13*, e0202683. [CrossRef]
65. Ledford, H. How Obesity Could Create Problems for a COVID Vaccine. *Nature* **2020**, *586*, 488–489. [CrossRef] [PubMed]
66. Sukkar, S.G.; Bassetti, M. Induction of Ketosis as a Potential Therapeutic Option to Limit Hyperglycemia and Prevent Cytokine Storm in COVID-19. *Nutrition* **2020**, *79–80*, 110967. [CrossRef] [PubMed]
67. Paoli, A.; Gorini, S.; Caprio, M. The Dark Side of the Spoon—Glucose, Ketones and COVID-19: A Possible Role for Ketogenic Diet? *J. Transl. Med.* **2020**, *18*, 1–9. [CrossRef] [PubMed]
68. Stam, H.J.; Stucki, G.; Bickenbach, J. European Academy of Rehabilitation Medicine Covid-19 and Post Intensive Care Syndrome: A Call for Action. *J. Rehabil. Med.* **2020**, *52*, jrm00044. [CrossRef]
69. Lubrano, C.; Masi, D.; Risi, R.; Balena, A.; Watanabe, M.; Mariani, S.; Gnessi, L. Is Growth Hormone Insufficiency the Missing Link Between Obesity, Male Gender, Age, and COVID-19 Severity? *Obesity* **2020**, *28*, 2038–2039. [CrossRef]
70. Basciani, S.; Camajani, E.; Contini, S.; Persichetti, A.; Risi, R.; Bertoldi, L.; Strigari, L.; Prossomariti, G.; Watanabe, M.; Mariani, S.; et al. Very-Low-Calorie Ketogenic Diets With Whey, Vegetable, or Animal Protein in Patients With Obesity: A Randomized Pilot Study. *J. Clin. Endocrinol. Metab.* **2020**, *105*, 2939–2949. [CrossRef] [PubMed]
71. Bruci, A.; Tuccinardi, D.; Tozzi, R.; Balena, A.; Santucci, S.; Frontani, R.; Mariani, S.; Basciani, S.; Spera, G.; Gnessi, L.; et al. Very Low-Calorie Ketogenic Diet: A Safe and Effective Tool for Weight Loss in Patients With Obesity and Mild Kidney Failure. *Nutrients* **2020**, *12*, 333. [CrossRef]
72. Benlloch, M.; López-Rodríguez, M.M.; Cuerda-Ballester, M.; Drehmer, E.; Carrera, S.; Ceron, J.J.; Tvarijonaviciute, A.; Chirivella, J.; Fernández-García, D.; de La Rubia Ortí, J.E. Satiating Effect of a Ketogenic Diet and Its Impact on Muscle Improvement and Oxidation State in Multiple Sclerosis Patients. *Nutrients* **2019**, *11*, 1156. [CrossRef] [PubMed]
73. Klement, R.J.; Weigel, M.M.; Sweeney, R.A. A Ketogenic Diet Consumed during Radiotherapy Improves Several Aspects of Quality of Life and Metabolic Health in Women with Breast Cancer. *Clin. Nutr.* **2021**, in press. [CrossRef] [PubMed]

MDPI
St. Alban-Anlage 66
4052 Basel
Switzerland
Tel. +41 61 683 77 34
Fax +41 61 302 89 18
www.mdpi.com

Nutrients Editorial Office
E-mail: nutrients@mdpi.com
www.mdpi.com/journal/nutrients

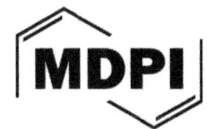

www.ingramcontent.com/pod-product-compliance
Lightning Source LLC
LaVergne TN
LVHW070638100526
838202LV00012B/834